Acta Neurochirurgica
Supplements

Editor: H.-J. Reulen
Assistant Editor: H.-J. Steiger

Advances in Stereotactic and Functional Neurosurgery 12

Proceedings of the 12th Meeting
of the European Society for Stereotactic
and Functional Neurosurgery,
Milan 1996

Edited by
C. B. Ostertag, D. G. T. Thomas,
A. Bosch, B. Linderoth, G. Broggi

Acta Neurochirurgica
Supplement 68

Springer-Verlag Wien GmbH

Originally published by Springer-Verlag/Wien in 1997
Softcover reprint of the hardcover 1st edition 1997

Typesetting: ASCO Trade Typesetting Ltd., Hong Kong

Printed on acid-free and chlorine free bleached paper

With 59 Figures

Die Deutsche Bibliothek - CIP-Einheitsaufnahme

[Acta neurochirurgica / Supplement]
Acta neurochirurgica. Supplement. - Wien ; New York : Springer
Früher Schriftenreihe
Früher u.d.T.: Acta neurochirurgica / Supplementum

68. Advances in stereotactic and functional neurosurgery
12 . - 1997

Advances in stereotactic and functional neurosurgery. - Wien ;
New York : Springer
(Acta neurochirurgica ; ...)
ISSN 0720-2972

12 1997
(Acta neurochirurgica ; 68)
ISBN 978-3-7091-7341-1 ISBN 978-3-7091-6513-3 (eBook)
DOI 10.1007/978-3-7091-6513-3

Cataloging-in-Publication Data applied for

ISSN 0065-1419 (Acta Neurochirurgica/Suppl.)
ISSN 0720-7972 (Advances in Stereotactic and Functional Neurosurgery)

ISBN 978-3-7091-7341-1

Foreword

Neurosurgery of the Future: Computers and Robots in Clinical Neurosurgical Practice and in Training – a Philosophical Journey into the Future

Many present day neurosurgeons believe that they already obtain good results in operative surgery with the benefit of the operating microscope and other aids which have become available in the last three decades and that the introduction of computers and robots to the operating theatre is superfluous. However, it is clear from analogy with the function of the airline pilot, another profession where there are great demands on manual skill and on spatial awareness, that these devices do have much to offer neurosurgery.

Classical neurosurgery, in the time of Cushing, Dandy and Scarff, was based on a three dimensional picture of the patient's brain formed in the surgeon's mind and often illustrated in elegant drawings. Such pictures were based on neuroradiological studies by pneumoencephalography, ventriculography or by angiography. Generally these studies showed the presence and position of a lesion by displacement of normal brain structures and the picture was built up by interference. This was then converted by the experienced neurosurgeon into a plan for the craniotomy site and the trajectory of the surgical approach. Once the brain was exposed further pre-operative information was obtained by visual inspection and by palpation with the brain needle. These classical forms of neuroradiology have largely been superseded by computerised tomography and by magnetic resonance imaging. The mental process which the neurosurgeon must follow to make use of these newer forms of imaging are different. Thus, CT and MR images are conventionally presented as axial images seen viewed from the patient's feet. Occasional errors are made in planning the position of the patient's head on the operating table, on the site and trajectory of the approach (a 15 degree error will cause 1.5 cm displacement at a depth of 5 cm) and even on the side of the brain which is to be operated.

Such errors should not be tolerated when there are now technical adjuncts available to help the neurosurgeon avoid them. Several forms of neuro-navigation systems for computerised image directed brain surgery, including wand based, microscope based and robot based systems. The author uses the robotic "Surgiscope" system. In this the imaging data of several modalities are transmitted through Dicon compatible channels to the work station in the operating theatre. There image fusion and preplanning of the surgery is done before the equipment is used to mark out the skull entry and to guide the surgeon accurately to the deeply sited planned target. Control of the accuracy of the surgery is provided by checking on the position of fixed points in the head and by following a check list in the computer menu.

A distinguished Scandinavian neurosurgeon, Professor Lars Leksell, himself a pioneer in stereotactic surgery, stated "A fool with a tool is still a fool". You have to be a master in stereotactic surgery to become a master in image-guided surgery. Education of neurosurgeons in the use of the modern computer and robotic neurosurgical equipment is clearly vital. As the pilot learns in the flight simulator so must the neurosurgeon rehearse and practice. Indeed, the equipment makes it possible for neurosurgical trainees to learn from operations by their seniors in a much more direct way than by referring to a text book. In future the possibility of tele-conferencing and tele-monitoring procedures can take this a step further.

It is clear that the expectations of the public and healthcare providers are for continued improvement and progress in neurosurgery. It is also clear throughout Europe the experience and the exposure of individual neurosurgeons to clinical cases while they are training, as well as when they are independent practitioners, are diminishing. It is probable that increasing use of computers and robots will help in reconciling these two conflicting trends.

Jens Haase, M. D.

Preface

The current changes in neurosurgery are equalized historically only by the period earlier in this century when Harvey Cushing introduced the methods of modern general neurosurgery. Even the interested observer feels amazement. The last decade has seen not only the acceptance of digital imaging into the daily routine but also the incorporation of achievements in basic biologic sciences which have been termed as "molecular neurosurgery" or "reconstructive neurology". Perhaps without recognizing it stereotactic neurosurgery has played a leading role in promoting the new developments, and transforming them into useful instruments for the whole field of neurosurgery. The stereotactic methodology – not long ago considered a physiologic subspeciality for functional neurological disorders – now pervades all aspects of neurosurgery. These proceedings from the *XIIth Meeting of the European Society for Stereotactic and Functional Neurosurgery* in Milan reflect the topics of the meeting and the impact on the field.

The major aim of the meeting and of the publication is an update of information. This compilation of selected abstracts therefore may serve the reader for both information and judgement. The contents is subdivided into sections on *Surgical Treatments of Parkinson's Disease, Pain, Psychosurgery, Epilepsy, Frameless Stereotaxy, Functional Imaging, Methodology, Gene Therapy, Radiosurgery and Tumours*. Necessarily this volume contains a mixture of various topics. Although rather eclectic the series of papers, however, reflects the current status and progress in the field. Abilities do not exist in the abstract but in individual examples (M. Oakeshott). Each individual example has what maybe called a style or idiom of its own which cannot be specified in propositions. The editors are immensely indebted to *Dr. Hazel Cockburn* (London) for undertaking the linguistic editing and proofreading of the manuscripts.

The most astounding development in neurosurgery is the general acceptance of "stereotactic space" what is now called "neuronavigation". The congress in Milan had the privilege to listen to one of the pioneers and proponents of the method namely *Jens Haase* from Aaalborg who with great enthusiasm unifies the views of both stereotactic and general neurosurgeons. For the editors this contribution was of such high significance as to place it as a foreword of this volume.

The Editors

Contents

Functional Imaging

Methodology

Gene Therapy

Radiosurgery

Tumours

Listed in Current Contents

Acta Neurochir (1997) [Suppl] 68: 1–10

Controversies in Pallidal Surgery

M. I. Hariz

Department of Neurosurgery, University Hospital, Umeå, Sweden

Summary

Posteroventral pallidotomy (PVP) has gained a worldwide acceptance after its reintroduction by Laitinen *et al.* in 1992 (56) and many studies have since been published. A review of the recent literature reveals that there is variation in the clinical indications for this procedure, the surgical technique used and the assessment of results. There is no uniform practice in the choice of the anatomical target point within the globus pallidus, the imaging of the target structure, the intraoperative assessment of the physiological target and the mode of evaluation of the surgical results. Although some neurosurgeons advocate that the lesion should be in the lateral pallidum, the majority insist it should be in the medial pallidum. It is shown here that, as long as the lesion is made at the posterior and ventral parts of the globus pallidus, it will necessarily include aspects of both medial and lateral posteroventral pallidum. There is a common agreement on the effectiveness of pallidal surgery on the L-dopa induced dyskinesias, but, its long-term effects on tremor, akinesia, freezing of the gait and other genuine parkinsonian symptoms need more extensive evaluation. The assessment of the outcome of pallidal surgery in terms of the patient's disability, quality of life and coping abilities following surgery seems to have been neglected.

Keywords: Parkinson's disease; stereotactic surgery; pallidotomy.

Introduction

Since the publication of the paper by Laitinen *et al.* in January 1992 [56], re-introducing posteroventral pallidotomy (PVP) for Parkinson's disease (PD), this procedure has generated many publications and presentations. Various opinions and ideas have been presented concerning mainly the following issues: What are the most appropriate indications for pallidotomy? Where is the ideal anatomical and physiological location of the target within the globus pallidus? Which radiological means are most suitable for imaging the target area? Which are the most appropriate methods for intra-operative assessment of the physiological target? Is chronic stimulation or radiofrequency (RF) lesion or even Gamma Knife radiation the most appropriate method for interrupting the pathological pathways within the globus pallidus? How to assess the clinical results of pallidal surgery?

In this paper, the controversies of the literature about these aspects of pallidal surgery will be reviewed and addressed in the light of the present author's experience in this field.

Indications for Pallidal Surgery

Posteroventral pallidotomy (PVP) is, just like any other treatment for PD, a symptomatic treatment. It is in the first place the pattern of symptoms of the patient and the degree of his/her disability that will decide whether surgery is to be recommended. If surgery is indeed to be performed, there are various options available, the most established of which are thalamotomy, pallidotomy and thalamic stimulation. While thalamotomy or thalamic stimulation is performed on patients whose main symptom is tremor, PVP is being performed mainly on Parkinonian patients exhibiting the full range of parkinsonian symptoms, including those due to the long standing L-dopa treatment. Therefore, many workers consider PVP to be indicated in patients with so-called "advanced" PD [3, 17, 40, 43, 45, 56–58, 69, 78, 81]. In a period of enthusiasm, PVP has even been tried on patients with the so called Parkinson Plus Syndrome [19], but the results were disappointing [21, 60, 62].

PD is generally considered "advanced" in terms of high Hoehn and Yahr staging [38], although this staging, which was introduced prior to L-dopa treatment, may be considered too inexact to classify the disease in patients on long term L-dopa therapy. Therefore, "advanced" PD generally means patients whose disease has evolved to a state of continuous fluctuations including various severe symptoms both in "on" and "off" phases. Thus, some authors insist that the procedure should be reserved for patients with L-dopa-induced fluctuations, since the best effects of pallidotomy are on the dyskinesias of the patient who exhibits "on-off" phenomena [3, 46, 50, 81]. Most authors, however, consider that pallidotomy is equally suitable for tremor, rigor, bradykinesia, dyskinesias and painful dystonia. Laitinen recommends pallidotomy to be performed even before dyskinesias are established [60]. Although, there appears to be no rigid age limit, provided the patient is in good mental condition [60, 62], nevertheless, it is more or less agreed upon that younger patients have a better outcome [3, 17, 60, 68]. In the present author's experience, elderly patients who exhibit the so-called non-fluctuating rigid-akinetic syndrome, especially those patients with severe freezing of the gait, do not respond as well to pallidotomy, as patients with fluctuations (46). In these patients, Benabid *et al.* have indicated that chronic subthalamic stimulation might be a more appropriate method to improve the mobility of the patient, although these results are still preliminary [5].

In the final analysis, it will be the overall long-term results of pallidotomy, performed and assessed uniformly in several centres and in a large number of patients exhibiting various symptoms of the disease, that will determine the final indications for this surgery and determine its place in the treatment of patients with Parkinson's disease [50].

Location of the "Best" Anatomical Target

In the original paper of Svennilson *et al.* in 1960 [82], assessing the results of Leksell's pallidotomies, it was mentioned that Leksell "moved" his target to a more postero-ventral direction, compared to the classical antero-dorsal target position then prevalent. It was further stated that the results of pallidotomies performed at this new target were even better than those performed on the previous antero-dorsal target [56, 82]. Leksell's lesion was centred at the ventralmost area of the posterior pallidum, 2 mm anterior to the mid-commissural point, 3 mm below the intercommissural line (ICL), and 20 mm lateral from the midline of the third ventricle. In 1960 ventriculography was the only means of calculating the coordinates of the target during surgery. This target point, projected on the corresponding plates (plates 27, 54 and 55) of the atlas of Schaltenbrand and Wahren [74], is situated in the ventroposteromedial (VPM) pallidum, just dorsal to the exit of tha ansa lenticularis, and just medial to the nucleus basalis. Gradually, Laitinen "moved" that target laterally, and insisted that pallidotomy should be done in the ventroposterolateral (VPL) pallidum, instead of in the VPM pallidum [58, 60, 62]. Meanwhile, basic research on animals revealed that it was indeed in the medial pallidum that the increased inhibitory activity of PD took place [1, 7, 12, 23]. This was confirmed by several authors performing microelectrode recording during human pallidotomy procedures [9, 16, 17, 39, 63, 67–69, 79, 80, 81]. These authors therefore advocated that pallidotomy should be aimed at interruption of this overactive medial pallidum. Laitinen continued to advocate the surgical interruption of the pathway in the lateral pallidum, because this would "release" the overactive medial pallidum and re-establish more normal activity in the medial pallidum [60, 62]. According to the scheme of de Long and others [12], it is primarily the medial pallidum, receiving input from the inhibitory subthalamic nucleus, that ought to be targeted in pallidotomy, while the lateral pallidum plays a secondary role in the inhibition of movements in PD. Therefore the common target of surgeons today is VPM pallidotomy, although VPL pallidotomy is advocated by Laitinen and several others [51, 58, 60, 62, 71, 85].

In this author's opinion, this is not an important issue, because as long as the pallidotomy is performed at the ventral posterior part of the pallidum, the radiofrequency (RF) lesion itself will include aspects of both medial pallidum and lateral pallidum (Fig. 1). If one looks carefully at the plates 27, 54 and 55 in the Atlas of Schaltenbrand and Wahren [74], one can clearly see that the shape of the pallidum is such that more posteriorly and the more ventrally it is more narrow and at this posterior ventral level, a pallidal lesion of the advocated diameter of 6 mm [68] will necessarily encompass a brain volume belonging to both pallidum medialis pars interna, pallidum medialis pars externa and pallidum lateralis (Fig. 1). It must be remembered that a stereotactic target point is only a point to be aimed at, while a stereotactic RF lesion is a volume of brain that is destroyed by RF heat. This volume, unless extremely tiny, which is not the case for pallidal RF lesions, will indeed comprise in itself both medial and lateral parts of the postero-ventral portion of the pallidum. Some published MR figures of reports describing posterior ventral medial

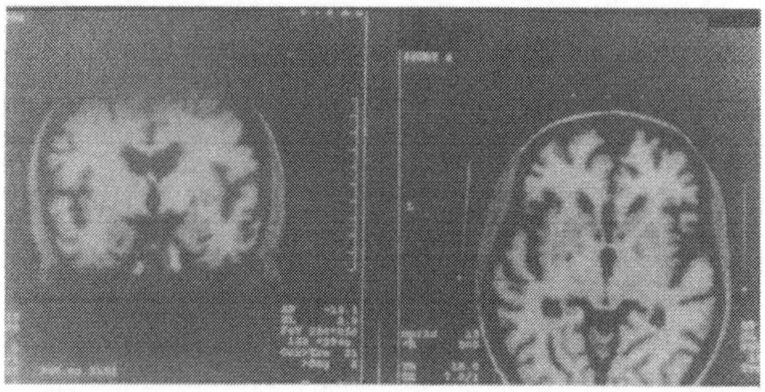

Fig. 1. A stereotactic MRI study, performed 6 months after surgery. A 2 mm-thick axial slice and a 2 mm-thick coronal slice at the level of a left pallidotomy lesion are shown. The lesion lies at the ventralmost area of the posterior pallidum, just medial to the internal border of the putamen, just lateral to the external edge of the internal capsule, just above the dorsal amygdala, and lateral and dorsal from the ambient cistern and the optic tract. On the axial slice one can clearly see that the lesion encompasses both medial and lateral pallidum as these structures converge at the posteroventral aspects of the pallidum

pallidotomy, show that the pallidal lesion if located strictly medial will lie too anterior and too dorsal in the pallidum [17, 67], and if it lies posteroventrally in the pallidum, it will definitely encompass both medial and lateral aspects [58, 60].

Therefore, it is even more impossible to imagine a stereotactic lesion confined solely to the internal part of the medial globus pallidus at its posteroventral aspects, as advocated by some [39]. Recently, some authors have questioned whether the lesion should lie in the posteroventral pallidal area of Leksell. Lozano stated in 1995 that his successful lesions lay more anterior and more dorsal than the target point of Leksell-Laitinen [68]. Iacono, however, states that although the classical target of Leksell-Laitinen is suitable for ablative pallidal lesion, neuro-augmentive chronic stimulation should rather be performed on the anterior-medial parts of the pallidum, because stimulation of the more anterior level yields better clinical results [42, 44].

It seems therefore that as the practice of pallidotomy spreads differences of opinion on the ideal target are increasing, as happened in the past with ventrolateral thalamotomy [59]. The present author believes that these varying opinions on the ideal locations of pallidal lesions may be partly due to inconsistent results of the "Laitinen-Leksell" pallidotomy as performed by different stereotactic surgeons and partly due to difficulties in interpreting the findings obtained during micro-electrode exploration of the pallidum.

Imaging of the Pallidal Target

Whatever the site of the target it has to be defined on a radiological study, by ventriculography (VG), CT or MRI. The author and others [2, 33–35] consider ventriculography obsolete, although it is still used by some surgeons [45]. CT target determination was used in the first papers of Laitinen *et al.* [56, 57], and is still used by others although it is now agreed that MRI is the best means of visualising the target area [53], nevertheless MRI has been reported to provoke such distortions on the image that several authors do not recommend it as the sole means of identifying the stereotactic target [2, 45]. Rather, methods combining MRI with VG [45] or MRI with CT [2] are used in order to obtain adequate geometrical accuracy. Some authors use additionally computerized atlas charts that can be adjusted to the individual patient's third ventricular dimensions [2, 17]. In the author's experience, 2 mm-thick axial and coronal stereotactic MRI study is superior to any other means, not only to visualize the target but also the optic tract and the internal capsule. The eventual distortions are of no clinically significant relevance if the MRI machine is properly calibrated for minimizing distortion, and if the frame fiducials lie as close as possible to the head, for example as is the case with the Laitinen Stereoadapter system [58, 61]. Furthermore, a high definition axial MRI image actually depicts the edges of the posterior ventral pallidum in relation to the medial border of the putamen and the lateral border of the internal capsule (Fig. 1). This contributes to further tuning the position of the classical Leksell target point obtained in relation to the commissures of the third ventricle. A thin high-resolution coronal MRI slice obtained perpendicular to the intercommissural line and lying some 10–12 mm behind the anterior commissure (Fig. 1), makes it possible to assess very accurately the depth of the target in relation to the ambient cistern, to the dorsal amygdala and to the optic tract [37]. In some patients, it appeared that the classical target depth of 6 mm ventral to the intercommissural line, as previously advocated by Leksell and Laitinen [56, 82], was too deep. Thus, coronal stereotactic MRI as described here, together with a dorsal to ventral intraoperative stimulation procedure as described by Laitinen [58, 60, 62], has practically eliminated the risk for scotoma, the incidence of which has dropped from the published 14% incidence in 1992 [56, 57], to less than 1% [32, 58, 60].

Intraoperative Assessment of the Physiological Target

Nearly all neurosurgeons (except those using Gamma Knife) agree that the anatomical target must be physiologically corroborated before any lesioning can take place. While some believe that macrostimulation is enough for physiological confirmation of the target, other feel that unless microelectrodes are used for recording and/or stimulation, the pallidotomy cannot be safely and efficiently performed [3, 9, 68]. There has been a clear tendency on the part of surgeons used to performing microelectrode investigations during ventral intermedius (Vim) thalamotomy [83] to transpose this experience to pallidotomy. The author agrees with Laitinen that the first anatomical corroboration of the target takes place during impedance measurement while introducing the probe to the target. The impedance value clearly differentiates between grey matter, white matter and CSF spaces [54, 58], provided the tip of the measuring probe is very small in surface area in relation to a large indifferent electrode. It is also important to observe carefully if the tremor, rigidity or bradykinesia are modified by the mere mechanical injury effect of the probe. This mechanical effect, however, is less evident than during thalamotomy, where the tremor can be completely stopped when the probe hits the "right" physiological target in the Vim nucleus of the thalamus.

Electrical macrostimulation of the target area is an excellent method for checking the position of the stereotactic probe. Here also, it is important that the probe tip is small. This guarantees that the stimulation effects are local-specific. For pallidal stimulation, using 1 msec in pulse length, the current threshold intensities are 8–10 mA at 5–6 Hz and 4–5 mA at 50–60 Hz, respectively. The interpretation of the stimulation responses during pallidotomy is not as straightforward as during thalamotomy, since there is no evident or consistent stimulation response to either high frequency or low frequency stimulation and no consistent effect of the acute stimulation on any of the parkinsonian symptoms [56]. The main aim of the stimulation thresholds during pallidotomy is to avoid harm to the internal capsule and the optic tract.

A careful study of microelectrode recording did not appear to improve the clinical effect of thalamotomy for parkinsonian tremor, or to reduce the incidence of side-effects [47]. The same may be true for pallidal surgery. Microelectrode recordings during pallidotomy is of great scientific importance, because the pallidum has never been previously mapped. Microrecording and microstimulation can confirm the existence and orientation of the somatomotor homunculus in the posteroventral pallidum [80], a fact that had already been empirically verified by Laitinen *et al.* during macrostimulation and staged coagulation of the posteroventral pallidum [58, 60]. However, microelectrode recording during pallidotomy increases the duration of surgery. The patient becomes tired, can no longer cooperate, and can no longer be assessable or reliable upon stimulation [68]. In addition, the infection risk may increase as may the risks of bleeding due to multiple electrode penetrations [65]. It seems therefore debatable whether the microcelectrode technique in comparison to impedance recording and electrical stimulation will improve the results of pallidotomy or reduce its side-effects. There is no evidence yet that micro-electrode-guided pallidotomy improves the effect of surgery or decreases the complication rate compared to macrostimulation-based pallidotomy [11, 28, 52].

By contrast, there are some neurosurgeons advocating or actually performing pallidotomy with radiosurgery without any physiological assessment of the target area [24, 25, 73]. However, in a recent paper it was shown that Gamma Knife radiosurgery was not suitable for pallidotomy [24]. It is the opinion of the author, since that neither stimulation nor recording are applicable, since that the physiological target might differ from the anatomical target, since that there might be inherent inaccuracies of the stereotactic frame and/or the radiological study and finally, since that lesioning cannot be stopped should adverse effects appear pallidotomy by radiosurgery is not only risky but also ethically questionable [15].

Ablation or Stimulation of the Pallidum

Nearly all pallidotomies are performed with radiofrequency (RF) current. The lesion is usually made incrementally, after appropriate stimulation, to encompass the posteroventral pallidum, and results in a lesion averaging 75–150 mm^3 [60, 67]. The pallidotomy lesion is typically 2–3 times larger than the vim thalamotomy lesion, more evidence that the lesion cannot be restricted solely to the medial pallidum at its posteroventral extent. It is a clinical advantage for the patient if the lesion extends into the external pallidum laterally rather than into the internal capsule medially.

In 1994, Siegfried *et al.* were the first to report that chronic pallidal stimulation was as successful as pallidotomy [76]. Chronic thalamic stimulation is now an established method for treating the tremor of PD [77], since Benabid *et al.* showed that this method is at least as effective as thalamotomy, carries less risks than thalamotomy and can safely be used bilaterally in the brain [6]. While the rationale for using chronic thalamic stimulation can easily be understood given the mode of action of high frequency stimulation on the low-frequent tremor oscillations, and given the risks inherent to thalamotomy, the rationale for using chronic pallidal stimulation is less obvious. In the pallidum there is no consistent evidence for the existence of "tremor cells" with tremor synchronous bursting, nor has it been shown that acute high frequency stimulation of the target during pallidotomy consistently blocks eventual tremor or other parkinsonian symptoms. In addition, the risks of bilateral staged pallidotomy are not as great as the risks of bilateral staged thalamotomy in terms of dysarthria, dysphasia, dysphonia, balance or memory impairment. Nevertheless the non-ablative mode and reversibility of the stimulation method have tempted some workers to use pallidal chronic stimulation rather than ablation, notwithstanding the greater cost [4, 27, 77]. It remains to be proven whether stimulation is better than ablation, even bilateral staged ablation, in increased effectiveness on the symptoms and decreased risks for the patient.

Staged bilateral pallidotomy is being performed more frequently as many patients desire soon after a successful pallidotomy, a similar procedure on the contralateral brain. Although in the author's and Laitinen's experience [58, 60] there is no evidence as yet that staged bilateral pallidotomy carries more risks for the patient's cognitive functions as long as the pallidotomies are carried out in the ventral posterior area of the pallidum, others have noted cognitive decline after bilateral staged or contemporaneous pallidotomy [10, 26, 28, 78]. Perhaps the pallidal lesions in these cases lay too medial [10, 26, 28]. Other workers have found no disadvantage in performing even contemporaneous bilateral pallidotomies [9, 43, 45].

The present author does not advocate that bilateral posteroventral pallidotomy be performed in one session for safety reasons, to allow the brain and the patient to recover after the first surgery and to give some time for assessment of the results of the first procedure. A wait of at least 6 months is advised before performing the pallidotomy on the other hemisphere.

Assessment of the Radiofrequency Lesion

In order to gain more knowledge about the ideal target to be lesioned, the ideal size of the lesion, the proper correlation between the site and size of the lesion and clinical results and eventual side-effects, it is mandatory to have an accurate image of the RF lesion. Some workers perform MRI within a few hours or days of the surgery [13, 14, 17]. While this may well tell the surgeon that he/she has hit the intended target, it gives no information about the "final" size of the lesion, due to the presence of massive local oedema. In addition, it is known that the lesion may well shrink over the first few months following surgery, and, since the clinical assessment of surgery may not be relevant before at least the resolution of oedema, an immediate postoperative MRI cannot prove that the clinical results do indeed correlate with the size or site of the final pallidal lesion [36]. Therefore the present author does not perform MRI – or CT – for lesion control before at least three months after surgery.

In imaging stereotactic pallidal lesions, it is mandatory to correlate accurately the lesion to the anatomical target and to the ventricular landmarks on the basis of which the target coordinates were defined. For this, the ideal is to perform contiguous 2 mm-thin MRI scans, with axial slices parallel to the intercommissural line (ICL) of the third ventricle and coronal slices perpendicular to the ICL (Fig. 1). Hereby, the size of the lesion can be accurately measured, its volume calculated and the accurate location of the lesion in relation to the target area and to the ventricular landmarks be properly assessed.

While it is generally agreed that the stereotactic pallidal lesion, in order to be effective, needs to lie at the ventralmost area of the posterior pallidum [58, 60, 87]. The author believes that there is no definite answer to what is the optimal size of a pallidal RF lesion. In addition, the target area in many patients with advanced PD exhibits small lacunas which might interfere with and influence the final size of the RF lesion. A review performed by the author of a small number of pallidotomies showed that, within certain extremes, there is no clear correlation between lesion size and clinical results [36]. Further studies are needed to establish the relationship, if any, between the final site and size of the lesion and the clinical results of pallidotomy.

Clinical Evaluation of Pallidal Surgery Results

For thalamotomy, there has been for a long time agreement among neurologists and neurosurgeons about the indications for and results of this procedure. Thus, thalamotomy is fairly effective against the tremor and the rigidity of Parkinson's disease and ineffective for akinesia [48, 49, 55, 83].

Pallidotomy has provoked more debate among neurosurgeons, neurologists and patients than any other previous surgical treatment for PD. The literature, whether scientific or journalistic, bears witness to the difficulties and sometimes discrepancies in judging the effects of pallidotomy. It is obvious that the results of pallidotomy are not as easily assessable as those of thalamotomy and its place in the treatment of PD patients is still under discussion [50]. The reasons may be that the patients undergoing pallidotomy are often in a multi-symptomatic advanced stage of the disease; the expectations may have been overestimated, and the quality of the assessments performed may have been questionable. Thus, the attitude towards pallidotomy, especially among neurologists, is equivocal [72]. To explain the complexity and diversity in assessment of pallidotomy results one must consider when the assessments are done, what is assessed, how, where and by whom.

When the assessment is done too early (within days or weeks from pallidotomy) most patients are usually doing well. This may be a genuine effect. It may also be a placebo effect, or the reversible effect of oedema around the RF lesion. When performed late, i.e., months or year(s) after surgery, the disease progression of these patients (who often are in a very advanced state of the disease) should be taken into account [22, 30]. One method to assess the proper effect of pallidotomy is to have a control group of matching patients, as described by Dogali *et al.* [17], or to have blinded assessments as described by Lozano *et al.* [69].

What should be assessed: The World Health Organisation emphasised in 1980 the importance of demarcating the three different entities of a disease, namely impairment, disability, handicap [88]. These entities cannot be better illustrated than in patients suffering from PD where impairment and disability may not always correlate [38, 64, 75, 84, 86]. Therefore, the results of pallidotomy may well differ if one assesses the patient's neurological symptoms, e.g., tremor, bradykinesia, rigidity, dyskinesia, dystonia, the patient's disability, i.e. talking, walking, feeding, dressing and other activities of daily living (ADL) or the patient's adaptation to his/her milieu and in society (coping ability, handicap). It should also be remembered that the psychological aspects in a patient with PD, such as depression and anxiety, must be taken into account.

How is the assessment done? If carried out on an out-patient basis, the assessment may vary from no effect to excellent effect depending on what state the patient happens to be in while in the neurologist's office. A quick neurological examination will tell nothing definite. An interview of the patient or relatives may be misleading, since the results of surgery may be totally different from one patient to another, or that symptom. A quick video or timed test of the patient before and after surgery will certainly not cover all aspects of the disease and definitely not the subjective feeling of the patient or his/her performances in ADL. An opto-electronic assessment using advanced computer programs is not physiological and stresses the patient whose symptoms are very sensitive to stressful situations. The use of scales, especially the widely used Unified Parkinson Disease Rating Scale (UPDRS) [20], gives a fair overall idea of the patient's disability, but does not address the very important aspect of the patient's coping abilities and quality of life. However, the UPDRS is currently the best available tool for routine monitoring of a patient's condition before and after surgery. Furthermore, the occurrence of "on-off" phenomena, with periods of severe akinesia and periods of dyskinesias, in the patients undergoing pallidotomy indicates assessment of the patient both in "off" and in "on" conditions and requires at least two spaced assessments for preoperative and postoperative evaluation [17, 69]. Other workers choose to have the patients assessed every hour throughout one day, both pre and postoperatively, to cover the whole fluctuations of the patient, but this may be time consuming, stressful for the patient and applicable only in small series of patients [46].

Where is the assessment done? The most common place where patients are assessed most commonly on an out-patient basis in a busy clinic, which may not be valid as far as pallidotomy cases are concerned. In-hospital assessment is expensive and may not show accurately how the patient is behaving at home or in the community. Assessment conducted at the patient's home by a therapist living with the patient may not be feasible.

Who is conducts the assessment? The neurosurgeon may be biased in assessing his/her results [75], and the patient might be tempted not to deceive his/her surgeon by complaining of the lack of effect of surgery. The neurologist is no neutral either and might consider that "the bottle is half empty" instead of considering it "half full", when making the assessment. The family doctor may lack a detailed neurological knowledge about the surgery or the disease. The physiotherapist may focus only on the impairment of the patient and on the function of this or that group of muscles, while the occupational therapist may focus only on assessing disability items in ADL. The psychologist may detect sub-clinical cognitive impairments while using sophisticated test, while the radiologist may find increased basal ganglia metabolism on the PET study [18, 31]. The nurse may focus on the behaviour of the patient in strictly nursing situations. The patient him- or herself may complain about issues totally different from the cardinal symptoms of the disease, or may be happy with the results despite no obvious clinical improvement. The patient's own assessment may be considered reliable [8, 66] or unreliable [29], according to what the patient is actually assessing.

In summary, in assessment of pallidotomy results there are at least four kinds of evaluation: that of the the neurosurgeon, that of the the neurologist, that of the patient and his family and some further objective assessment [58]. As outlined above these vary what has been stated above. However, in the opinion of the author, if the patient is coping better with the disease after surgery than before, the main goal of pallidotomy has been reached. The question remains how to document this coping ability and how long will the eventual improvement last?

Concluding Remarks

Undoubtedly, the modern pallidotomy has become an accepted part of modern neurosurgery. Its pathophysiological substrate is still not fully understood, and its effect may be considered paradoxical [70]. Its indications, however, are not as easy to define as has been the case for thalamotomy. Furthermore, pallidal surgery is not uniformly technically conducted in terms of anatomical targetting, intraoperative physiological assessment, and stimulation or lesioning parameters. Most patients undergoing pallidotomy are not in controlled clinical trials.

The results will need long time to be properly assessed because the patients undergoing pallidotomy are much more heterogeneous than those undergoing thalamotomy. Besides this, there are difficulties in assessing results of surgery that is non-uniformly performed, non-uniformly evaluated, and conducted on a non-homogeneous patient group [50]. Everybody in the neurological and neurosurgical community agrees today that pallidotomy is very effective for L-dopa induced dyskinesias, in the medium long term. As for its long-term effect on tremor, bradykinesia, freezing of the gait and other genuine Parkinsonian symptoms, the consensus amongst neurosurgeons, and especially amongst neurologists is far from being achieved. In the final analysis, it is indeed the result of a surgical procedure that will set its indications. Therefore, the real and strict indications of pallidotomy will have to wait a comprehensive assessment of its long-term results before being generally agreed upon by neurologists, by neurosurgeons and by all those who care for patients with Parkinson's disease.

References

1. Albin RL, Young AB, Penney JB (1989) The functional anatomy of basal ganglia disorders. Trends Neurosci 12: 366–375
2. Alterman RL, Kall BA, Cohen H, Kelly PJ (1995) Stereotactic ventrdateral thalamotomy: Is ventriculography necessary? Neurosurgery 37: 717–722
3. Alterman R, Kelly P, Beric A, Eidelberg D, Fazzini E, Perrine K, Sterio D (1996) Selection criteria for posteroventral pallidotomy (Abstract). Acta Neurochir (Wien) 138: 636
4. Barcia-Salorio JL, Pascual-Leone A, Barcia JA, Garcia-March G, López-Gómez L, Roldán P, Llácer JL (1996) Deep brain stimulation (DBS) of the posteroventral globus pallidus internus (GPi) and of the nucleus ventro-oralis posterior (Vop) in movement disorders. (Abstract) Acta Neurochir (Wien) 138: 637
5. Benabid AL, Pollak P, Gross C, Hoffman D, Benazzouz A, Gao DM, Laurent A, Gentil M, Perret J (1994) Acute and long-term effects of subthalamic nucleus stimulation in Parkinson's disease. Stereotact Funct Neurosurg 62: 76–84
6. Benabid AL, Pollak P, Gervason C, Hoffmann D, Gao DM, Hommel M, Perret JE, De Rougemont J (1991) Long-term suppression of tremor by chronic stimulation of the ventral intermediate thalamic nucleus. Lancet 337: 403–406
7. Blanchet PJ, Boucher R, Bedard PJ (1994) Exeitotoxic lateral pallidotomy does not relieve L-dopa induced dyskinesia in MPTP parkinsonian monkeys. Brain Res 650: 32–39
8. Brown RG, MacCarthy B, Jahanshahi M, Marsden CD (1989) Accuracy of self-reported disability in patients with Parkinsonism. Arch Neurol 46: 955–959
9. Burchiel KJ, Favre J, Taha J (1996) Pallidotomy for Parkinson's disease: surgical technique and results (abstract). J Neurosurg 84: 336A

10. Burzaco J (1985) Stereotactic pallidotomy in extrapyramidal disorders. Appl Neurophysiol 48: 283–287
11. De Lotbinière ACJ (1996) Microelectrode recording: essential for the optimal placement of radiofrequency pallidotomy? (Abstract). Acta Neurochir (Wien) 138: 636
12. DeLong MR (1990) Primate models of movement disorders of basal ganglia origin. Trends Neurosci 13: 281–285
13. DeSalles AAF, Brekhus SD, DeSouza EC, Behnke EJ, Farahani K, Anzai Y, Lufkin R (1995) Early postoperative appearance of radiofrequency lesions on magnetic resonance imaging. Neurosurgery 36: 932–937
14. DeSalles AAF, Behnke E, Bronstein J, Masteman D, Vassilev V, Cabatan-Awang C, Medin P (1996) MRI guided pallidotomy and acute radiofrequency lesion aspect (abstract). Acta Neurochir (Wien) 138: 642
15. DeSalles AAF, Hariz M (1993) Functional Radiosurgery. In: DeSalles AAF, Goetsch S (eds) Stereotactic surgery and radiosurgery. Medical Physics Publishing, Madison, Wisconsin, pp 389–406
16. Dogali M, Beric A, Sterio D, Eidelberg D, Fazzini S, Takikawa S, Samelson DR, Devinski O, Kolodny EH (1995) Anatomic and physiologic considerations in pallidotomy for Parkinson's disease. Acta Neurochir (Wien) [Suppl] 64: 9–12
17. Dogali M, Fazzini E, Kolodny E, Eidelberg D, Sterio D, Devinski O, Beric A (1995) Stereotactic ventral pallidotomy for Parkinson's disease. Neurology 45: 753–761
18. Eidelberg D, Moeller JR, Ishikawa T, Dhawan V, Spetsieris P, Silbersweig D, Stern E, Woods RP, Fazzini E, Dogali M, Beric A (1996) Regional metabolic correlates of surgical outcome following unilateral pallidotomy for Parkinson's disease. Ann Neurol 39: 450–459
19. Eidelberg D, Takikawa S, Moeller JR, Dhawan V, Redington K, Chaly T, Robeson W, Dahl JR, Margouleff D, Fazzini E, Przedborski S, Fahn S (1993) Striatal hypometabolism distinguishes striatonigral degeneration from Parkinson's disease. Ann Neurol 33: 518–527
20. Fahn S, Elton RL Members of the UPDRS Development Committee (1987) Unitied Parkinson's disease rating scale. In: Fahn S, Marsden CD, Calne DB, Goldstein M, (eds) Recent developments in Parkinson's disease, vol 2. Macmillan Health Care Information, Florham Park, NJ, pp 153–163
21. Fazzini E, Dogali M, Berich A, Chin L, Eidelberg D, Sterio G, Samelson D, Loftus S, Gianutsos B, Newman B, Kolodny E, Laitinen L (1993) Ventral pallidotomy operations in patients with Parkinson's plus syndromes (abstract). Ann Neurol 34: 266
22. Fazzini E, Dogali M, Eidelberg D, Beric A, Sterio G, Perrine K, Kolodny E (1996) Three-year follow up following unilateral pallidotomy in Parkinson's disease (abstract). Neurology 46: A200
23. Filion M, Boucher R, Bedard P (1985) Globus pallidus unit activity in the monkey during the induction of parkinsonism by 1-methyl-4-phenyl-1,2,3,6-tetrahydropyridine (MPTP). Soc Neurosci Abstr 11: 1160
24. Friedman JH, Epstein M, Sanes JN, Lieberman P, Cullen K, Lindquist C, Daamen M (1996) Gamma knife pallidotomy in advanced Parkinson's disease. Ann Neurol 39: 535–538
25. Frichs GM, Norén GC (1996) Neurosurgical treatment of parkinsonism with the Leksell Gamma Knife (abstract). Mov Disord 11 [Suppl 1]: 242
26. Galvéz-Jiménez N, Lozano AM, Duff J, Trépanier L, Saint-Cyr JA, Lang AE (1996) Bilateral pallidotomy: pronounced amelioration of incapacitating levodopa-induced dyskinesias but accompanying cognitive decline (abstract). Mov Disord 11 [Suppl 1]: 242
27. Galvéz-Jiménez N, Lang AE, Lozano A, Tasker R, Duff J, Hutchinson W, Ashby P, Dostrovsky O (1996) Deep brain stimulation in Parkinson's disease: new methods of tailoring functional surgery to patient needs and response (abstract). Neurology 46: A402
28. Ghika J, Favre J, Frankhauser H, Regli F (1996) Neurological and neuropsychological complications of bilateral contemporaneous pallidotomy in Parkinson's disease (abstract). Neurology 46: A417
29. Golbe LI, Pae J (1988) Validity of a mailed epidemiological questionnaire and physical self-assessment in Parkinson's disease. Mov Disord 3: 245–254
30. Green J, Vitek JL, Baron M, Bakey RAE, DeLong MR (1996) Neuropsychological sequelae of pallidotomy for treatment of Parkinson's disease: one year pilot findings (abstract). Neurology 46: A200
31. Grafton ST, Waters C, Sutton J, Lew MF, Couldwell W (1995) Pallidotomy increases activity of motor association cortex in Parkinson's disease: a positron emission tomographic study. Ann Neurol 37: 776–783
32. Hariz MI, DeSalles AAF (1996) The side-effects and complications of posteroventral pallidotomy (abstract). Acta Neurochir (Wien) 138: 643
33. Hariz MI, Bergenheim AT, Fodstad H (1993) Air-ventriculography provokes an anterior displacement of the third ventricle during functional stereotactic surgery. Acta Neurochir (Wien) 123: 147–152
34. Hariz MI, Bergenheim AT (1990) A comparative study on ventriculographic and computed tomography-guided determinations of brain targets in functional stereotaxis. J Neurosurg 73: 565–571
35. Hariz MI, Bergenheim AT (1993) Clinical evaluation of CT-guided versus ventriculography-guided thalamotomy for movement disorders. Acta Neurochir (Wien) [Suppl] 58: 53–55
36. Hariz MI (1990) Correlation between clinical outcome and size and site of the lesion in CT-guided thalamotomy and pallidotomy. Stereotact Funct Neurosurg 54 and 55: 172–185
37. Hariz MI (in press) Image-guided functional ablation of the brain. In: DeSalles AAF, Lufkin R (eds) Minimally invasive therapy of the brain. Thieme, Stuttgart
38. Hoehn MM, Yahr MD (1967) Parkinsonism: onset, progression, and mortality. Neurology 17: 427–442
39. Hutchison WD, Lozano AM, Davis KD, Saint-Cyr JA, Lang AE, Dostrovsky JO (1994) Differential neuronal activity in segments of globus pallidus in Parkinson's disease patients. NeuroReport 5: 1533–1537
40. Iacono RP, Lonser RR, Mandybur G, Morenski JD, Yamada S, Shima F (1994) Stereotactic pallidotomy results for Parkinson's exceed those of fetal graft. Am Surg 60: 777–782
41. Iacono RP, Lonser RR (1994) Reversal of Parkinson's akinesia by pallidotomy (letter). Lancet 343: 418–419
42. Iacono RP, Lonser RR, Mandybur G, Yamada S (1995) Stimulation of the globus pallidus in Parkinson's disease. Br J Neurosurg 9: 505–510
43. Iacono RP, Lonser RR, Yamada Sh (1994) Contemporaneous bilateral postero-ventral pallidotomy for early onset "juvenile type" Parkinson's disease. Case report. Acta Neurochir (Wien) 131: 247–252
44. Iacono RP, Lonser RR, Maeda G, Kuniyoshi S, Warner D, Mandybur G, Yamada Sh (1995) Chronic anterior pallidal stimulation for Parkinson's disease. Acta Neurochir (Wien) 137: 106–112
45. Iacono RP, Shima F, Lonser RR, Kuniyoshi S, Maeda G, Yamada S (1995) The results, indications and physiology of

posteroventral pallidotomy for patients with Parkinson's disease. Neurosurgery 36: 1118–1127
46. Johansson F, Malm J, Nordh E, Hariz M (in press) The usefulness of pallidotomy in advanced Parkinson's disease. J Neurosurg Neurol Psychiatry
47. Jones MW, Tasker RR (1990) The relationship of documented destruction of specific cell types to complications and effectiveness in thalamotomy for tremor in Parkinson's disease. Stereotact Funct Neurosurg 54 and 55: 207–211
48. Kelly PJ, Gillingham FJ (1980) The long-term results of stereotaxic surgery and L-dopa therapy in patients with Parkinson's disease. A 10-year follow-up study. J Neurosurg 53: 332–337
49. Kelly PJ (1988) Contempory Stereotactic Ventralis Lateral Thalamotomy in the Treatment of Parkinsonian Tremor and Other Movement Disorders. In: Heilbrun MP (ed) Stereotactic neurosurgery, vol 2. Willliams and Wilkins, Baltimore, pp 133–147
50. Kelly PJ (1995) Pallidotomy in Parkinson's disease (editorial comment). Neurosurgery 36: 1154–1157
51. Kishore A, Turnbull I, de la Fuente-Fernandez R, Schulzer M, Calne DB, Snow BJ (1996) Ventral pallidotomy improves motor signs and dyskinesias in Parkinson's disease (abstract). Mov Disord 11 [Suppl 1]: 240
52. Kondziolka D, Bonaroti EA, Lunsford LD (1996) Pallidotomy for Parkinson's disease. Contemp Neurosurg 18(6): 1–7
53. Kondziolka D, Dempsey PK, Lunsford LD, Kestle JRW, Dolan EJ, Kanal E, Tasker RR (1992) A comparison between magnetic resonance imaging and computed tomography for stereotactic coordinate determination. Neurosurgery 30: 402–407
54. Laitinen L, Johansson GG, Sipponen P (1966) Impedance and phase angle as a locating method in human stercotaxic surgery. J Neurosurg 25: 628–633
55. Laitinen L, Vilkki J (1973) Measurement of parkinsonian hypokinesia with Purdue pegboard and motor reaction time tests. In: Siegfried J (ed) Parkinson's disease, vol 1. Hans Huber, Berlin, pp 185–192
56. Laitinen LV, Bergenheim AT, Hariz MI (1992) Leksell's posteroventral pallidotomy in the treatment of Parkinson's disease. J Neurosurg 76: 53–61
57. Laitinen LV, Bergenheim AT, Hariz MI (1992) Ventroposterolateral pallidotomy can abolish all parkinsonian symptoms. Stereotact Funct Neurosurg 58: 14–21
58. Laitinen LV, Hariz MI (1996) Movement disorders. In: JR Youmans (ed) Neurological surgery, 4th ed. Saunders, Philadelphia, pp 3575–3609
59. Laitinen LV (1985) Brain targets in surgery for Parkinson's disease. J Neurosurg 62: 349–351
60. Laitinen LV (1995) Pallidotomy for Parkinson's disease. Neurosurgery Clin North Am 6: 105–112
61. Laitinen LV (1988) The Laitinen system. In: Lunsford LD (ed) Modern stereotactic neurosurgery. Nijhoff, Boston, pp 99–116
62. Laitinen LV (1994) Ventroposterolateral pallidotomy. Stereotact Funct Neurosurg 62: 41–52
63. Lang AE, Lozano A, Duff J, Miyasaki J, Galvez-Jiminez N, Hutchison W, Tasker R, Dostrovsky J (1995) Posteroventral medial pallidotomy in Parkinson's disease (abstract). Mov Disord 10: 691
64. Lang, AET, Fahn S (1989) Assessment of Parkinson's disease. In: Munsat TL (ed) Quantification of neurologic deficit. Butterworths, Boston, pp 285–301
65. Linazasoro G, Guridi J, Gorospe A, Ramos E, Mozo A, Obeso JA (1996) Posteroventral pallidotomy in Parkinson's disease. Clinical results in 27 patients (abstract). Mov Disord 11 [Suppl 1]: 240
66. Louis ED, Lynch T, Marder K, Fahn S (1996) Reliability of patient completion of the historical section of the unified Parkinson's disease rating scale. Mov Disord 11: 185–192
67. Lozano AM, Hutchison WD, Dostrovsky JO (1995) Microelectrode monitoring of cortical and subeortical structures during stereotactie surgery. Acta Neurochir (Wien) [Suppl] 64: 30–34
68. Lozano A, Hutchison W, Kiss Z, Tasker R, Davis K, Dostrovsky J (1996) Methods for microelectrode-guided posteroventral pallidotomy. J Neurosury 84: 194–202
69. Lozano AM, Lang AE, Galvez-Jimenez N, Miyasaki J, Duff J, Hutchison WD, Dostrovsky JO (1995) Effect of GPi pallidotomy on motor function in Parkinson's disease. Lancet 346: 1383–1387
70. Marsden CD, Obeso JA (1994) The functions of the basal ganglia and the paradox of stereotaxic surgery in Parkinson's disease. Review article. Brain 117: 877–897
71. Mcyer CHA (1996) Pallidotomy for Parkinson's disease promptly improves a wide range of voluntary activities – especially gait and trunk movements. (abstract) Acta Neurochir (Wien) 138: 635
72. Quinn N (1994) Reversal of Parkinson's akinesia by pallidotomy (letter). Lancet 343: 1095–1096
73. Rand RW, Jacques DB, Mclbye RW, Copcull BG, Fisher MR, Levenick MN (1993) Gamma knife thalamotomy and pallidotomy in patients with movement disorders: preliminary results. Stereotact Funct Neurosurg 61: 65–92
74. Schaltenbrand G, Wahren W (1977) Atlas for stereotaxy of the human brain, 2nd ed. Thieme, Stuttgart
75. Schwab RS, England AC Jr (1969) Projection technique for evaluating surgery in Parkinson's disease. In: Gillingham FJ, Donaldson JM (eds) Third symposium on Parkinson's disease. Livingstone, Edingburgh, pp 152–157
76. Siegfried J, Lippitz B (1994) Bilateral chronic electrostimulation of ventroposterolateral pallidum: a new therapeutic approach for alleviating all parkinsonian symptoms. Neurosurgery 35: 1126–1130
77. Siegfried J, Lippitz B (1994) Chronic clectrical stimulation of the VL-VPL complex and of the pallidum in the treatment of movement disorders: personal experience since 1982. Stereotact Funct Neurosurg 62: 71–75
78. Spiegelmann R, Chasin S (1996) Posteroventral pallidotomy: experience with 100 cases (abstract). Acta Neurochir (Wien) 138: 644
79. Sterio D, Beric A, Dogali M, Fazzini E, Alfaro G, Devinsky O (1994) Neurophysiological properties of pallidal neurons in Parkinson's disease. Ann Neurol 35: 586–591
80. Sterio D, Markovic Lj, Kelly P, Beric A (1996) Activity of globus pallidus neurons in Parkinson's disease (abstract). Mov Disord 11 [Suppl 1]: 78
81. Sutton JP, Coulwell W, Lew MF, Mallory L, Grafton S, DeGiorgio C, Welsh M, Apuzzo MLJ, Ahmadi J, Waters CH (1995) Ventroposterior medial pallidotomy in patients with advanced Parkinson's disease. Neurosurgery 36: 1112–1117
82. Svennilson E, Torvik A, Lowe R, Leksell L (1960) Treatment of Parkinsonism by stereotactic thermolesions in the pallidal region. Acta Psychiatr Neurol Scand 35: 358–377
83. Tasker RR, Yamashiro K, Lenz F (1988) Thalamotomy for Parkinson's Disease: Microelectrode Technique. In: Lunsford LD (ed) Modern stereotactic neurosurgery. Nijhoff, Boston, pp 297–314

84. Tourtellotte WW, Syndulko K (1989) Quantifying the neurologic examination: principles, constraints, and opportunities. In: Munsat TL (ed) Quantification of neurologic deficit. Butterworths, Boston, pp 7–16
85. Tsubokawa T, Moriyasu N (1975) Lateral pallidotomy for relief of ballistic movement – its basic evidences and clinical application. Confin Neurol 37: 10–15
86. Van Manen J (1969) Postural instability after ventrolateral thalamic lesions. In: Gillingham FJ, Donaldson IML (eds) Third symposium on Parkinson's disease. Livingstone, London, pp 237–241
87. Vitek JL, Hashimoto T, Baron M, Kaneoke Y, Turner R, Bakay R, DeLong MR (1994) Pallidotomy in Parkinson's disease: correlation of lesion location to clinical outcome. (abstract). Mov Disord 9: 477–478
88. World Health Organization (1980) International classification on impairments, disability, and handicaps. World Health Organization, Geneva

Correspondence: Marwan I. Hariz, M.D., Ph.D., Department of Neurosurgery, University Hospital, S-901 85 Umea, Sweden.

Acta Neurochir (1997) [Suppl] 68: 11–13

Chronic Electrostimulation of Ventroposterolateral Pallidum: Follow-up

J. Siegfried and **G. Wellis**

Department of Neurosurgery, Klinik Im Park, Zurich, Switzerland

Summary

Introduced in 1992, and first published with report of 3 cases in 1994, the ventroposterolateral electrostimulation of the pallidum raised exciting prospects. The follow-up of this new approach will be presented in 19 cases with at least 6 months control, and up to 42 months. The very favorable effects observed in the first series could be confirmed and extended to a larger group of patients during a longer period.

Keywords: Neurostimulation; pallidal stimulation; Parkinson's disease; movement disorders.

Introduction

Following the very encouraging results of ventroposterolateral pallidotomy in all symptoms of Parkinson's disease [4], by renewing an old stereotactic method [8] and precising the best target in the pallidum internum [5], an alternative technique has been introduced in 1992 [6,7] with permanent electrostimulation achieved bilaterally in one session. The present report analyses the authors' experience of this promising method with longer follow-up.

Material

From November 17, 1992 to March 7, 1996, 21 patients were considered as suitable candidates for permanent ventroposterolateral pallidal stimulation. In 18 cases, the operation was performed bilaterally in one session, and in 3 cases unilaterally, with a total of 39 neurostimulations of the pallidum.

The clinical features of the patients are summarized in Table 1. The severity of the diseases was in almost all cases at stage IV in the classification of Hoehn and Yahr [2]; only 2 cases operated unilaterally, and 1 case of multiple system atrophy, were at stage III. The diagnosis of Parkinson's disease has been reconsidered subsequently in 2 cases, and the diagnosis of multiple system atrophy suggested. All other cases were typical, and in 5 cases a juvenile form of Parkinson's disease was evident. All cases showed a severe on-off phenomenon under Levodopa treatment.

The assessment of patients using the Webster Rating Scale [9] was performed before the operation in the on stage, and then at least every 3 months postoperatively. This scale has been a standard method of the authors since 1968; it is easy to apply, and can be performed by different examiners with comparable results, which is not the case for other standardized evaluations (New York University Scale, Northwestern University Scale, UCLA Scale) [1]. The Unified Rating Scale for Parkinsonism, Version 2.0 has been applied in only a few cases and will not be analysed here [3].

Method

The stereotactic technique of implantation of electrodes in the ventroposterolateral part of the pallidum internum has been described in detail elsewhere [6]. The target coordinates were 3 mm in front of the midcommissural point; 3 mm below the intercommissural line (the ventralmost position of the electrode tip); and 20 mm lateral to the midline of the third ventricle. A monopolar electrode (Medtronic, Inc., Minneapolis) was used 31 times, and a quadripolar one 8 times. After a short test of 48 hours or more, programmable pulse generators (ITREL, Medtronic Inc., Minneapolis) were implanted subcutaneously under the clavicles, and connected to the intracerebral electrodes. The best programme of stimulation was tested. With 130 Hz and 210 microseconds duration, the amplitude was increased until the appearance of scotomas or corticospinal reactions, and stopped just before. The amplitude at 6 months had a range of 1.0 to 3.1 volts, with a mean of 2.46 V.

Results

The most dramatic effect of permanent ventroposterolateral stimulation bilaterally in cases of Parkinson's disease is the disappearance or the marked attenuation of severe iatrogenic dyskinesias. However, akinesia or hypokinesia is clearly improved, as well as rigidity. The tremor, which was before the operation never severe, improves or even almost disappears. Substantial improvement is also observed in walking ability, postural stability, and to a lesser and variable degree on speech (Tables 2 and 3). In 3 other cases, unilateral pallidal stimulation was performed, but in one of these the follow up is missing. The reason for unilateral stimulation was, in one case, the simultaneous implantation of an electrode in the ventrolateral thalamus for very strong tremor in the opposite side, and in the other a previous thalamotomy has been performed 4 years before for the opposite side. The improvement with unilateral stimulation is shown in Table 4. The effect of bilateral pallidal stimulation in cases of multiple system atrophy was poor (Table 5).

No neurological complications have to be reported.

Table 1. *Clinical Features at the Time of Operation of 21 Patients Treated by Chronic Electrostimulation of the Ventroposterolateral Pallidum*

Sex	Age (years)	Stage Hoehn/Yahr	Webster rating
Male 12	Mean 62	IV 18	Mean 20.5
Female 9	Range 51–75	III 3	Range 14.0–26.0

In all cases, the medical treatment became easier, and dopamine agonists as well as anticholinergic drugs could be decreased.

Table 2. *Effects of the Permanent Chronic Electrostimulation of the Ventroposterolateral Pallidum bilaterally in Parkinson's Disease, inclusive Juvenile Form*

	Before 16 cases	6 mo. 16 cases	9 mo. 13 cases	12 mo. 12 cases	18 mo. 9 cases	24 mo. 3 cases	30 mo. 2 cases	36 mo. 2 cases	42 mo. 1 case
Akinesia	16 cases	+++	+++	++	++	++	++	++	++
Rigidity	16 cases	+++	+++	+++	+++	+++	+++	+++	+++
Tremor	14 cases	++	++	++	++	++	++	++	++
Dyskinesias	16 cases	+++	+++	+++	+++	+++	+++	+++	+++
Speech	16 cases	+	+	+	+	–	–	–	–
Gait	16 cases	++	++	+	+	+	+	+	–
Postural stability	16 cases	++	++	++	+	+	+	+	–

+++ very marked; ++ marked; + slight; – none. *mo.* months.

Table 3. *Effect of the Permanent Chronic Electrostimulation of the Ventroposterolateral Pallidum Bilaterally on the Webster Rating Scale in Parkinson's Disease*

	No. of cases	Webster rating scale score	
		Range	Mean
Before	14	14.0–26.0	20.5
6 months	13	6.5–14.5	10.5
12 months	10	7.0–14.5	11.0
18 months	7	7.0–14.5	11.0
24 months	3	9.0–14.5	12.0
36 months	2	9.0–14.5	12.0

Table 4. *Effect of the Permanent Chronic Electrostimulation of the Ventroposterolateral Pallidum Unilaterally on the Webster Rating Scale in Parkinson's Disease*

	No. of cases	Webster rating scale score	
		Range	Mean
Before	3	16.0–22.0	19.0
6 months	2	7.0–12.0	9.5
20 months	2	7.0–12.0	10.0
27 months	1	12.0	12.0

No follow-up in 1 case, 1 case after thalamotomy on opposite side 4 years earlier, 1 case with simultaneous VL thalamus stimulation on opposite side.

Discussion

The marked improvement of permanent ventroposterolateral stimulation on akinesia, rigidity and iatrogenic dyskinesias is clearly demonstrated. An improvement is also observed in the majority of cases on postural stability, walking ability and tremor; this last symptom was, however, never strongly marked before the operation. In many cases, the speech becomes clearer, less dysphonic or dysarthric, better understood, but to a moderate degree. This global improvement results in an amelioration of the quality of life with a return to active social life; the disappearance of dyskinesias is for the patient and his family of great significance. The selection of patients for this new technique has to be carefully analysed; considering only the implanted material, the treatment is expensive. However, the sometimes dramatic improvement in quality of life has to be taken in consideration in the evaluation of costs to clinical benefit.

Table 5. *Effects of Permanent Chronic Electrostimulation of the Ventroposterolateral Pallidum Bilaterally in Multiple System Atrophy*

	Before 2 cases	3 months 2 cases	12 months 2 cases	18 months 2 cases	24 months 1 case	42 months 1 case
Akinesia	2 cases	+	+	+	+	+
Rigidity	2 cases	±	±	±	±	±
Tremor	–	–	–	–	–	–
Dyskinesias	1 case	++	++	++	++	++
Speech	2 cases	–	–	–	–	–
Gait	1 case	–	–	–	–	–
Postural stability	1 case	–	–	–	–	–
Poor response to Levodopa	2 cases	±	±	±	±	±
Blepharospasm	1 case	–	–	–	–	–
Supranuclear palsy	1 case	–	–	–	–	–
Dementia	1 case	–	–	–	–	–

++ marked; + slight; ± very slight; – none.

References

1. Diamond SG, Markham CH (1983) Evaluating the evaluations: or how to weigh the scales of parkinsonian disability. Neurology 33: 1098–1099
2. Hoehn MM, Yahr MD (1967) Parkinsonism: onset, progression and mortality. Neurology 17: 427–442
3. Koller WC (1987) Handbook of Parkinson's disease. Marcel Dekker Press, New York, pp 482–488
4. Laitinen LV, Bergenheim AT, Hariz MI (1992) Leksell's posteroventral pallidotomy in the treatment of Parkinson's disease. J Neurosurg 76: 53 61
5. Laitinen LV (1994) Ventroposterolateral pallidotomy. Stereotact Funct Neurosurg 62: 41–52
6. Siegfried J, Lippitz B (1994) Bilateral chronic stimulation of ventroposterolateral pallidum: a new therapeutic approach for alleviating all parkinsonian symptoms. Neurosurgery 35: 1126–1130
7. Siegfried J, Lippitz B (1994) Chronic electrical stimulation of the VL-VPL complex and of the pallidum in the treatment of movement disorders: personal experience since 1982. Stereotact Funct Neurosurg 62: 71–75
8. Svennilson E, Torvik A, Lowe R *et al* (1960) Treatment of parkinsonism by stereotactic thermolesions in the pallidal region. A clinical evaluation of 81 cases. Acta Psychiatr Neurol Scand 35: 358–377
9. Webster DD (1968) Clinical analysis of the disability in Parkinson's disease. Mod Treat 5: 257–282

Correspondence: J. Siegfried, M.D., Department of Neurosurgery, Klinik Im Park, Seestr. 220, CH-8002 Zurich, Switzerland.

Acta Neurochir (1997) [Suppl] 68: 14–17

Posteroventral Pallidotomy in Movement Disorders

P. R. Schuurman[1], **R. M. A. de Bie**[2], **J. D. Speelman**[2], and **D. A. Bosch**[1]

Departments of Neurosurgery[1] and Neurology[2], Academic Medical Centre, University of Amsterdam, Amsterdam, The Netherlands

Summary

Since 1992 there has been renewed interest in pallidotomy now that the limitations and adverse effects of long-term dopaminergic therapy have become more apparent and more difficult to control in patients with advanced Parkinson's disease.

The authors describe the effect of pallidotomy in 19 patients, sixteen of whom had advanced Parkinson's disease with painful dystonia and/or response fluctuations with severe akinesia while in "off" and dyskinesias while in "on". One patient had cortico-basal degeneration with rigidity, one patient had secondary dystonia and one had dystonic posturing due to Wilson's disease. Fifteen patients underwent unilateral pallidotomy; four patients had a staged bilateral procedure.

Follow-up ranged from 3 to 42 months (mean 18 months). All patients with peak-dose dyskinesias and/or dystonia had marked reduction of symptoms, including the cases of Wilson's disease and secondary dystonia. The akinesia and rigidity scores of Parkinson-patients in "off" were greatly reduced, mainly but not only on the contralateral side. Evaluation by the patients showed remarkable improvement of symptoms in 79%, leading to substantially improved functional abilities in 68%.

In this series the decrease in dopamine-response fluctuations, dystonia, hypokinesia and rigidity with functional improvement as judged by examiners and patients reflect a significant regain of independence.

Keywords: Pallidotomy; Parkinson's disease; movement disorders; stereotaxy.

Introduction

Stereotactic pallidotomy was used in attempts to abolish the hypokinesia, rigidity and tremor of Parkinson's disease (PD) as early as the 1950's [4], later to be replaced largely by thalamotomy [5] which was reported to have a more permanent effect, though mainly on tremor. With the introduction of levodopa, surgical therapy almost disappeared except for the most severe cases of medically refractory PD.

After two decades of widespread experience with levodopa, the limitations and adverse effects of long-term dopaminergic treatment became more apparent and harder to deal with, which led to a revival of interest in pallidotomy. The renaissance was started by Laitinen describing Leksell's pallidotomy in 38 patients [8], after which many others reported favourable effects of the procedure not only on the cardinal symptoms of PD but also on response fluctuations and dyskinesias induced by L-dopa [3, 6, 7, 9].

In this paper the authors describe the effect of posteroventral pallidotomy on akinesia, rigidity, dyskinesias and dystonia in 19 patients with various extrapyramidal movement disorders.

Material and Methods

Patients

Fifteen patients had advanced Parkinson's disease with painful dystonia and/or dopamine response fluctuations with hypokinesia and rigidity in the "off"-phase and dyskinesias in the "on"-phase. One patient with PD was totally unresponsive to L-dopa with permanent akinesia, rigidity and tremor. In one patient with cortico-basal degeneration, rigidity was the target symptom. One case had secondary dystonia of the left arm due to a cavernous haemangioma in the right thalamus. One patient had Wilson's disease with generalized dystonic posturing and anarthria. Age ranged from 17 to 74 yrs. (mean: 53 yrs., Table 1).

Fifteen patients underwent unilateral pallidotomy, two of whom had had a contralateral thalamotomy for tremor reduction in the past. Four patients received staged bilateral pallidotomies, two of whom had had a previous thalamotomy.

Surgical Technique

Patients were held off drugs 12 hours before surgery. The target-coordinates of the posteroventral globus pallidus at the border of the medial and lateral segments according to Leksell were 2–3 mm. anterior to the midcommissural point, 5 mm. below the inter-commissural line and 22 mm. lateral to the midline of the third ventricle [8], visualized by positive contrast ventriculography. Electrical

Table 1. *Baseline Patient Characteristics (n = 19)*

Patient	Age	Sex	Diagnosis	Duration (yrs.)	UPDRS motor (PD, off)	Hoehn & Yahr (PD, off)	Pallidotomy side
1	46	F	PD	11	73	5	Bilat
2	54	M	PD	11	53	4	L
3	57	F	PD	10	27	4	R
4	51	M	PD	14	32	3	L
5	41	M	PD	15	38	3	L
6	46	M	PD	5	34	1	L
7	61	M	PD	19	44	2	R
8	60	M	PD	29	72	5	R
9	56	M	PD	20	97	5	Bilat
10	70	F	PD	8	27	1	R
11	58	F	PD	29	50	3	L
12	66	M	PD	8	51	5	R
13	50	F	PD	13	63	5	Bilat
14	47	M	PD	17	53	5	Bilat
15	74	F	PD	23	65	5	R
16	57	M	PD	19	51	4	L
17	17	F	dystonia	5	—	—	R
18	63	M	CBD	3	—	—	L
19	41	F	Wilson	22	—	—	R

PD Parkinson's disease, *CBD* cortico-basal degeneration.

monopolar stimulation was carried out using a Fisher electrode with a 1.8 × 4.0 mm. uninsulated tip. In the trajectory towards the calculated target point, low (2 Hz.) and high (130 Hz.) frequency stimulation was performed in 2 mm. steps starting 8 mm. from the target, to determine proximity of the internal capsule and optic tract, and to verify the target structure as judged by the clinical effect. Microelectrode recording or stimulation was not used. Radiofrequency thermolesions were produced at 80C. for 60 seconds directly after stimulation at each 2 mm. step and were not postponed until after trial-stimulation of the entire tract because of the possibility of entering the cisterna ambiens just below the target, thereafter rendering coagulation ineffective due to energy dispersion through the cerebrospinal fluid.

Pre- and Postoperative Assessment

The Unified Parkinson's Disease Rating Scale (UPDRS) motor score, Hoehn & Yahr Staging, Schwab & England Functional Scale, videotapes of the patients and subjective evaluations by the patients were used to determine the clinical condition pre- and postoperatively. Follow-up ranged from 3 to 42 months (mean: 18 months). Statistical analysis was performed using sign rank tests for the mentioned clinical scales in the group of Parkinson patients.

Results

The average pre-operative and post-operative UPDRS scores, Hoehn & Yahr staging and Schwab & England functional scores of the Parkinson patients are presented in Table 2, along with standard deviations and 95% confidence intervals for the change from baseline to last follow-up. For the four patients with bilateral procedures, the results after the first pallidotomy are used for tabulation. All Parkinson patients with peak-dose dyskinesias and/or (painful) dystonia in the "on"-phase had marked reduction of these symptoms, and total "off"-time was reduced, although the latter was not recorded accurately. The hypokinesia and rigidity of Parkinson patients in "off" was reduced in all cases except for one patient who developed a severe complication. Tremor was also reduced, but to a lesser extent than the hypokinesia, rigidity and dyskinesias.

After unilateral pallidotomy, a bilateral effect was seen in most patients, though the effect was much stronger on the contralateral side. There was a disturbing imbalance between the two sides of the body in rigidity and hypokinesia in four cases, one of whom also had residual ipsilateral dyskinesias. A second contralateral pallidotomy was performed in these patients, after which there was satisfying bilateral symptom reduction.

The case of cortico-basal degeneration was unimproved. The patient with Wilson's disease had decreased dystonic posturing and reversal of anarthria. In the case of isolated dystonia of the arm, there was marked reduction of the involuntary movements.

In the subjective evaluation of the results of surgery, patients were asked to give a separate score for the change in motor-symptoms and the change in func-

Table 2. *Effects of Pallidotomy in the Patients with Parkinson's Disease* (n = 16)

	Pre-op (SD) off	Post-op (SD) off	Change	95% Confidence interval	P
UPDRS motor score	51.13 (19.63)	27.67 (17.78)	24.47	(13.24–33.70)	0.001
Total rigidity	9.93 (4.08)	4.53 (5.00)	5.40	(2.46–8.33)	0.001
Rigidity ipsilat.	3.00 (1.89)	2.07 (2.15)	0.93	(−0.64–2.03)	0.012
Rigidity contralat.	5.07 (1.91)	1.53 (2.10)	3.53	(2.09–4.98)	0.002
Total hypokinesia	19.33 (6.59)	11.13 (7.28)	8.20	(4.52–11.88)	0.007
Hypokinesia ipsilat.	8.20 (4.13)	6.37 (4.19)	1.83	(−0.09–3.76)	0.039
Hypokinesia contralat.	11.13 (3.68)	4.77 (3.42)	6.37	(4.10–8.63)	0.001
Total resting tremor	4.07 (4.13)	0.80 (1.42)	3.27	(1.38–5.16)	0.001
Tremor ipsilat.	1.60 (2.23)	0.80 (1.42)	0.80	(−0.68–1.67)	0.068
Tremor contralat.	2.27 (2.09)	0.07 (0.26)	2.20	(0.97–3.30)	0.001
Posture	2.47 (1.19)	1.47 (1.36)	1.00	(0.53–1.47)	0.005
Gait	2.40 (1.24)	1.47 (1.36)	0.93	(0.36–1.50)	0.005
Balance	2.13 (1.30)	1.33 (1.29)	0.80	(0.04–1.56)	0.056
Hoehn & Yahr	3.67 (1.45)	2.90 (1.15)	0.77	(0.26–1.28)	0.012
Schwab & England	52.67 (19.45)	74.00 (17.65)	21.33	(12.49–30.18)	0.002

UPDRS motor score: items 18–31, total rigidity: item 22, total hypokinesia: items 23–26, total rest-tremor: item 20, posture: item 28, gait: item 29, balance: item 30.
For the patients with bilateral surgery, values after the first procedure are used.

Table 3. *Patient Evaluation of Outcome* (n = 19)

	Symptomatic	Functional
++	15	13(3*)
+	2	4
0	1	1
−	0	0
−−	1	1*

++ total or remarkable improvement; + some improvement; 0 unchanged; − mild worsening; −− substantially worse; * bilateral surgery.

tional abilities in general daily life, as presented in Table 3. Total alleviation or marked improvement of symptoms was reported by 79% (15/19) of the patients, mild improvement by 11% (2/19). In 68% (13/19) there was substantial improvement in overall functional abilities, and an additional 21% (4/19) of patients reported some benefit. The patient with corticobasal degeneration had no benefit from the operation. One Parkinson patient, who was initially in excellent condition after staged bilateral surgery, developed a delayed stroke two weeks after the second procedure, with a small hypointense area on MRI (presumably due to infarction) partially involving the internal capsule, producing a worse clinical and functional condition than before surgery. Transient complications were slight facial paresis (2), slight dysarthria (1) and loss of orientation and concentration (1). Permanent complications were quadrantanopia (1), slight dysarthria (1), loss of initiative and slight disequilibrium (1) and the delayed stroke (1).

Discussion

Symptomatic improvement by pallidotomy in the condition of Parkinsonian patients in all stages of their disease has been reported by many authors [3, 6, 8, 9]. Symptoms responding well are hypokinesia, rigidity, dyskinesia and (painful) dystonia, as is confirmed by the authors data. In our tabulated results, the improvement in rigidity and hypokinesia is underestimated, as some patients did not have rigidity or hypokinesia as target symptom, thereby reducing overall changes.

Thalamotomy or thalamic stimulation is generally considered superior to pallidotomy for abolishing tremor. The effect of pallidotomy on tremor in this group is subject to negative selection bias, as tremor-dominant cases are preferably treated by thalamic surgery, giving this group lower baseline tremor scores.

Improvement in motor function after unilateral pallidotomy is predominantly contralateral, but there is also an ipsilateral effect in most patients. The reason for this is not clear, although bilateral cortical projections onto the striatal-pallidal-thalamocortical loop and bilateral pallidothalamic projections have been suggested as a possible explanations [9, 10]. This observation of a bilateral effect should induce caution in performing simultaneous bilateral pallidotomy, as this might not be necessary for the patient and the relative risk is at least twice as high.

Akineto-rigid states due to multiple system degeneration are reported to respond poorly to stereotactic surgery [1, 2], as was again seen in the present case with cortico-basal degeneration. The favourable effect on dystonia in secondary segmental dystonia and Wilson's disease has not been reported before in recent literature. As these are single cases, however, general conclusions cannot be drawn.

Due to the proximity of the optic tract to the target, visual field deficit can occur if the lesion expands too far ventrally. During trial high- and low-frequency stimulation, visual sensations reported by the patient should indicate that the electrode is too close to the optic tract. However, in the authors' case where this complication occurred, no such sensations were reported during surgery. Permanent dysarthria might occur if the lesion involves part of the internal capsule, damaging corticobulbar fibers, as was seen in one of the earlier cases. Cognitive deterioration after pallidotomy has recently been described by others, whereby those patients who already have mild cognitive dysfunction are especially at risk [1], even more so after bilateral surgery. Loss of initiative in one patient after unilateral surgery, but formal preoperative neuropsychological testing had not been performed other than the MMSE-score. It seems prudent to do neuropsychological evaluation pre-operatively, especially in older patients or those whose baseline cognitive status is dubious.

Delayed stroke has not been reported before, but from personal communications is known to have occurred in more patients. It is possible that this is due to damage to the wall of a terminal branch of the lenticulostriate artery, giving rise to infarction or bleeding at a later time, possibly connected to a period of hypo- or hypertension. If this is the case, it seems hard to develop a strategy to avoid this – hopefully rare – complication.

In this series, the subjects the decrease in dopamine-response fluctuations, dystonia, hypokinesia and rigidity with functional improvement as judged by examiners and patients reflects a significant recovery of independence.

References

1. Alterman R, Kelly P, Beric A, Eidelberg D, Fazzini E, Perrine K, Sterio D (1996) Selection criteria for posteroventral pallidotomy. Acta Neurochir (Wien) 138: 636
2. De Salles AAF, Bronstein J, Masterman D (1996) Living with Parkinson's disease. [Correspondence] New Engl J Med 335: 130–131
3. Dogali M, Fazzini E, Kolodny E, Eidelberg D, Sterio D, Devinsky O (1995) Stereotactic ventral pallidotomy for Parkinson's disease. Neurology 45: 753–761
4. Guiot G, Brion S (1953) Traitement des mouvements anormaux par la coagulation pallidale. Technique et résultats. Rev Neurol 89: 578–580
5. Hassler R, Riechert T (1954) Indikationen und Lokalisationsmethode der gezielten Hirnoperationen. Nervenarzt 25: 441–447
6. Iacono RP, Shima F, Lonser RR, Kuniyoshi S, Maeda G, Yamada S (1995) The results, indications, and physiology of posteroventral pallidotomy for patients with Parkinson's disease. Neurosurgery 36: 1118–1125
7. Klockgether T, Loschmann PA, Wullner U (1994) New medical and surgical treatments for Parkinson's disease. [Review]. Curr Opin Neurol 7: 346–352
8. Laitinen LV, Bergenheim AT, Hariz MI (1992) Leksell's posteroventral pallidotomy in the treatment of Parkinson's disease. J Neurosurg 76: 53–61
9. Lozano AM, Lang AE, Galvez-Jimenez N, Miyasaki J, Duff J, Hutchinson WD (1995) Effect of GPi pallidotomy on motor function in Parkinson's disease. Lancet 346: 1383–1387
10. Parent A, Hazrati LN (1995) Functional anatomy of the basal ganglia. I. The cortico-basalganglia-thalamo-cortical loop. Brain Res Rev 20: 91–127

Correspondence: P. R. Schuurman, M. D., Department of Neurosurgery, Academic Medical Center, Meibergdreef 9, 1105 AZ Amsterdam, The Netherlands.

Acta Neurochir (1997) [Suppl] 68: 18–23

Selection Criteria for Unilateral Posteroventral Pallidotomy

R. L. Alterman[1], P. Kelly[1], D. Sterio[1], E. Fazzini[1], D. Eidelberg[2], K. Perrine[1], and A. Beric[1]

[1]New York University Center for the Study and Treatment of Movement Disorders and [2]North Shore University Hospital, Manhasset, NY, USA

Summary

In an attempt to refine the indications for posteroventral pallidotomy (PVP) the authors instituted strict selection criteria which are based on the experience gained from the first 60 pallidotomy patients treated at their institution. In addition to clinical evaluation, all pallidotomy candidates undergo neuropsychological testing and ^{18}F-fluoro-deoxyglucose utilization positron emission tomography (FDG/PET). The data from which these criteria were developed are presented as are early clinical results. The authors demonstrate that these criteria enhance the efficacy of the procedure by assuring therapeutic response and reducing the incidence of post-operative dementia. Their indications and contraindications for pallidotomy are discussed.

Keywords: Parkinson's disease; pallidotomy; stereotaxis; dementia.

Introduction

Posteroventral pallidotomy (PVP) has re-emerged as an effective treatment for medically refractory Parkinson's disease (PD) [23]. A number of groups have now reported excellent short-term responses in many patients [8, 9, 21–24, 27]. In particular, patients with rigidity, bradykinesia and DOPA-induced dyskinesiae seem to derive the greatest benefit, though the longevity of response remains to be determined.

PVP is not for everyone. As with any surgical procedure, selection criteria for pallidotomy must be refined in order to maximize efficacy and minimize complications. Injuries to the optic tract and internal capsule have been all but eliminated by image-guided, computer-assisted targetting and electrophysiological monitoring with micro- and macroelectrodes; however, the ability to predict response and eliminate the minority of patients who will develop rapidly progressive dementia would greatly improve the efficacy of the procedure. Towards this end, the authors have developed a strict set of selection criteria for performing PVP. In this discussion they present the data from which their criteria are derived and preliminary clinical results which support the validity of their approach to the pallidotomy candidate.

Clinical Methodology

Pallidotomy has been performed at NYU since December 1991. At the time of writing of this manuscript, 130 patients have undergone 143 pallidotomies at this centre. During this time the surgical technique has changed little though our selection criteria have narrowed.

Preoperative Assessment

All candidates for pallidotomy are examined by one neurologist (EF), one of the neurosurgeons (PJK; RLA) and, in some cases, the neurophysiologist (AB). Ideal candidates have asymmetric, bradykinetic PD with severe "on-off" fluctuations. "Off" periods are characterized by rigidity and bradykinesia, with or without tremor. "On" states find the patient less rigid, but DOPA-induced dyskinesiae predominate and are often worse than the PD itself. Medication response is inconsistent and "off" periods are lengthening. Painful muscle cramping and dystonia may also be present.

Patients with "mid-line" symptoms (ie. swallowing difficulty, hypophonic speech, postural instability and freezing) respond less well to pallidotomy. Patients in whom tremor predominates may be better suited for thalamotomy. Obviously, each PD patient is a unique mosaic of "good" and "bad" symptoms and much experience must be gained in selecting appropriate surgical candidates.

An MRI is obtained in order to rule out significant cerebral atrophy, the presence of which increases the risk of intraoperative haemorrhage.

Those who are considered to be good candidates by clinical examination are referred to the neuropsychologist (KP) who administers a battery of tests which are listed in Table 1. The goal of neuropsychological testing is to detect pre-clinical dementias as well as to provide a baseline with which to compare post-operative

Table 1. *Neuropsychological Tests Administered to Pallidotomy Candidates*

Test	Ref.
Beck Depression Inventory (BDI)	1
Controlled Oral Word Association Test (COWT)	2
California Verbal Learning Test (CVLT)	6
Mini-Mental State (MMS)	15
Stroop Test (Stroop)	16
Boston Naming Test (BNT)	17
Wisconsin Card Sorting (WCST)	19
Hooper Visual Organization Test (Hooper)	20
Trail Making Test (Trails)	28
Symbol Digit Modalities Test (SDMT)	29

cognitive function. Neuropsychological testing is performed in the mid-morning with the patient on medications (i.e. best possible "on" state).

Those who pass their neuropsychological evaluation are referred to the positron emission tomography (PET) facility at North Shore University Hospital on Long Island, New York. There, patients undergo ^{18}F-fluorodeoxyglucose utilization PET (FDG/PET) as well as ^{18}F-fluoro-DOPA binding PET. Details of the PET technique have been published previously [11–13].

Prior studies have demonstrated PET's ability to distinguish true idiopathic PD from striato-nigral degeneration (SND) [11]. Patients with PD exhibit lentiform hypermetabolism on FDG/PET as well as reduced fluoro-DOPA binding. In contrast, patients with SND and other so called "Parkinson's Plus Syndromes" (PPS) exhibit reduced lentiform metabolism on FDG/PET [11].

Only those patients who meet the authors' clinical criteria, have no evidence of dementia on neuropsychological testing, and exhibit lentiform hypermetabolism on FDG/PET are recommended for pallidotomy.

The Unified Parkinson's Disease Rating Scale (UPDRS) [14] and the three upper extremity timed motor tasks of the Core Assessment Program for Intracerebral Transplantation (CAPIT) [25] are administered to each surgical candidate, on and off medications, on the day prior to surgery.

Surgical Technique

Pallidotomy is performed on awake patients who have been off their Parkinson's medications for at least 12 hours. The authors employ the Leksell G frame, magnetic resonance imaging, and computer assistance (CASS System, Midco, San Diego, California) to derive their anatomical target. Leksell's coordinates for PVP are employed.

Final target selection is based on microelectrode recording (MER). MER is performed with a 1 micron tungsten tipped microelectrode which is advanced with an hydraulic microdriver. The details of the electronic equipment we employ have been published previously as have the electrophysiological properties of the internal and external segments of globus pallidus [4, 27, 30]. In addition to defining target laterality, MER determines lesion depth by unequivocally defining the floor of GPi.

Once a satisfactory trajectory has been identified by MER, macroelectrode stimulation is performed with a 0.2 ms biphasic wave at 5 & 50 Hz, from 0–10 volts. The electrode is advanced to the floor of GPi as defined by MER. As a general rule, it has been found that it is safe to make lesions if the motor threshold is greater than 2 volts and the visual threshold is greater than 3 volts given the authors' stimulation parameters.

Lesions are made by heating the electrode to 80°C for 60 seconds. After cooling to 39°C, the electrode is backed up 2 mm and another lesion is made. Typically 4–5 lesions are made at 2 mm intervals along the trajectory, spanning GPi as determined by MER. Motor strength and speech are checked after each lesion. A CT scan is obtained immediately after surgery to rule out haemorrhage. Patients are observed overnight and discharged on the first or second postoperative day.

Post-operative Follow-up

An MRI is obtained within the first postoperative week to evaluate lesion placement. After that, patients are followed by the neurologist every 3 months for the first year, every four months for the second year and then annually. At each visit, the UPDRS and upper extremity CAPIT tests are performed. All scores reported here are those achieved with the patient off medications for 12 hours. Differences in the median pre- and post-operative scores were tested for statistical significance by the Wilcoxon Rank Sums Test.

At 6 months and 1 year, neuropsychological testing and PET are repeated. In those cases where bilateral procedures are to be performed, there is a wait of at least 6 months before deciding about the second lesion and employ the 6 month PET and neuropsychological evaluations are used to help determine the appropriateness of further intervention.

Results

At the time this manuscript was prepared, 130 patients had undergone pallidotomy at NYU medical center. Sixty patients were operated on from 1991 through November 1994. This early series of patients has the longest follow-up and it is from their results that selection criteria have been developed. Of those 60, 6 patients had Parkinson's Plus syndromes. These patients exhibited lentiform hypometabolism on FDG/PET and did not respond to PVP. Eight patients underwent staged bilateral pallidotomy and are excluded from this analysis. Eleven patients had inadequate follow-up. One patient died of a myocardial infarction 6 months after surgery. Our analysis therefore consists of 34 patients with true idiopathic PD who underwent unilateral PVP with microelectrode recording and who have at least 6 months of follow-up.

The median UPDRS scores for these 34 patients are demonstrated in Table 2. At 6 months post-op, the median motor and ADL scores of the UPDRS were

Table 2. *Median UPDRS Scores Following Unilateral Pallidotomy*

	No.	Motor	ADL
Baseline	34	31	16
6 months	34	9	7.5
12 months	22	9.5	4
24 months	15	7	4
36 months	7	3	2

Median pre- and post-operative UPDRS scores in 34 patients with idiopathic Parkinson's disease who underwent unilateral posteroventral pallidotomy with microelectrode recording. These scores demonstrate a dramatic functional improvement 6 months post operatively which is maintained for up to three years. Testing is performed by the same examiner, in the mid-morning, with the patient off anti-parkinsonian medications for 12 hours. The difference between baseline and postoperative scores in all instances are statistically significant to $P < 0.001$ by the Wilcoxon Rank Sums Test.

Table 3. *Mini-Mental State Scores in 5 Patients Who Developed Progressive Dementia Following Unilateral Pallidotomy*

Patient	Mini-mental state (normal range: 24–30)	Neuropsychological tests performed worse than other pallidotomy patients
1	27	BNT, COWT, Trails
2	27	Stroop, Trails, WCST
3	23	CVLT
4	11	COWT, Hooper, Stroop, Trails, CVLT
5	28	N/A

Preoperative mini-mental state scroes in 5 patients who developed progressive dementia following unilateral pallidotomy. Only 1 of 5 was demented by MMS criteria. An additional patient was borderline. These patients performed poorly on other tests administered (ie. >1.5 standard deviations from the mean for PD patients), some of which are indicative of early Alzheimer's dementia. Patient 5 refused more extensive testing.

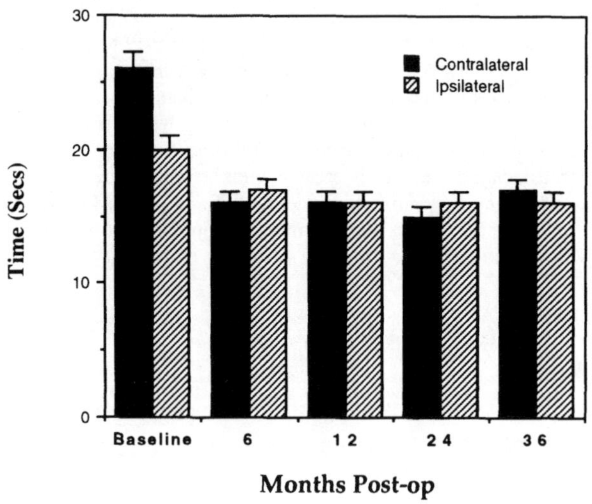

Fig. 1. CAPIT finger tap scores following unilateral pallidotomy. Median pre- and post-operative CAPIT finger tap scores for 34 patients who underwent unilateral pallidotomy. Contralateral extremity scores improved approximately 50% while ipsilateral scores improved 15%. These improvements have persisted in 5 patients who are 36 months post-pallidotomy

improved 70% and 50%, respectively ($p < 0.001$ at all time points). Furthermore, these improvements are maintained for up to 3 years. While the data in Table 2 would suggest that the UPDRS scores continue to improve over time, the authors believe this is an artifact resulting from the small number of patients with long-term follow-up. It does appear, however, that improved function can be expected for up to 3 years (possibly more) following unilateral pallidotomy.

Performance of the 3 upper extremity timed motor tasks of the CAPIT was also dramatically improved. Finger tap scores are depicted in Fig. 1 and are representative of the results observed with all 3 tasks. Function improved approximately 50% in the extremity contralateral to the lesion while ipsilateral extremity function improved 15%. Again, these differences are statistically significant and are maintained for up to 3 years.

The sole surgical complication in these 60 patients was a haemorrhage which required evacuation. There were no capsular strokes, optic tract injuries, speech difficulties or infections.

Five patients (8%) exhibited progressive dementia following their procedure. Table 3 demonstrates that only one of the 5 would have been characterized as obviously demented on their preoperative Mini-Mental State exam (patient 4); one patient would have been graded as borderline (patient 3). Other tests, however, uncovered cognitive deficits consistent with early comorbid Alzheimer's dementia. Specifically, these patients scored poorly (i.e. >1.5 standard deviations off the norm for PD patients [26]) in exercises which test naming, verbal fluency, and verbal learning (eg. Boston Naming Test [17], Controlled Oral Word Association Test [2]). As a result, patients with similar profiles are no longer offered pallidotomy at this institution.

Results of the authors' FDG/PET studies in pallidotomy patients have already been published [12, 13] but the salient points will be reviewed here. More than just a qualitative examination, FDG/PET quantita-

Table 4. *Preliminary Pallidotomy Results in 15 Patients Operated on After the Institution of Strict Selection Criteria*

	No.	Motor	*P	ADL	*P
Baseline	15	26	—	14	—
6 months	15	8.5	0.0008	4.5	0.002

Median pre- and post-operative UPDRS scores in the first 15 patients operated on subsequent to the institution of stricter selection criteria. * The difference in scores is significant by the Wilcoxon Rank Sums Test.

tively predicts response to surgical intervention. Eidelberg *et al.* have demonstrated that the degree of preoperative lentiform hypermetabolism correlates with functional improvement following pallidotomy [12]. Furthermore, post-pallidotomy FDG/PET studies reveal profound physiological changes which support clinical observations. Lesioning the internal segment of globus pallidus reduces the excessive inhibitory input of the pallidothalamic projection which results from PD [3, 7]. Reduced afferent input to the thalamus leads to a reduction in thalamic glucose utilization as less energy for processing information is required [13]. This "normalization" of inhibitory input from GPi to ventrolateral thalamus translates into bilaterally enhanced activity in the primary and supplementary motor cortices [5, 13, 18], corroborating the clinical observation of bilateral improvement in CAPIT performance. These results demonstrate that preoperative FDG/PET results can guide surgical decision making and permit an estimation of expected therapeutic results, while post-operative PET studies can enhance understanding of the pathophysiology of PD and the physiologic impact of lesioning procedures.

Table 4 demonstrates preliminary results on the first 15 patients operated on subsequent to the institution of the authors' stricter selection criteria who have at least 6 months of follow-up. Again, dramatic, statistically significant reductions in ADL and motor scores of the UPDRS are noted. Dyskinesiae and/or dystonias, when present, were eliminated or markedly reduced.

No haemorrhages, strokes, optic tract injuries, infections or speech deficits occurred in these 70 patients. Two elderly patients experienced temporary confusion post-operatively which cleared with reductions in their dose of L-DOPA. No patient has exhibited evidence of progressive dementia at this time. All patients have enjoyed a therapeutic response.

Discussion

There is broad consensus that posteroventral pallidotomy effectively relieves rigidity, bradykinesia and DOPA-induced dyskinesiae in a subset of Parkinson's disease patients whose response to medication is waning [8, 9, 21–24, 27]. Beyond this general agreement many points of contention arise. Controversies include: (1) the proper indications for the procedure; (2) the best method for anatomical targeting; (3) the need for microelectrode recording; (4) the proper site, size and configuration of the lesion; and (5) the advisability of performing bilateral lesions. These issues will only be resolved with accurate, very specific descriptions of technique, long-term results and complication rates.

In this report the authors have described their selection criteria for performing unilateral pallidotomy and provided the data from which these criteria were developed. Institution of these criteria as of November 1994 has resulted in more consistent responses among those who are operated on and reduced the incidence of complications, specifically by eliminating post-operative dementias. Though these criteria are somewhat strict, they believe their results justify their continued use. The criteria assure therapeutic responses in those who have surgery, avoid unwarranted surgery in those who will not respond and minimize avoidable complications.

The PET findings which have arisen from this work and that of other groups highlight the need to further incorporate functional imaging into the daily practice of neurology and neurosurgery. FDG/PET accurately identifies patients with Parkinson's Plus syndromes who will not respond to pallidotomy, predicts response to pallidotomy in those with lentiform hypermetabolism and demonstrates the profound metabolic changes which result [5, 10–13, 18]. We believe its role is invaluable in both the clinical and research spheres, providing an objective means with which to evaluate pallidotomy patients pre- and post-operatively while advancing our understanding of the physiology of PD and the effects of lesioning procedures.

Detailed neuropsychological testing demonstrates that the Mini-Mental State alone insufficiently detects patients who are at risk of developing post-operative dementia. Deficiencies in verbal learning, verbal fluency and naming which are indicative of early Alzheimer's dementia can be detected by neuropsychological testing in those with normal MMS scores. This experience suggests that such patients should not undergo pallidotomy.

Based on this data and the experience of others we submit the following list of indications and contra-indications for unilateral stereotactic posteroventral pallidotomy is submitted. The age cut-off recommended is a relative yardstick. Response to pallidotomy may decrease with age; however, many patients over the age of 65 exhibit symptoms which are well-suited to pallidotomy and lead more active lives following the procedure. The authors simply believe that after the age of 65, only ideal candidates should undergo surgery.

Indications for Pallidotomy

(1) DOPA-induced dyskinesia; (2) Rigidity; (3) Bradykinesia; (4) Severe "on-off" fluctuations; (5) Dystonia/muscular spasms; (6) Predominance of appendicular symptoms; (7) Lentiform hypermetabolism on FDG/PET.

Contra-indications for Pallidotomy

(1) Age greater than 65 years (relative); (2) Dementia; (3) Predominance of axial symptoms; (4) Postural instability; (5) Severe contractures; (6) Lentiform hypometabolism on FDG/PET.

Employing these guidelines, the authors find unilateral pallidotomy to be a safe and effective procedure for medically refractory PD when MRI localization, computer guidance and neurophysiologic monitoring are employed.

References

1. Beck AT (1987) Beck depression inventory: manual. The Psychological Corporation, San Antonio, TX
2. Benton AL, Hamsher KS, Varney NR, Spreen O (1983) Contributions to neuropsychological assessment. Oxford University Press, New York
3. Bergman H, Wichamann T, DeLong MR (1990) Reversal of experimental parkinsonism by lesions of the subthalamic nucleus. Science 249: 1436–1438
4. Beric A, Sterio D, Dogali M, Fazzini E, Eidelberg D, Kolodny E (1996) Characteristics of pallidal neuronal discharges in Parkinson's disease patients. Adv Neurol 69: 123–128
5. Ceballos-Baumann AO, Obeso JA, Vitek JL, DeLong MR, Bakay R, Linazasoro G, Brooks DJ (1994) Restoration of thalamocortical activity after posteroventral pallidotomy in Parkinson's disease. Lancet 344: 814
6. Delis DC, Kramer JH, Kaplan E, Ober BA (1987) California verbal learning test: adult version. The Psychological Corporation, San Antonio, TX
7. DeLong MR, Crutcher MD, Georgopoulos AP (1985) Primate globus pallidus and subthalamic nucleus functional organization. J Neurophysiol 53: 530–543
8. Dogali M, Fazzini E, Kolodny E, Eidelberg D, Sterio D, Devinsky O, Beric A (1995) Stereotactic ventral pallidotomy for Parkinson's disease. Neurology 45: 753–761
9. Dogali M, Sterio D, Fazzini E, Kolodny E, Eidelberg D, Beric A (1996) Effects of posteroventral pallidotomy on Parkinson's disease. Adv Neurol 69: 585–590
10. Eidelberg D (1992) Positron emission tomography studies in parkinsonism. Neurol Clin North Am 10: 421–433
11. Eidelberg D, Takikawa S, Moeller JR, Dhawan V, Redington K, Chaly T, Robeson W, Dahl JR, Margouleff D, Fazzini E, Przedborski S, Fahn S (1993) Striatal hypometabolism distinguishes striatonigral degeneration from Parkinson's disease. Ann Neurol 33: 518–527
12. Eidelberg D, Moeller JR, Ishikawa T, Dhawan V, Spetsieris P, Chaly T, Robeson W, Dahl JR, Margouleff D (1995) Assessment of disease severity in parkinsonism with Fluorine-18-fluorodeoxyglucose and PET. J Nucl Med 36: 378–383
13. Eidelberg D, Moeller JR, Ishikawa T, Dhawan V, Spetsieris P, Silbersweig D, Stern E, Woods RP, Fazzini E, Dogali M, Beric A (1996) Regional metabolic correlates of surgical outcome following unilateral pallidotomy for Parkinson's disease. Ann Neurol 39: 450–459
14. Fahn S, Elton RL, members of the UPDRS development committee (1987) Unified Parkinson's disease rating scale. In: Fahn S, Marsden CD, Calne DB, Goldstein M (eds) Recent developments in Parkinson's disease, vol 2. MacMillan Health Care Information, Florham Park, NJ, pp 153–164
15. Folstein M, Folstein S, McHugh PJ (1975) "Mini-mental state," a practical method for grading the cognitive state of patients for the clinician. J Psych Res 12: 189–198
16. Golden CJ (1978) Stroop color and word test. Stoelting, Chicago, Ill
17. Goodglass H, Kaplan E (1983) The assessment of aphasia and related disorders, 2nd ed. Lea and Febiger, Philadelphia PA
18. Grafton ST, Waters C, Sutton J, Lew MF, Couldwell W (1995) Pallidotomy increases activity of motor association cortex in Parkinson's disease: a positron emission tomographic study. Ann Neurol 37: 776–783
19. Heaton RK (1981) Wisconsin card sorting test: manual. Psychological Assessment Resources, Odessa, Florida
20. Hooper HE (1983) Hooper visual organization test (VOT). Western Psychological Services, Los Angeles, CA
21. Iacono RP, Lonser RR (1994) Reversal of Parkinson's akinesia by pallidotomy. Lancet 343: 418–419
22. Iacono RP, Shima F, Lonser RR, Kuniyoshi S, Maeda G, Yamada S (1995) The results, indications, and physiology of posteroventral pallidotomy for patients with Parkinson's disease. Neurosurgery 36: 1118–1127
23. Laitinen LV, Bergenheim AT, Hariz MI (1992) Leksell's posteroventral pallidotomy in the treatment of Parkinson's disease. J Neurosurg 76: 53–61
24. Laitinen LV, Bergenheim AT, Hariz MI (1992) Ventroposterolateral pallidotomy can abolish all parkinsonian symptoms. Stereotact Funct Neurosurg 58: 14–21
25. Langston JW, Widner H, Goetz CG, Brooks D, Fahn S, Freeman T, Watts R (1992) Core assessment program for intracerebral transplantation (CAPIT). Mov Disord 7: 2–13
26. Lezak MD (1995) Neuropsychological assessment, 3rd ed. Oxford University Press, New York, NY

27. Lozano AM, Lang AE, Galvez-Jimenez N, Miyasaki J, Duff J, Hutchinson WD, Dostrovsky JO (1995) Effect of GPi pallidotomy on motor function in Parkinson's disease. Lancet 346: 1383–1387
28. Reitan RM, Wolfson D (1985) The Halstead-Reitan neuropsychological test battery: theory and interpretation. Neuropsychology Press, Tucson, AZ
29. Smith A (1968) The symbol digit modalities test: a neuropsychologic test for economic screening of learning and other cerebral disorders. Learning Disorders 3: 83–91
30. Sterio D, Beric A, Dogali M, Fazzini E, Alfaro G, Devinsky O (1994) Neurophysiological properties of pallidal neurons in Parkinson's disease. Ann Neurol 35: 586–591

Correspondence: Ron L. Alterman, M.D., NYU Medical Center, 530 1st Avenue, 8R, New York, NY 10016, USA.

Acta Neurochir (1997) [Suppl] 68: 24–28

The Effects of Pallidotomy on Parkinson's Disease: Study Design and Assessment Techniques

R. E. Gross[1], A. M. Lozano[1], A. E. Lang[2], R. R. Tasker[1], W. D. Hutchison[1], and J. O. Dostrovsky[3]

[1] Division of Neurosurgery, Department of Surgery, [2]Division of Neurology, Department of Medicine, Morton and Gloria Shulman Movement Disorders Centre, and [3]Department of Physiology, The Toronto Hospital Neurological Centre and The University of Toronto, Toronto, Canada

Summary

Lesions of the internal segment of the globus pallidus are increasingly being utilized in the surgical treatment of advanced Parkinson's disease, yet studies to demonstrate the safety and efficacy of these procedures are only now being completed. The importance of procedural variations between centres in the outcome of pallidotomy is not yet known. In order to compare accurately results between centres, carefully designed, prospective studies are needed. The authors utilized blinded, randomly evaluated videotaped examinations of pre- and post-operative patients undergoing microelectrode-guided GP_i pallidotomy. Their results demonstrate significant effects on contralateral akinesia and tremor in the "off" state, and striking attenuation of levodopa-induced dyskinesias in the "on" state. More modest effects on postural stability and gait disturbance were seen only in non-blinded evaluations. This type of study design should enable many of the outstanding issues related to pallidotomy indications, procedures and outcomes to be addressed.

Keywords: Parkinson's disease; pallidotomy; movement disorders; stereotaxy.

Introduction

Since the resurgence of pallidotomy with the landmark paper of Laitinen *et al.* [6], reports have shown variable results for this procedure in medically-refractory Parkinson's disease (PD). There may be multiple sources for this variability. First, patient selection criteria may differ between centres. Second, procedural variations, with resultant discrepancies in lesion location and size, may contribute to differences in outcome. Centres differ in the use of: imaging modalities (MRI, CT, MRI/CT co-registration, ventriculography); stereotactic localization systems (e.g., Leksell, Codman-Roberts-Wells, Laitinen stereoadapter); physiological techniques to select final lesion target (impedance monitoring, macrostimulation, semi-microelectrode recording, high-impedance microelectrode recording and stimulation); target selection (the recommended co-ordinates of Laitinen *et al.* [6]; direct targetting of the medial pallidum based on MRI; or the use of microelectrode recording to determine the location of the sensorimotor portion of the internal segment of the globus pallidus, GP_i); and parameters used for final lesion creation (electrode diameter and exposed tip length; temperature and duration of lesion; number of lesions and inter-lesion spacing). Finally, there are significant differences between centres in the selection of pre- and post-operative assessment tools and the manner in which the data are collected (e.g. blinded versus non-blinded assessments).

The sources of variability can account for significant inter-centre differences in outcome results, and make comparisons of results between centers very difficult. Further, inadequate assessment techniques make the arguments for the validity of pallidotomy in the treatment of PD prone to similar types of criticisms that were responsible for the demise of procedures that were prematurely advocated as efficacious in PD (e.g. adrenal medullary transplantation). Failure to apply valid and reliable target identification techniques and outcome measures in studies of the results of pallidotomy also impairs the ability to make scientifically sound conclusions on the role of specific regions of the internal portion of the globus pallidus (GP_i) in the pathophysiology of Parkinson's disease. Previous reports have emphasized the importance of microelectrode recording of single unit responses in target localization within the globus pallidus [1, 4, 9, 10].

Table 1. *Patient Characteristics*

	Value (SE)	Range
No.	14	
Age	58.9 (7.9)	44–71
Sex	8M : 6F	
Duration	13.9 (5.1)	7–25
Drug dose: L-dopa	1260.7 (685.9)	400–2600
Drug dose: L-dopa equiv.	1367.3 (x)	
H&Y: off	3.9 (0.9)	2.5–5
H&Y: on	2.9 (0.9)	1.5–5
Lesion side	7R : 7L	

The techniques used for the pre- and post-operative assessment of GP_i pallidotomy will be the focus of this report.

Patients and Surgical Procedures

The authors have previously reported 14 patients with Parkinson's disease treated with GP_i pallidotomy [9]. All had advanced Parkinson's disease of mean duration of 13.9 years (± 5.1; range 7–25 years), and were 44 to 71 years of age (mean 58.9 ± 7.9) (Table 1). All had severe motor fluctuations, manifested as bad "off" states, with Hoehn and Yahr scores of 3.9 ± 0.9 (range 2.5–5). All were levo-dopa responsive (Hoehn and Yahr 2.9 ± 0.9 while"on") but suffered from disabling drug-induced dyskinesias. Patients gave informed consent for the study, which was approved by the Toronto Hospital Committee for Research on Human Subjects. Pre-surgical evaluatios are discussed below.

The surgical procedures have been described elsewhere [10]. Briefly, patients were off their medications from the night before surgery so that they were in the "off" state, to obtain direct measures of abnormal cellular activity and to allow the observation of the immediate clinical effects of GP_i lesions on the "off" symptoms. A Leksell G frame was applied with local anaesthetic, and a stereotactic MRI was obtained. On the T1-weighted 1 mm thick axial images, the co-ordinates of the anterior and posterior commissures were obtained, and inputted into a computer program which stretched or shrank the sagittal 20 or 22 mm Schaltenbrand and Wahren map according the patients' intercommissural distance. The tentative target was chosen using this map, at a point 1mm dorsal to the inferior margin of the internal segment of the globus pallidus (GP_i), in the anterior-posterior midportion of the nucleus 20 mm lateral to the intercommissural line. This tentative target roughly corresponded to the target recommended by Laitinen *et al.* [6].

A single twist drill hole (3 mm) was made under local anaesthesia, 2 cm from the midline over the coronal suture. A high impedance ($\sim$1 megaohm) tungsten microelectrode with a 20–30 μm exposed tip was introduced through a guide cannula to a point 15 mm above the presumptive target, as previously described. Single-unit activity was recorded along the trajectory which was characteristic of the external segment of the globus pallidus (GP_e), followed by firing patterns characteristic of GP_i [1, 4, 10]. Lying between these nuclei, adjacent to the white matter laminae that separate GP_e from GP_i (lamina pallidi medialis) and GP_{ie} from GP_{ii} (lamina pallidi incompleta), were often found cells with characteristic firing patterns, called border cells [2]. The sensorimotor segment of GP_i was identified by the presence of cells with movement (active or passive) – evoked changes in firing rate. Recording was continued along a trajectory until cellular activity was no longer detected. Strobe light-evoked responses, characteristic of the optic tract, were sought at the ventral-most aspect of the trajectory, using microelectrode recording. The optic tract was usually identified with microstimulation through the same electrode tip (1–100 μA, 300 Hz, 200 μs pulse-width), which elicited phosphenes in the contralateral visual field. The internal capsule was also identified by the low noise level and of occasional recording of short duration axonal spikes and more importantly by the presence of microstimulation elicited contralateral motor contractions. Additional trajectories were made, adjusted based on the results of previous trajectories, until the GP_i, optic tract and internal capsule were definitively identified.

Lesions were created in GP_i using a radiofrequency lesioning electrode with a 1 mm diameter and a 3 mm exposed tip. Lesions were targetted to a region where movement-related cells were identified, 3 mm away from microstimulation-induced visual, somatosensory or motor responses (with 200 μA current using the above parameters). This target usually differed from the tentative target [10]. Speech, vision and motor function were repeatedly assessed during lesioning at 60°, 70°, 80° and, finally, 90° (60 seconds each). Improvements in bradykinesia and rigidity were immediately evident. During lesioning dystonic or choreoathetotic movements were often noted contralateral to the lesion, which invariably resolved (within 30 min to 6 hr). Medications were resumed post-operatively at pre-operative dose levels. Patients were monitored in hospital for one to five days, and at intervals after discharge (see below).

Study Design and Patient Assessment

The gold standard of any "drug" study is the placebo-controlled, randomized, double-blinded design with between-subjects comparisons. For a number of reasons, such a design is usually not possible, especially when evaluating surgical therapies. An adequate placebo group may not be available. For a surgical treatment, this would require a "sham" operation. Since these procedures are done with awake patients and take approximately four hours for mapping, this would in fact involve an elaborate process with "sham" microelectrode recordings, which is practically difficult. A non-operated group may be used instead of a placebo group. However, patients would need to be randomized into treatment or non-treatment arms. It may be difficult to find patients willing to be randomly assigned to surgical or non-surgical therapies. The use of a control, non-operated group that was collected without randomization introduces selection bias into the analysis. The authors therefore chose a within-subjects design, comparing patients before and after GP_i pallidotomy. They used videotaped recordings of the neurologic evaluations to blind the examiners to: (1) "on" or "off" states, (2) pre- or post-operative status, and (3) time after surgery. During videotaping, all patients wore hospital gowns and caps to mask pre- and post-operative status. Certain aspects of the clinical examination that require examiner/patient contact (e.g. rigidity) could not be assessed in this manner. "on" and "off" states were randomly evaluated by examiners not directly involved in the care of the patients, for items of the UPDRS that did not require examiner/ patient contact.

Pre- and Post-operative Assessment

Since the recommendations of the Core Assessment Program for Intracerebral Transplantation (CAPIT) committee were published [8], the core assessment program has been extensively utilized in controlled trials of PD therapies. The utility of CAPIT is that it provides a necessary means by which results can be compared between centres. The recommendations cover both the particular assessment tools to be used and their timing with respect to the patient's functional state (on or off medications). The authors will comment on the particular details of the CAPIT assessment, and how they modified them for use with blinded assessments.

Unified Parkinson's Disease Rating Scale

The Unified Parkinson's Disease Rating Scale (UPDRS), contained within CAPIT, provides an extensive objective and subjective assessment of the cardinal features of PD and the complications of treatment, as well as the impact on patients' quality of life. Although recent studies have yielded several recommendations for the modification of the UPDRS, the current 3.0 version is still in use. The UPDRS contains three subsections: mentation, behaviour and mood; activities of daily living; and motor examination. The first two subsections contain extensive information that cannot be blindly evaluated, as much of it is historical. The authors present pre-operative and post-operative total UPDRS scores for comparison with other studies, and in keeping with CAPIT recommendations. The motor subsection contains 14 questions of which only one (rigidity, score no. 22) cannot be rated using the videotaped recordings. They present overall motor subsection scores as "blinded" with this caveat. Individual are analysed scores from the motor examination on both the ipsilateral and contralateral sides. In addition, motor items were grouped to quantitate effects on the cardinal signs of PD, akinesia, tremor, postural stability, gait and rigidity. Values were obtained both contralaterally and ipsilaterally. Blinded evaluations of drug-induced dyskinesias were also obtained, with separate scores for right and left sides as well as a total score which assesses axial involvement. Finally, a simple timed manual task was assessed, the time to tap the index finger between two targets separated by 30 cm for ten successive cycles. Other timed tasks were excluded for reasons outlined previously [7].

Patients were evaluated two times pre-operatively, of which one was videotaped. Patients were again assessed at one week post-operatively, and at three month intervals thereafter. Only data from the 6 month time point is the subject of this report (see Lozano *et al.* [9] for time course). Separate assessments were performed, at each time point, in the practically-defined worst "off" state, and one hour after their morning medications during their typical best "on" state. Videotapes were randomized and scored by a neurologist experienced in the use of the above scales, who was not involved in the patients' pre- or post-operative care.

The non-blinded data were obtained form live assessments: UPDRS total score (including the blinded measures, above); ADL (activities of daily living); Schwab and England; rigidity, arm and leg rigidity components of UPDRS (score no. 22); postural instability/gait disorder (PIGD), walking, freezing and falling from the ADL scores [13–15]; and the tapping task. Since all of the assessments, except for the timed tapping test, yield non-parametric data, results were analysed with sign rank test statistics. Percentage changes from preoperative status were derived, however, from calculated means. The timed tapping task was analyzed by use of the t statistic.

Results

Because changes in medication dosages may confound pre- versus post-operative comparisons, dosages were changed as little as possible through the course of the study. Nevertheless, while total levodopa dosage levels were unchanged, a comparison of total levodopa and agonist dosages, converted to equivalent levodopa dose, revealed a small but significant decrease (1367.3 mg to 1221.1 mg, $p < 0.02$).

Blinded Assessments

Off State (off medications for 12 hours)

Blinded evaluations of pre- and post-operative videotapes of UPDRS subscales revealed significant differences at 6 months in the "off" state [9]. The total motor UPDRS subscale, which includes all items except for the rigidity item (no. 22), improved by 30% in the "off" state ($p = 0.004$), whereas there was an insignificant increase while on. The authors performed further analyses of motor items, covering the range of cardinal signs of PD (except for rigidity). During the "off" state, significant improvements were seen in the values for total akinesia (22%, $p = 0.007$). Significant improvements in contralateral tremor were also observed, with a difference between pre-operative and six month post-operative scores of 60% ($p = 0.03$). There was, however, no significant effect of pallidotomy on ipsilateral or total tremor scores. Neither gait nor postural stability improved in the blinded evaluations.

On State

The most striking change in the "on" state was seen in the contralateral dyskinesia scores, which improved by 90% after six months ($p = 0.008$). This was reflected also in an improvement in the total dyskinesia score. There was a small but insignificant improvement in the ipsilateral dyskinesia score.

Non-blinded Assessments

The non-blinded scores confirmed the findings above. Total UPDRS, which contains a few additional motor scores (e.g. rigidity), as well as activities of daily living, mentation and complications of medication, was significantly improved in the "off" state (27%, $p = 0.002$). Total rigidity decreased (31%, $p = 0.0007$), which was due to a significant contralateral effect, without any ipsilateral change. In contrast to the blinded assessments, there was a significant improvement in the composite score for postural stability and gait disturbance, which includes the two blinded items (nos. 29 & 30) in addition to the walking, freezing and falling items (nos. 13, 14 & 15) from the ADL subscale of the UPDRS (23%, $p = 0.02$). As noted above, there were no significant changes in any of the "on" UPDRS scores at 6 months.

Finally, the timed tapping test, which is a quantitative measure of bradykinesia, improved contralaterally by 39% ($p = 0.02$) compared to 20% on the ipsilateral side ($p = 0.002$). Interestingly, this was the only measure that significantly improved in the "on" state, although the magnitude of the changes were modest (contra: 17%, $p = 0.0006$; ipsi: 14%, $p = 0.005$).

Discussion

The authors have utilized blinded assessments, using videotaped examinations, to document the post-operative improvements in the cardinal signs of Parkinson's disease six months following microelectrode-guided stereotactic GP_i pallidotomy. Independent examiners familiar with the evaluation scales blindly and randomly (vis a vis pre- versus post-operative videotapes and "on" versus "off" medications) scored those items in the motor subscale of the UPDRS amenable to blinded evaluation. Using this methodology, which they believe removes as much bias as possible in the context of the surgical nature of the intervention, the authors have demonstrated clear improvements in akinesia, dyskinesia and tremor on the contralateral side to the surgery during the "off" state. More modest improvements were demonstrated on the ipsilateral side on the akinesia and dyskinesia scales. These results were corroborated by the non-blinded assessments and extended to include rigidity, which could not be evaluated in a blinded fashion. The tapping test which was used also demonstrated improvements both contralaterally and, more modestly, ipsilaterally. This was the only measure, other than dyskinesia, that was improved during the "on" state.

Changes in postural stability and gait were more problematic. The blinded assessments were unable to demonstrate a statistically significant improvement in gait, although there was a clear trend towards this. However, when combined with the unblinded assessment of these parameters derived from the activities of daily living subscale (item nos. 13, 14 and 15), there was a statistically significant improvement in "postural stability and gait disturbance". This difference may be related to the nature of the ADL subscale, which relies on patient self-reporting. Changes in postural stability and gait disturbance may be subtly improved, below the sensitivity of the motor subscale, yet be sufficient to impart improvements in quality of life as reflected, for example, in decreased falling. Yet this type of information may be subject to patient and family bias. As assessed using these instruments, the effect of unilateral GP_i on postural stability and gait is more modest than on akinesia and dyskinesia.

The results reported in the current study, and other recent studies [1, 3, 5], reveal a statistically-significant improvement in drug-induced dyskinesia, bradykinesia, rigidity and tremor on the side contralateral to posteroventral pallidotomy at 6 months to one year. The authors have found more modest effects on postural stability and gait using blinded assessments, in contrast to the results using non-blinded techniques, to evaluate these signs. In contrast to the work of others [1, 3, 5], they did not find a substantial benefit of pallidotomy on the best "on" state, except for a striking effect on dyskinesias.

Important issues that need to be addressed in future studies include: (1) the optimal location and size of the pallidal lesion, (2) the duration of clinical improvements, (3) when to operate during the course of the illness, and, (4) because the effects are predominantly contralateral, the safety and efficacy of bilateral surgery.

Given the variability of the disease course, surgical variations and day-to-day fluctuations in patient performances, as well as the effects of patient and physician expectations on clinical evaluations, the authors recommend the adoption of blinded and randomized assessments of videotaped UPDRS examinations in the evaluation of the outcome of surgical interventions for PD. The elimination of as many sources of bias as possible is necessary in the critical evaluation of these interventions. Although more time-consuming in the short run, ultimately the use of defined, blinded study designs will lead to the generation of data that will be less ambiguous. This will lead to more rapid acceptance (or rejection) of new surgical procedures by the medical and scientific communities, patient groups and health management organizations.

Acknowledgment

This work was supported by the Medical Research Council of Canada and Parkinson's Foundation of Canada (A. M. L.), and the National Parkinsons Foundation (A. E. L.).

References

1. Baron MS, Vitek JL, Bakay RAE, *et al* (1996) Treatment of advanced Parkinson's disease by posterior GP_i pallidotomy: 1-year results of a pilot study. Ann Neurol 40: 355–366
2. DeLong MR (1971) Activity of pallidal neurons during movement. J Neurophysiol 34: 414–427
3. Dogali M, Fazzini E, Kolodny E, *et al* (1995) Stereotactic ventral pallidotomy for Parkinson's disease. Neurology 45: 753–761
4. Hutchison WD, Lozano AM, Davis KD, *et al* (1994) Differential neuronal activity in segments of globus pallidus in Parkinson's disease patients. NeuroReport 5: 1533–1537
5. Iacono RP, Shima F, Lonser RR, *et al* (1995) The results, indications, and physiology of posteroventral pallidotomy for patients with Parkinson's disease. Neurosurgery 36: 1118–1127
6. Laitinen LV, Bergenheim AT, Hariz MI (1992) Leksell's posteroventral palllidotomy in the treatment of Parkinson's disease. J Neurosurg 76: 53–61
7. Lang AE, Benabid A-L, Koller WC, *et al* (1994) Core assessment program for intracerebral transplantation (letter). Mov Disord 10: 527–529
8. Langston JW, Widner H, Goetz CG, *et al* (1992) Core assessment program for intracerebral transplantation (CAPIT). Mov Disord 7: 2–13
9. Lozano AM, Lang AE, Galvez-Jimenez N, *et al* (1995) Effect of GP_i pallidotomy on motor function in Parkinson's disease. Lancet 346: 1383–1387
10. Lozano A, Hutchison W, Kiss Z, *et al* (1996) Methods for microelectrode-guided posteroventral palllidotomy. J Neurosurg 84: 194–202

Correspondence: Dr. Andres M. Lozano, Division of Neurosurgery, 2-433 McLaughlin Pavilion, The Toronto Hospital, Toronto Western Division, 399 Bathurst Street, Toronto, Ontario M5T 2S8, Canada.

Acta Neurochir (1997) [Suppl] 68: 29–36

Frameless 3D Volume Registration of MR Data Sets For Stereotactic Pallidotomy

R. M. Lehman[1], R. Kumar[2], R. S. Mezrich[3], and S. Negin[3]

[1] Division of Neurosurgery, UMDNJ-Robert Wood Johnson Medical School, New Brunswick, NJ, [2]David Sarnoff Research Institute, Princeton, NJ, and [3]Laurie Imaging Center, New Brunswick, NJ, USA

Summary

Frameless 3D volume registration of Magnetic Resonance (MR) and computed (CT) data sets has been described by Kummar *et al.* [11]. Its use in 3D volume registration for stereotactic planning in patients undergoing pallidotomy is presented. Pre-operative examinations with the stereotactic frame and postoperative examinations without the stereotactic frame can be co-registered and reviewed for accuracy of planned and lesional coordinates.

Keywords: Frameless 3D volume registration; CT; MRI; pallidotomy.

Introduction

Frameless 3D volume registration of Magnetic resonance (MR) and Computed (CT) data sets has been described by Kumar *et al.* [11]. Initially, patients at the authors' institution undergoing stereotactic pallid otomy were imaged with CT and MR. After a series of fifteen patients had undergone pallidotomy using these image techniques for localization of lesion, MR solely was used. This decision was based on finer anatomical detail and the ability to minimize error [13]. They present the use of 3D volume acquisition and the co-registration of the preoperative examinations with the stereotactic frame, and the postoperative examination without frame, to review the accuracy of the planned coordinates with the postoperative lesional coordinates.

Material and Methods

A series of fifteen patients undergoing CT and MR directed stereotactic pallidotomy using the Cosman-Roberts-Wells (CRW) frame, (Radionics, Randolph, Massachusetts) were reviewed.

The CT and MR images of three patients were selected for automated, volumetric frameless co-registration of their 3D data sets to assess accuracy of localization. The technique involves matching of MR and CT or pre- and postoperative MRI data sets by a direct optimization technique utilizing edge and internal volume structures with a gradient based descent approach and a coarse to fine control strategy over a 4D pyramid (Fig. 1).

Preoperative MR images were acquired with the patient in the stereotactic frame on a 1.5 Tesla system using the standard quadrature head coil (Signa operating with a 5.0 level software, GE Medical System Division, Milwaukee, Wisconsin). Preoperative images with the target (globus pallidus) close to the isocenter of the magnet were acquired in sagittal, axial and coronal projections parallel and perpendicular to the AC-PC line, as identified on the midsagittal image, using multiplanar spin-echo T1(TR/TE= 500/14) (Fig. 2).

In addition, a spoiled grass (SPGR) (TR/TE= 40/14, 30° flip angle) 3D volume acquisition was obtained. The image acquisition matrix was 256 × 256 with 124 axial slice spanning the head and the field of view was 24 cm. Postoperatively the patients were imaged in the first week and at six weeks on the same MRI system. The stereotactic frame was not used and the field of view reduced to 20 cm. This volume acquisition was identical to the pre-operative one, as was the multiplanar acquisition. The data was transferred by ethernet to several work stations including MacIntosh Power PC, GE Advantage Work Station, and the Princeton Engine, a parallel computer system capable of interactive volume rendering and segmentation (Fig. 3).

Results

Registration of pre- and postoperative MR images using this frameless 3D volumetric data set methodology achieves subpixel accuracy, i.e. submillimeter discrepancy. This is revealed by the cursor in the stereotactic preoperative volume axial image being superimposed upon the centre of the lesion in the identical postoperative, frameless axial image. Note should be taken of the exact edge match in this superimposed axial image (Fig. 4). This is further demonstrated in the 3D volume, surface-rendered images (Fig. 5).

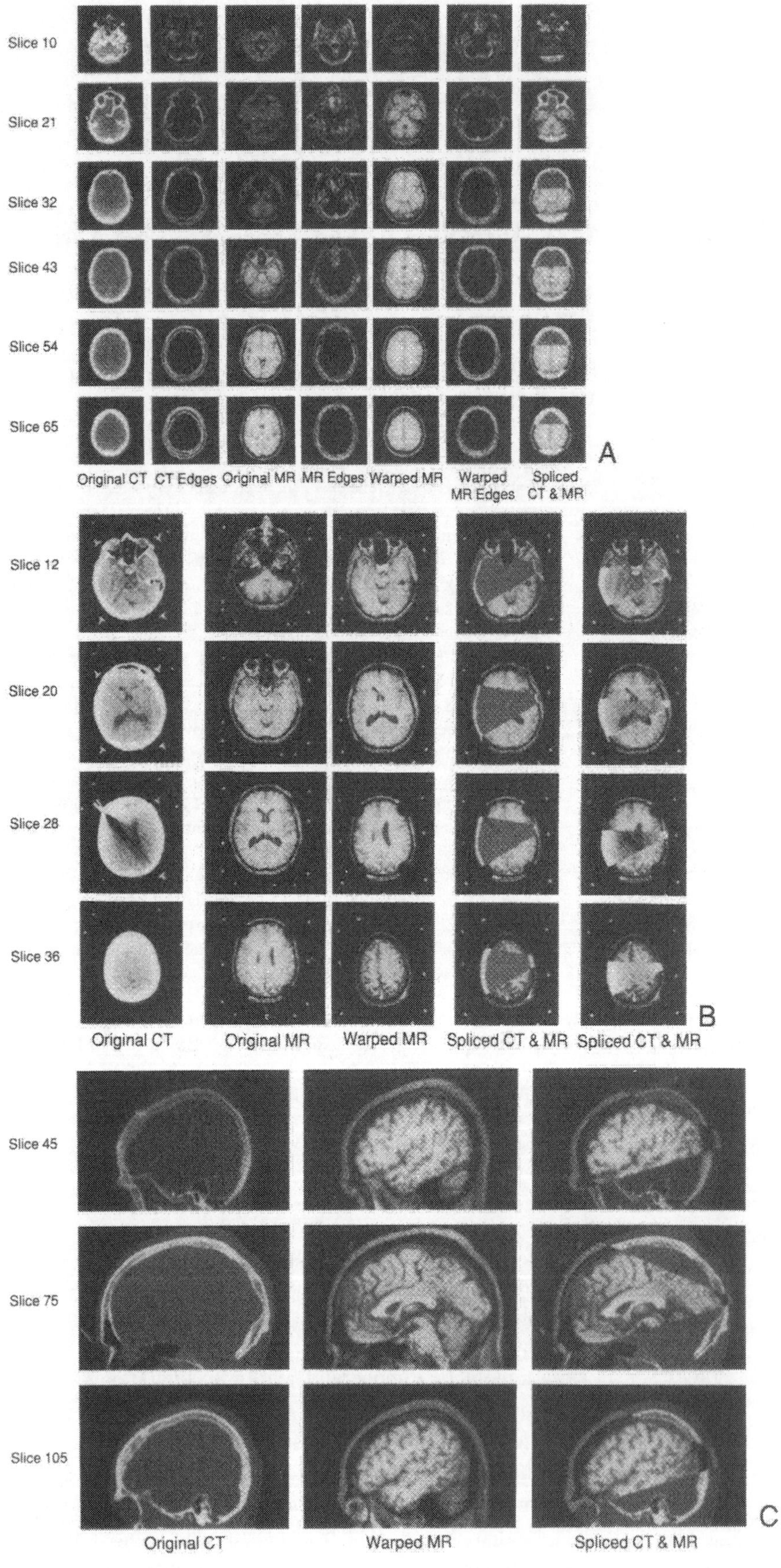

Fig. 1 (A–C). Multiple steps: Edge-based registration and warping of 3D MR data. (B) Axial view; (C) sagittal view

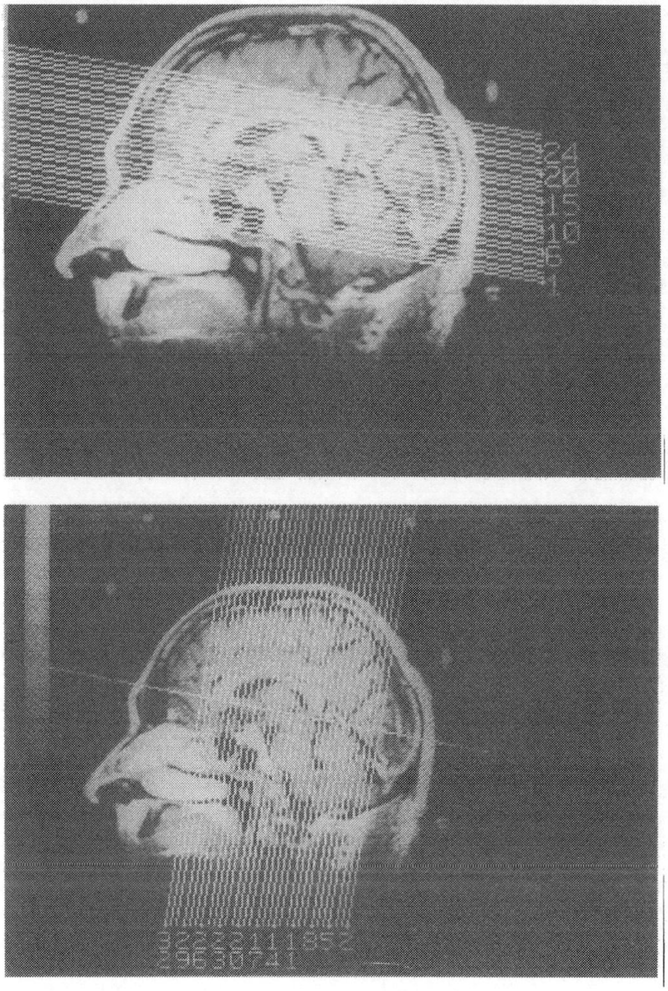

A

B

Fig. 2. (A, B) Axial images parallel to AC-PC line. Coronal acquisition perpendicular to AC-PC line

Discussion

Volume registration techniques involve a geometric transformation model, match measure and search or matching method [1]. A 4D pyramid is constructed from each of the two data sets, and the motion parameters are estimated in a coarse to fine detail within each pyramid. The sum of squared difference (SSD) measure is used as a match measure [2]. The SSD error must be minimized between the two data sets. At each pyramid level the solution from the previous pyramid level is used as an initial estimate. The algorithm computes 3D Laplacian, Gaussian or edge pyramids. A direct hierarchical method is used to do the minimization [5, 11, 15, 16] (Fig. 6).

There has been wide clinical application of interactive use of computed images. In previous work, three-point transformation of image data has been used in either pre-operative imaging with or without the stereotactic frame to be co-registered with perioperative images or to localize anatomical structures at the time of surgery [3, 4, 6, 9, 12]. Additionally, PET, functional MRI, MRS and SPECT with different resolutions can be co-registered [8]. This type of transformation of image data does not match voxel for voxel, and therefore inaccuracies of registration will occur.

Volumetric analysis within 3D image space is crucial to radiosurgery as well microsurgery [7, 10]. The authors feel the same concern for volumetric analysis in functional stereotaxy such as pallidotomy. The ability to superimpose the pre- and postoperative 3D volume data sets allows analysis of accuracy in the lesion location in relation to preoperative coordinates. Further, it permits localization of electrophysiological data in 3D volume. This has a particular implication for the number of electrode passes for recording the

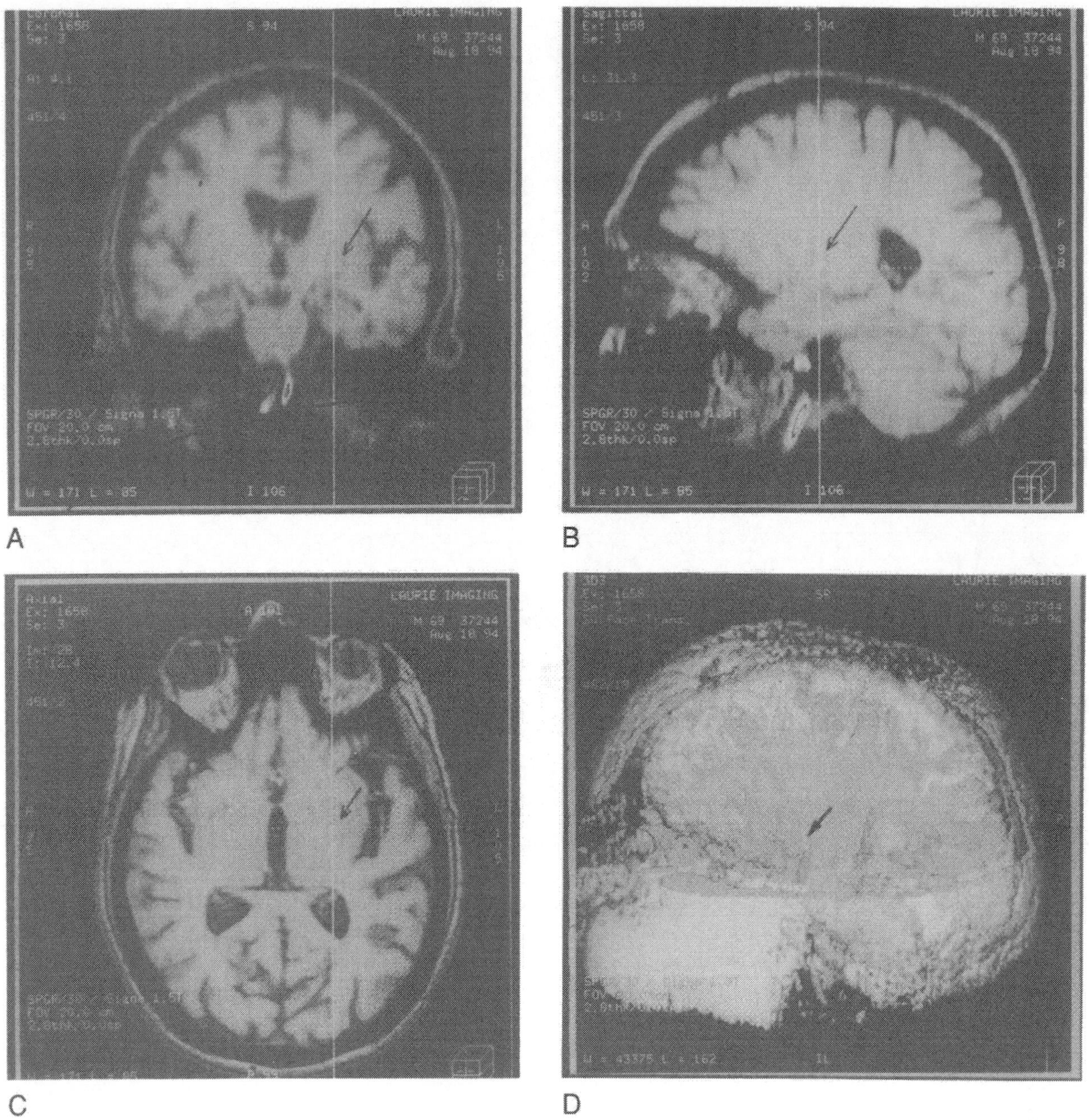

Fig. 3. (A–D) Post-operative MR images in multiplanar 2D and 3D volume surface rendered views. (Arrows: epicenter of lesion)

optimal site for lesion-making. Size of lesion, location and volume of electrophysiological data will further be determined more precisely by this analysis. Finally, this methodology may be the first step leading to frameless stereotactic pallidotomy with intraoperative MR imaging re-freshing the data [14].

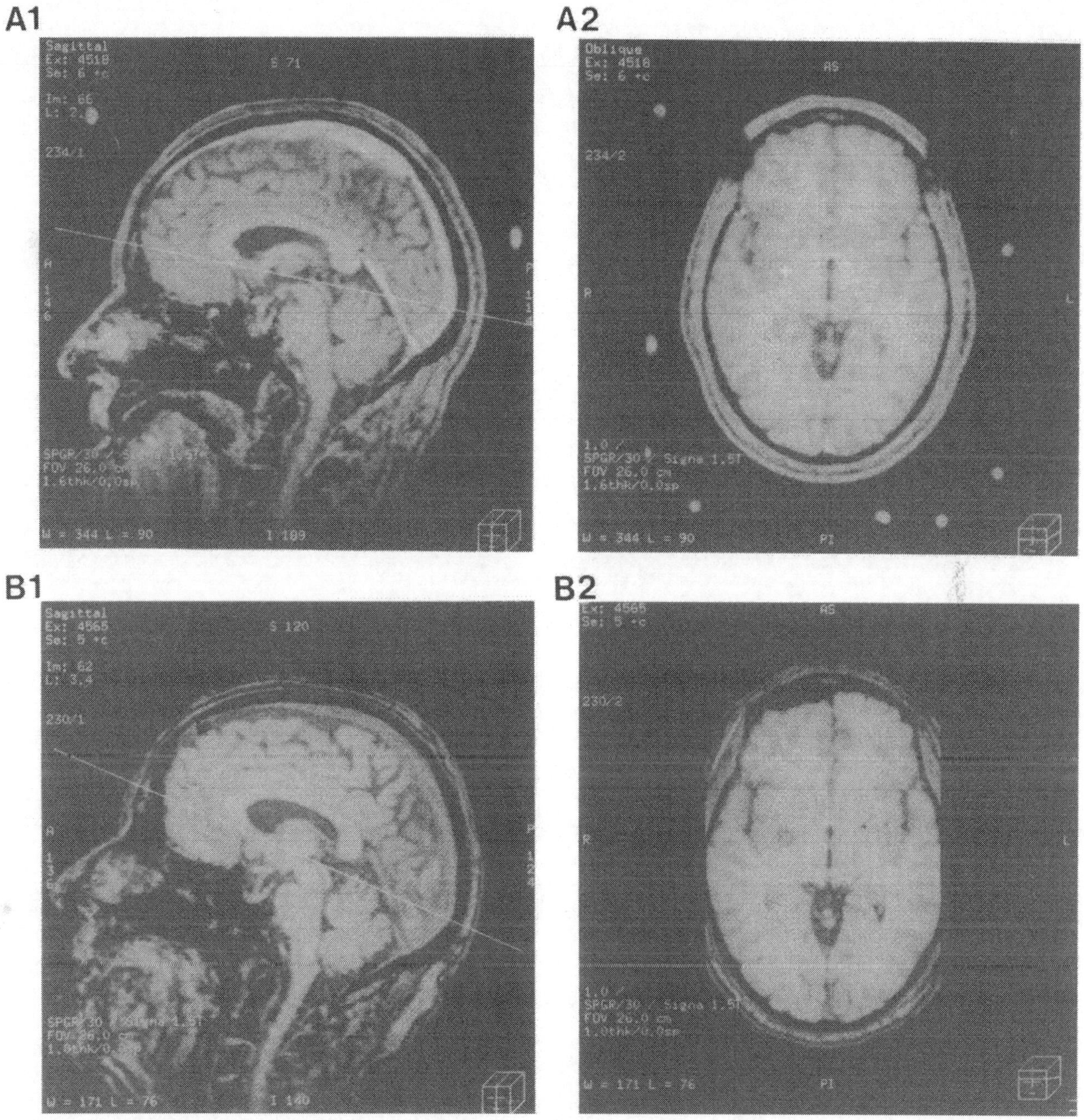

Fig. 4. (A) Pre-operative MRI. One axial slice through intercommissural plane of 60 slice volumetric study. Note target selection. (B) Post-pallidotomy MRI, same slice of volumetric study. (C) Difference (subtraction) image (A2-B2) (see p. 34). Lesion seen at superior extent of slice level readily confirmed, i.e. *intercommissural plane*

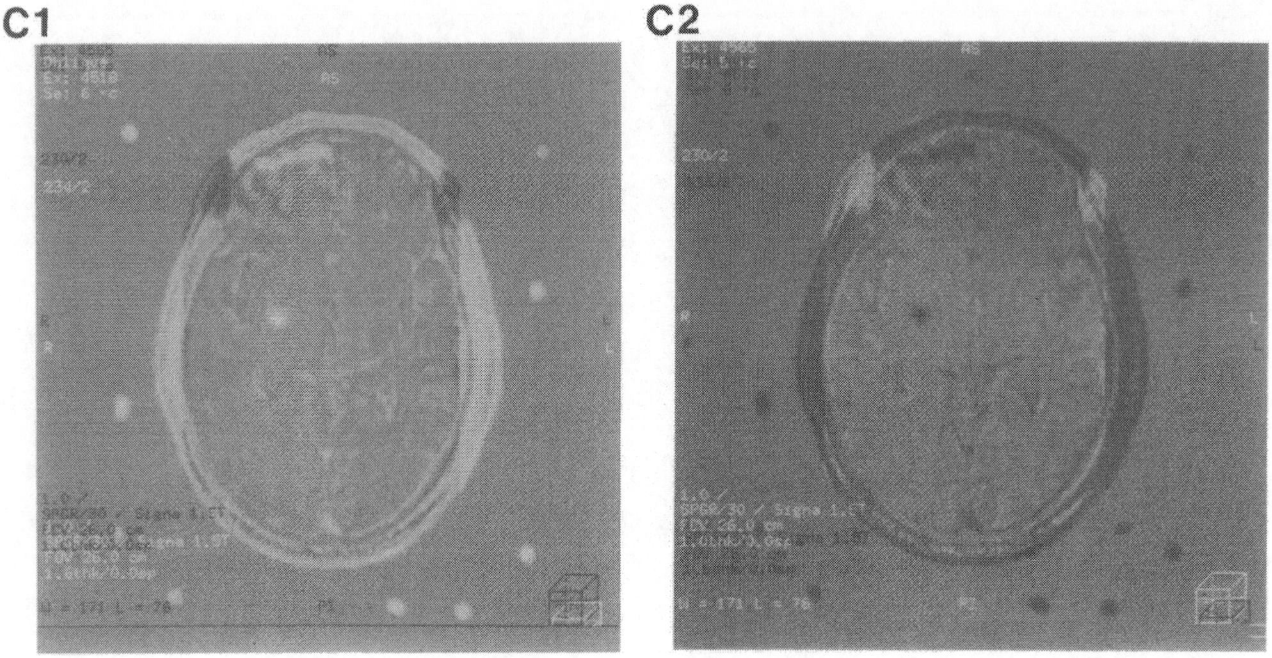

Fig. 4. (cont.)

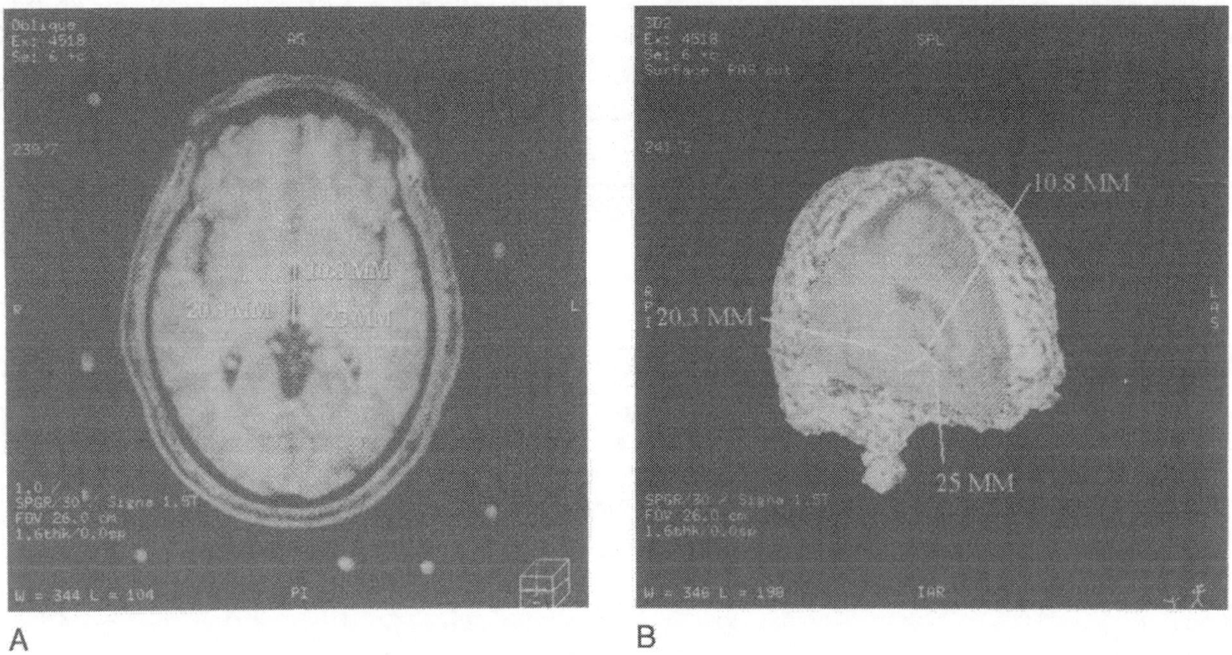

Fig. 5. (A) Pre-operative volumetric MRI with single slice for localization at intercommissural plane. (B) Pre-operative 3D volume surface-rendered study with cut-out at intercommissural plane. (C) Post-operative 3D volume surface-rendered study with cut-out at same level (see p. 35) (Arrow: epicenter of superior portion of lesion)

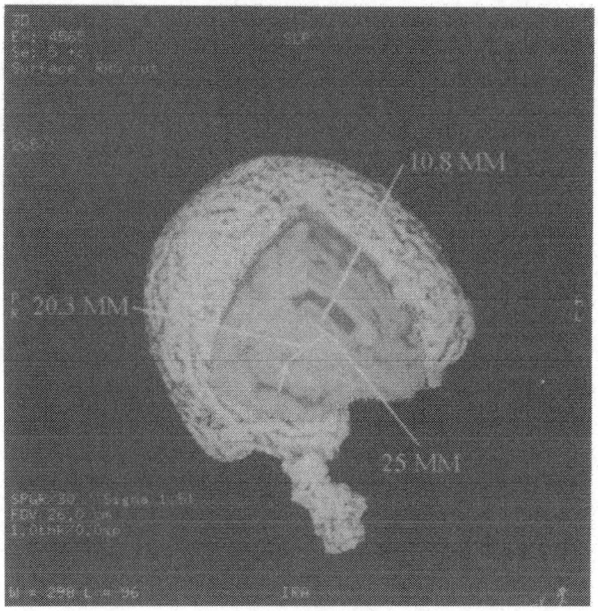

C

Fig. 5. (cont.)

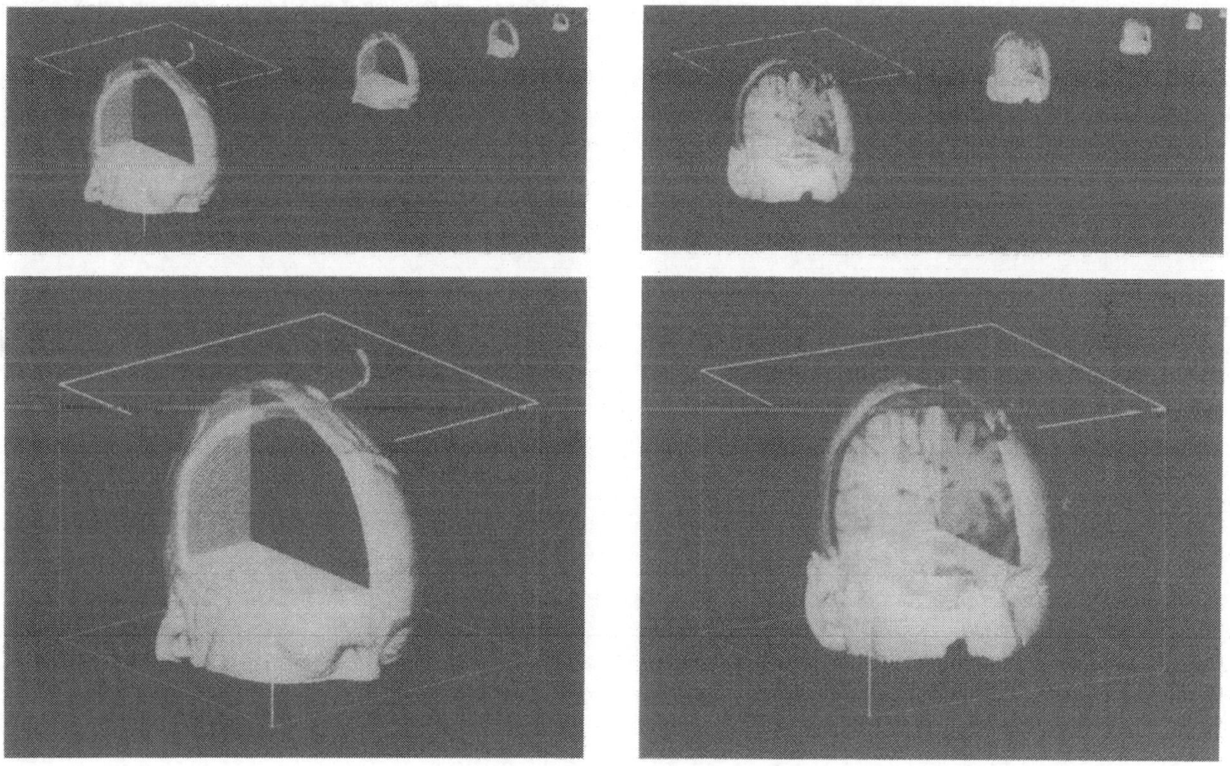

A B

Fig. 6 (A, B). Compression techniques using 4D pyramid to facilitate co-registration of the data sets, from most compressed (least detail) to least compressed (most detail)

References

1. Brown L (1992) A survey of image registration techniques, ACM Computing Surveys 24(4): 325–376
2. Burt P (1988) Smart sensing within a pyramid vision machine. Proceedings of the IEEE 76: 8
3. Cohen DS, Lustgarten JH, Miller E, Khandji AG, Goodman RR (1995) Effects of coregistration of MR to CT images on MR stereotactic accuracy. J Neurosurg 82: 772–779
4. Day R, Heilbrun MP, Koehler S, McDonald P, Peters W, Siemionow V (1994) Three-point transformation for integration of multiple coordinate systems: applications to tumor, functional and fractionated radiosurgery stereotactic planning. Stereotact Funct Neurosurg 63: 76–79
5. Freeborough PA, Fox AC (1996) Scaling compensation in the registration of serial 3D MRI of the brain. Proceedings of the International Society for Magnetic Resonance in Medicine, New York City, NY
6. Giorgi C (1994) Imaging techniques and computers. Stereotact Funct Neurosurg 63: 8–16
7. Guthrie BL, Adler JR, Jr (1992) Computer-assisted preoperative planning, interactive surgery and frameless stereotaxy. Clin Neurosurg 112–131
8. Itti L, Chang L, Ernst T (1996) Robust multimodality registration for neuroimaging. Proceedings of the International Society for Magnetic Resonance in Medicine, New York NY, 35
9. Kall BA, Goerss SJ, Kelly PJ (1992) Three-dimensional display in the evaluation and performance of neurosurgery without a stereotactic frame: more than a pretty picture? Stereotact Funct Neurosurg 58: 45–51
10. Kikinis R, Gleason PL, Moriarty TM, Moore MR, Alexander E, III, Stieg PE, Matsumae M, Lorensen WE, Cline HE, Black PM, Jolesz FA (1996) Computer-assisted interactive three-dimensional planning for neurosurgical procedures. Neurosurgery 38: 640–651
11. Kumar R, Dana K, Anandan P, Okamoto N, Bergen J, Hemler P, Sumanaweera TS, van den Elsen PA, Adler J (1994) Frameless registration of MR and CT 3D volumetric data sets. Proceedings, IEEE Workshop on Applications of Computer Vision, Sarasota, FL
12. Lehman RM, Mezrich RS, Kumar R, Dana K, Anandan P (1995) Frameless 3D volume registration for stereotactic planning. Proceedings of the 10th European Congress of Neurosurgery, Berlin, Germany
13. Lehman RM, Mezrich RS, Sage J, Goldbe L (1994) Peri- and postoperative magnetic resonance imaging localization of pallidotomy. Stereotact Funct Neurosurg 62: 61–70
14. Moriarty TM, Kikinis R, Jolesz FA, Black PM, Alexander E, III (1996) Magnetic Resonance Imaging Therapy. Neurosurgery Clinics of North America, Vol 7, No. 2. Saunders, Philadelphia
15. Unser M, Aldroubie A, Geifen CR (1993) SPIE mathematical imaging, vol 2034. San Diego, CA
16. Weaver JP, Kostelec PJ, Healy DM, Jr (1996) Elastic registration of MR images: the comparison of a feature matching algorithm and spine pyramid algorithm. Proceedings of the International Society for Magnetic Resonance in Medicine, New York, NY

Correspondence: Richard M. Lehman, M.D., Division of Neurosurgery, UMDNJ-RWJMS, 125 Paterson Street, Suite 2100, New Brunswick, NJ 08901-1977, USA.

Acta Neurochir (1997) [Suppl] 68: 37–41

Unilateral Pallidotomy for Parkinson's Disease Promptly Improves a Wide Range of Voluntary Activities – Especially Gait and Trunk Movements

C. H. A. Meyer

Queen Elizabeth Neuroscience Center, Birmingham, U.K.

Summary

26 patients with Parkinson's disease were assessed in the OFF state 2–3 days before and one week after pallidotomy for the time to complete each of 25 standardized motor tasks testing a wide range of voluntary activities important for daily living. After pallidotomy there were substantial improvements across this wide range of activities. Patients completed tasks that they could not perform preoperatively. In general for individual tasks (a) preoperative and postoperative scores were directly related, and (b) the absolute improvement (preop time – postop time) was directly related to preoperative performance: numerical improvements were greater in patients who were worse preoperatively. When the 25 tasks were ranked according to improvement relative to preoperative performance postoperative improvements were successively greater for (a) limbs ipsilateral to pallidotomy, (b) contralateral limbs, and (c) standing and walking. The best results were for activities in which the trunk plays a large part.

Keywords: Pallidotomy; bradykinesia; Parkinson's disease.

Introduction

Led by Laitinen's revival of pallidotomy at the site favoured by Leksell [3] neurosurgeons increasingly report that the operation improves many clinical features of Parkinson's disease including bradykinesia, the slowness of voluntary movement [1–3]. Assessment of bradykinesia has used rating scales (such as the UPDRS series) [4] and the time to complete standardized motor tasks. To date timed tasks have involved relatively few test activities, chiefly walking and movements of individual limbs. In the present study timed motor tasks record the early effect of unilateral pallidotomy on a wide range of voluntary actions relevant to everyday life – including actions in which the trunk plays a large part and which are the source of considerable disability in Parkinson's disease.

Methods

26 patients with dopa-sensitive idiopathic Parkinson's disease, age median 58 (range 36–74) years, were treated by stereotactic unilateral ablation, left sided in 15 patients, at the Leksell-Laitinen site in the ventroposterolateral globus pallidus. Operative details: Hitchcock frame; frontal burr hole; straight monopolar Fischer electrode 2 mms × 1.8 mms; radiofrequencey lesions 80°C for 60 seconds typically at the surgical target and 2 mms and 4 mms more superficially along the electrode's trajectory; lesion site confirmed by immediate post-op brain scanning.

Patients stayed on their established anti-parkinsonian medication before and after surgery.

Two-three days before and seven days after pallidotomy patients were assessed in the practically-defined OFF state, (i.e. having been OFF anti-parkinsonian medication for 12 hours overnight [4]), with respect to (i) UPDRS Motor Examination [4] and (ii) the time, to the nearest half second, to complete each of the standardized tasks of voluntary movement.

Standardized Motor Tasks

On each day of testing the patient performed each of the 25 tasks twice: the better performance was the one recorded for the day.

For scoring purposes the maximum time, used for patients unable to perform a task, was 120 seconds.

I. The Manual Tasks Comprised the Following

A. One Handed Tasks

Each one performed separately by hands contralateral (CON) and ipsilateral (IPSI) to the side of pallidotomy

Pronation supination:

(i) The number of successive cycles of forearm pronation-supination (UPDRS test) in 30 seconds, expressed as time to complete 10 cycles.
(ii) Finger taps: In 30 seconds, the number of cycles in each of which index, middle, ring and little fingers tap successively against thumb – expressed as time for 10 cycles.
(iii) 2-Point movement: In 30 seconds the number of cycles in each of which the hand moves from left to right and back to left between contact points 30 cm apart – expressed as time for 10 cycles.

Clothes pegs: The number of clothes pegs moved in 30 seconds (5 wire-sprung clothes pegs initially fastened to the edge of a thin vertical board are moved successively to and fro between fastening to this board and fastening to a similar one 20 cm away) – expressed as time to move 10 clothes pegs.

Pegboard: In 60 seconds, the number of smooth cylindrical metal pegs (diameter 1.5 mms, length 20 mm) moved from a cylindrical well (recess with diameter 50 mm, depth 18 mm) into holes in a pegboard – expressed as time to move 5 pegs.

B. Two Handed Tasks

(i) Pegboard: Two hands move pegs independently but simultaneously: score the number of peg pairs in 60 seconds, expressed as time for 5 pairs.
(ii) Bow: The time to fasten a limp cord into a bow with double loop.
(iii) Buttons: The time to fasten three buttons to join the flaps of a standard coat laid on a horizontal surface.

2. Non-Manual Tasks

(i) Foot taps contralateral: In 30 seconds the number of cycles of tapping by the foot contralateral to pallidotomy. In each cycle the patient while sitting with heel on ground and forefoot elevated lifts the foot until the toes contact a surface 10 cm above and returns heel to ground – expressed as time for 20 cycles.
(ii) Foot taps ipsilateral: Similar task by foot ipsilateral to pallidotomy.
(iii) Standing ×3: Three successive cycles, each of arising i.e. standing up from a chair and sitting down again.
(iv) Walk: From a standing position, walk 7 metres and return to start position.
(v) Sws (Standard-Walk-Sit): From sitting in a chair, stand, walk 7 metres, return to chair and sit.
(vi) Coat: While standing the patient dons a standard laboratory coat and pulls the lower lapels across in front.
(vii) Roll Towards: From a horizontal supine position on a bed the patient rolls over towards the side of brain surgery into a prone position with arms outstretched along side of trunk, hands towards feet.
(viii) Roll Away: Similar task, rolling from supine away from the side of surgery.
(ix) Arise Towards: From a supine position lying on bed near its edge the patient stands up unsupported beside bed, arising towards the side of brain surgery.
(x) Arise Away: Similar task, the patient moving away from side of brain surgery.
(xi) Bridge Towards: While supine the patient bridges, i.e., wriggles, across a firm hospital bed (90 cm wide) from one side to the other, moving towards the side of pallidotomy.
(xii) Bridge Away: Similar task, movement in direction away from side of pallidotomy.

Statistical test: Non-parametric two-tailed tests were used.

Results

UPDRS Motor Exam

For this composite assessment in the OFF state the patient group's preoperative rating, median 40 (quartile range 30, 56) improved postoperatively to median 27 [22, 35] (Sign test N26 $P < 0.001$).

Scoring in the OFF state of constituent items within the UPDRS showed improvements, each significant (Sign tests $P < 0.005$) after pallidotomy in contralateral arm and leg rigidity and resting tremor and in contralateral postural-action arm tremor. Ratings indicated smaller improvements ($P < 0.05$) in ipsilateral arm and leg rigidity and upper limb resting tremor.

For UPDRS ratings in the ON state pallidotomy had great success in eliminating contralateral limb dyskinesias ($P < 0.005$).

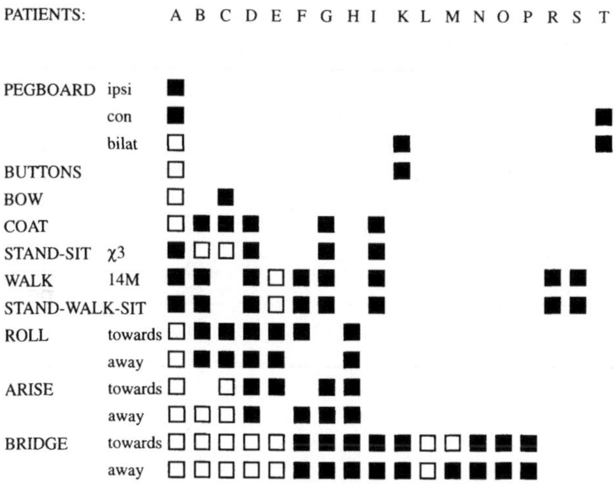

Fig. 1. Squares signifying individual patients unable to perform voluntary motor tasks in OFF state preoperatively. After pallidotomy these patients were able (shaded) or unable (unshaded) to complete the tasks

Standardized Motor Tasks

Preoperatively all hand tasks could be completed in the OFF state by all 26 patients apart from failure to complete pegboard tests by 3 patients and buttons and bow tests by 2 patients (Fig. 1). More patients were unable to perform non-manual tasks. Standing and sitting from a chair (stand ×3) could not be completed by 8 patients, walking by 9 patients, rolling over or arising from bed by 6 or 7 patients, and bridging (wriggling) across a bed by 15 patients.

In many cases, especially for walking and trunk movement tasks, pallidotomy restored independent mobility to patients unable to perform the tasks preoperatively. However, despite surgery some patients, e.g., 6 for trunk bridging, remained unable to complete certain tasks.

As a whole the patient group improved in the time to complete each of the 25 standardized tasks (Table 1). The change was statistically significant for all tasks except the pegboard test performed by the ipsilateral hand.

For each task, as exemplified in Fig. 2, preoperative and postoperative scores were directly related (Spearman r_s, for PRO-SUP (con) $P < 0.02$, for all other tasks $P < 0.01$).

For each task the Absolute Improvement i.e. (PREOP-POSTOP) seconds, was directly related to the preoperative time: Spearman r_s $P < 0.01$ for all tasks apart from arising from bed ($P < 0.05$) and trunk bridging (NS), the tasks for which correlations were influenced most by patients unable to perform the test before or after surgery, e.g. Fig. 2.

For each task there was a very strong association (r_s, $P < 0.01$) between Absolute Improvement and the change relative to the preoperative score, i.e. the Relative Improvement,

$$\frac{\text{(Preop-Postop)}}{\text{Preop}} \times 100\%$$

Overall the 25 tasks differed significantly (Friedman X_r^2 164 $P < 0.001$) in Relative Improvement after pallidotomy. For the order of tasks ranked according to Relative Improvement there is strong concordance among patients (Kendall W 0.27 $P < 0.001$). When tasks are plotted according to the sum of their rankings for Relative Improvement (Fig. 3) it appears that pallidotomy helps the ipsilateral hand movements least and the trunk movements most. For the patient group the median values of Relative Improvement for the different individual tasks (Table 1) were 8–18% for the hand and foot ipsilateral to pallidotomy, 18–27% for the contralateral hand or foot, 30–39% for standing and walking, and 45–58% for rolling over, arising and wriggling across a bed.

Discussion

For this group of patients who had postoperative improvements for dyskinesias, rigidity and tremor as reported by other surgeons [1–3], unilateral pallidotomy improved a wide range of voluntary movements relevant to everyday life. This extends previous reports of improvements in timed voluntary motor performance occurring immediately [2] and lasting 6 months or more [1] after pallidotomy.

The finding of voluntary motor improvements in ipsilateral limbs in these dopa-treated patients supports previous reports [1, 2] and recalls ipsilateral improvements found in the pre-dopa era by timed motor testing after unilateral thalamotomy-subthalamotomy for Parkinson's disease [5].

Of patients unable preoperatively to perform certain tasks concerning walking or trunk movement, some patients had striking improvement in these after pallidotomy though other patients remained unable to complete the task concerned. Apart from these ex-

Table 1. *Standard Motor Tasks (see Methods)*

		Pre sec		Post sec		(Pre-post)	(Pre-post)/pre %	
		Median	Quartile	Median	Quartile	Significance of change	Median	Quartile
One hand								
PRO-SUP	con	11.5	(10, 17)	8	(7, 9)	*	27	(18, 52)
	ipsi	11	(8.5, 14.5)	9	(7, 13)	*	18	(3.5, 31)
FING TAP	con	25	(16.5, 30)	18.5	(14.5, 21)	*	27	(5, 39)
	ipsi	21	(17, 27.5)	18.5	(16, 25)	*	18	(0, 20.5)
2-POINT	con	9	(8, 10)	7.5	(6.5, 8)	*	18	(9, 29)
	ipsi	8.5	(7, 11)	7.5	(6.5, 9)	*	9	(0, 21)
CLOTHES PEG	con	16.5	(13.5, 19)	12.5	(11.5, 16.5)	*	20	(10, 32)
	ipsi	14.5	(12, 19)	13.5	(11.5, 15)	*	11	(0, 21)
PEGBOARD	con	25	(23, 75)	22	(18, 30)	*	24	(7, 43)
	ipsi	25	(21.5, 37)	24	(17.5, 30)	ns	11	(−9, 19)
Two hands								
PEGBOARD		50	(33.5, 150)	37.5	(27.5, 50)	*	17	(0, 57)
TIE BOW		12.5	(10.5, 18)	8.5	(7.5, 12)	*	33	(11, 50)
BUTTONS		21	(14, 43)	17	(13, 23.5)	*	26	(7, 44)
Non-manual								
FOOT TAP	con	14.5	(11, 19)	11	(9, 12.5)	*	24	(14, 37)
	ipsi	14	(12, 19)	12.5	(10, 15.5)	*	11	(0, 19)
STAND x3		8	(6.5, 17)	6	(5, 8)	*	30	(16, 38)
WALK		28	(13, u)	12.5	(10.5, 35)	*	37	(12, 67)
S-W-S		38.5	(15, u)	16	(12.5, 40)	*	39	(14, 63)
COAT		13	(9, 44)	8	(6, 22)	*	33	(24, 54)
ROLL T		11	(5, u)	4	(3.5, 10)	*	45	(22, 71)
ROLL A		11.5	(6.5, 61)	5	(3, 8)	*	54	(33, 75)
STAND T		9.5	(5.5, 100)	5	(2.5, 13)	*	50	(17, 63)
STAND A		8	(5.5, u)	4	(3, 7)	*	45	(20, 69)
BRIDGE T		u	(20, u)	19.5	(7, u)	*	55	(0, 77)
BRIDGE A		u	(23, u)	15	(6, 50)	*	58	(22, 72)

For patient group, N26, in OFF state, table shows median and quartile ranges for time to nearest half second to complete each task pre- and post-operatively (significance of change, Wilcoxon 2-tail test, $^*P < 0.01$, NS not sig at P0.05) and for Relative Improvement, i.e., Improvement (PRE-POST) as percentage of PRE operative score.
U = Unable to perform.

treme cases the biggest improvements for individual tasks occurred in general in patients who were worst before surgery – though patients who were slowest preoperatively tended to remain slower than other patients after pallidotomy.

The present study indicates that in its immediate effect on voluntary movement in the OFF state pallidotomy helps the ipsilateral hand and foot least, the contralateral hand and foot more, and standing and walking a good deal. It emphasises the operation's immediate benefit for actions in which the trunk plays a relatively large part including donning a coat, rolling over, arising from bed and bridging (wriggling) across a bed. Pallidotomy can restore independent mobility to certain patients who are bed- or chair-fast when in the OFF state preoperatively.

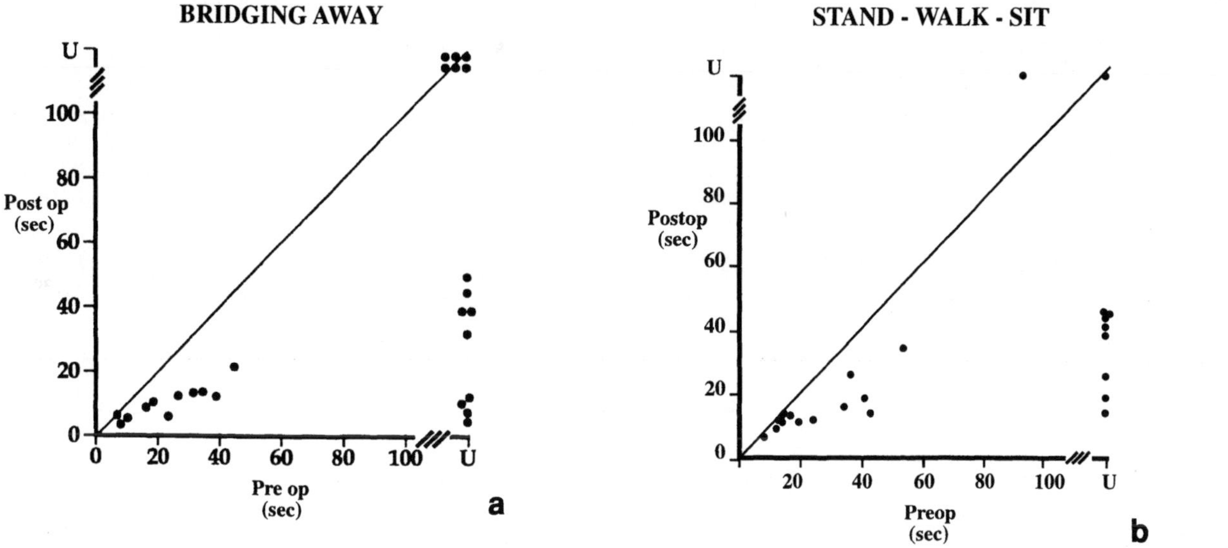

Fig. 2 (a, b). Patient are plotted by time to complete tasks in OFF state before and after pallidotomy. "U" signifies inability to complete the task. Improvements are plotted below, and deteriorations above, the oblique line

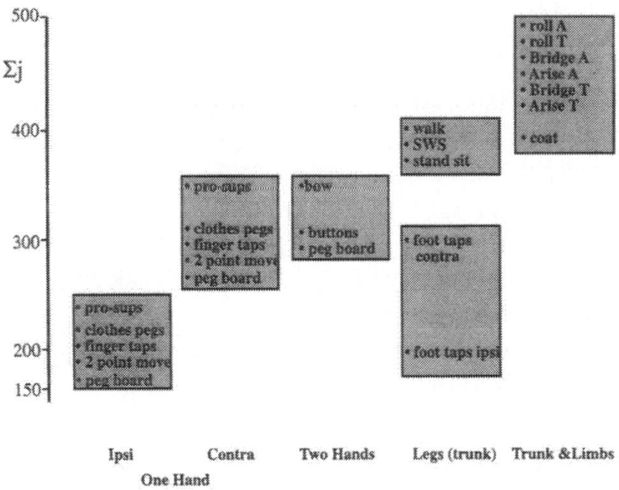

Fig. 3. 25 Standardized motor tasks (see Methods) plotted according to the sum of rankings (Ej) for each task – after all tasks had first been ranked for each separate patient according to the Relative Improvement of timed performance, i.e. (preop – postop)/preop. "*T*" and "*A*" signify movement towards or away from side of pallidotomy. Surgery had least benefit for ipsilateral hand/foot, most for actions of trunk and limbs

Acknowledgements

To Mrs Cheryl Bickerton for preparing the manuscript.

References

1. Fazzini E, Dogali M, Beric A *et al* (1995) The effects of unilateral ventral posterior medial pallidotomy in patients with Parkinson's disease and Parkinson's plus syndromes. In: Koller WC, Paulson G (eds) Therapy of Parkinson's disease, 2nd ed rev. and expanded. Marcel Dekker, New York, pp 353–379
2. Laitinen LV (1994) Ventroposterolateral pallidotomy. Stereotact Funct Neurosurg 62: 41–52
3. Laitinen LV, Hariz MI, Bergenheim AT (1992) Leksell's posteroventral pallidotomy in the treatment of Parkinson's disease. J Neurosurg 76: 53–61
4. Langston JW, Widner H, Brooks D *et al* (1991) Core assessment program for intracerebral transplantation (CAPIT). In: Lindvall O, Bjorklund A, Widner H (eds) Intracerebral transplantations in movement disorders. Elsevier, London, pp 227–241
5. Meyer CHA (1981) Bilateral improvement in voluntary movement after unilateral diencephalic lesions for parkinsonism. Appl Neurophysiol 44: 345–354

Correspondence: Carl H. A. Meyer, FRACS, Queen Elizabeth Neuroscience Centre, Queen Elizabeth Hospital, Edgbaston, Birmingham B 15 2TH, UK.

Acta Neurochir (1997) [Suppl] 68: 42–48

The Side-Effects and Complications of Posteroventral Pallidotomy

M. I. Hariz[1] and **A. A. F. De Salles**[2]

[1] Department of Neurosurgery, University of Umeå, Sweden and [2]Division of Neurosurgery, University of California at Los Angeles (UCLA), CA, USA

Summary

The side-effects and complications of posteroventral pallidotomy are analysed in 138 consecutive patients who underwent 152 pallidotomies. Transient side-effects, lasting less than three months, appeared in 18% of the patients, that is, 16.5% of the surgical procedures. Long term complications, lasting more than 6 months, were noted in 10% of the patients, that is, 9.2% of the surgical procedures. Sixteen complications occurred alone or in various combinations in 14 patients and included fatigue and sleepiness (2), worsening of memory (4), depression (1), aphonia (1), dysarthria (3), scotoma (1), slight facial and leg paresis (2) and delayed stroke (2). Complications such as dysarthria and paresis could be attributed to MR- or CT-verified pallidal lesions lying too medially and encroaching on the internal capsule. Two of the patients with deterioration in memory had some memory impairment before surgery, and the aphonic patient had dysphonia preoperatively. The study suggests that stereotactic MRI and careful impedance monitoring and macrostimulation of the posteroventral pallidum area should be sufficient for minimizing the risk of complications; the stereotactic lesion should be centreed within the posterior ventral pallidum without involvement of internal capsule. It is concluded that pallidotomy is a safe procedure if performed on cognitively alert patients, and it seems that both the incidence and especially the severity of complications are lower for posteroventral pallidotomy than for thalamotomy.

Keywords: Pallidotomy; Parkinson's disease.

Introduction

The modern posteroventral pallidotomy (PVP), reintroduced by Laitinen *et al.* in 1992 [20] has gained a worldwide spread in the surgical treatment of advanced Parkinson's disease (PD). While the benefit of this procedure for various Parkinsonian symptoms is being continuously evaluated [3, 5, 7, 8, 14, 17, 18, 22, 27, 29, 30, 32, 34, 37], the experience so far should disclose whether there is a specific morbidity inherent in this surgery. In this study, the experience of two stereotactic centres in the last 3 years is reviewed in order to assess the side effects and complications that occurred in patients following posteroventral pallidotomy.

Material and Methods

Patients

One hundred and thirty eight consecutive patients with Parkinson's disease were included in this study. The patients were operated on between June 1992 and December 1995. There were 85 men and 53 women, with a mean age of 66 years (range: 33 to 80 years). The patients underwent a total of 152 pallidotomies, 83 right-sided and 69 left-sided. Twelve patients had undergone staged bilateral pallidotomies with an interval of 3 months to one year between the two procedures. Two patients had a re-pallidotomy on the same side 6 months and 13 months, respectively, after the first surgery.

Surgical Procedure

Stereotactic CT and/or MRI were used for calculation of the pallidal target's coordinates. Either the Leksell apparatus [28] or the Laitinen apparatus [13, 20] was used for imaging studies and surgery. On the CT or MR scans, the target point was defined in the posterior-ventral pallidum; it lay 1–3 mm in front of the midpoint between anterior commissure (AC) and posterior commissure (PC) of the third ventricle, 20–22 mm lateral to the midline of the third ventricle and 3–6 mm ventral to the level of the AC-PC line.

At surgery, a monopolar electrode with a 2 mm-long and 1.8 mm thick non-insulated tip was used for impedance monitoring, monopolar stimulation and radiofrequency (RF) coagulation. For stimulation of the target area, the electrical thresholds for capsular or optic side-effects using a current of 1 msec in length were 8–10 mA at 6 Hz, and 5 mA at 60 Hz, or 2 V at 5 Hz and 50 Hz, respectively. If no untoward effects appeared at stimulation, the RF lesions were performed incrementally. There were generally 2–3 lesion points, and sometimes 4 lesion points lying 2 mm apart. Each lesion was made by heating the target area with 75–85°C for 60 sec. If untoward effects appeared upon electrical stimulation, the electrode was repositioned, or the lesion was made smaller than initially intended. The stimulation and coagulation through the target area were performed from ventral to dorsal in some patients, and from dorsal to ventral in the other patients.

Assessment Procedure

The patients were assessed up to 36 months after surgery (mean 12 months). In this paper, only the untowards and negative effects of surgery, i.e., side-effects and complications, will be reported. These were defined as new changes or deficits objectively assessable and observed by the surgeon in the immediate postoperative period and at the subsequent assessments in the out-patient department. The side-effects and complications included also any negative changes, attributed to the surgery, that the patients or the relatives subjectively experienced during the follow up period. The side-effects of surgery were classified into "transient", i.e. lasting less than three months, and "long term", i.e., lasting 6 months or more after surgery. For patients who underwent a second pallidotomy on the contralateral hemisphere, or a repeat pallidotomy on the same hemisphere, the eventual side-effects and complications were assessed separately for each of the two surgical procedures. When feasible, a CT or MRI scan of the brain was reviewed to document whether the side-effect could be related to a malplaced or a too large radiofrequency lesion.

Results

Transient or long term side-effects and complications occurred in a total of 39 patients (28.26% of patients).

The transient side-effects that appeared in 25 patients (18.11% of patients, 16.44% of pallidotomies) are shown in Table 1: the subcortical haematomas that appeared in two patients were located in the electrode track. One of these patients had also meningitis. Of the three patients who had facial paresis, one patient had also paresis of leg and dysarthria. Dysarthria occurred in additional 4 patients, all of whom had a lesion too medial within the pallidum. In another patient with paresis of leg, a CT scan performed 5 days after surgery revealed a lesion too anterior and too medial with significant surrounding oedema (Fig. 1). Two patients exhibited a dyspraxia of the foot upon walking. These patients had no sensory deficit, no pyramidal signs and no impairment of voluntary movements of leg and foot while sitting or lying in bed. Three patients experienced decreased effectiveness of L-dopa. A CT scan of one of these patients showed a lesion too small and restricted to the lateral and dorsal area of the pallidum. Two patients experienced epileptic fits in the first week following surgery. In one of these patients, an MRI scan performed three months after surgery revealed that the pallidal lesion encroached on the dorsal amygdala (Fig. 2). Four patients had increased drooling after surgery, two of them after the second contralateral pallidotomy. Five patients had transient confusion: in one of them the surgery was interrupted because of intra-operative confusion. In another patient, the reduction of the anticholinergic drug after surgery improved the patient; and in a third patient, there was a preoperative history of confusion that was worsened by surgery, but the patient returned to base-line as far as confusion episodes were concerned within three months after surgery.

Table 1. *The Nature and Incidence of Transient Side-Effects in Percent of Patients Operated Upon, and in Percent of Total Surgical Procedures*

Transient side-effects	Number of side-effects	Incidence in % of patients	Incidence in % of surgical procedures
Subcortical haematoma*	2	1.44	1.31
Meningitis*	1	0.72	0.65
Facial paresis*	3	2.17	1.97
Paresis of leg*	2	1.44	1.31
Dysarthria*	5	3.62	3.28
Dyspraxia of fot	2	1.44	1.31
Less effect of L-dopa	3	2.17	1.97
Epileptic fits	2	1.44	1.31
Increased drooling*	4	2.89	2.63
Extreme tiredness*	3	2.17	1.97
Confusion*	5	3.62	3.28
Total	25*	18.11	16.44

* Since one patient could have more than one transient side-effect (*), the total number of patients (*) with side-effects is less than the total sum of side-effects.

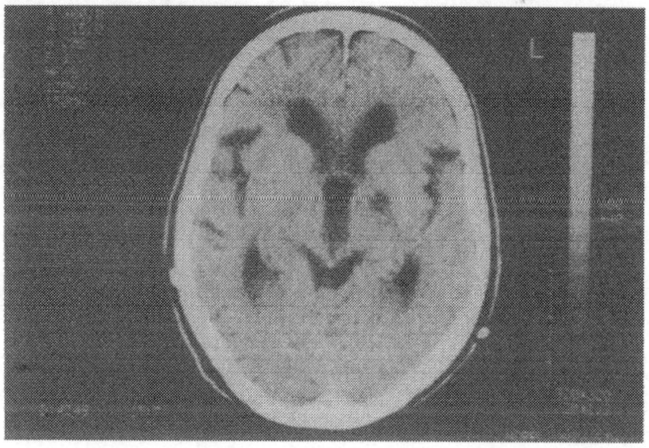

Fig. 1. CT scan showing a one week-old left pallidal RF lesion in a patient with dilated ventricles. The pallidal lesion lies 21 mm lateral to the midline of the third ventricle, and extends into the internal capsule

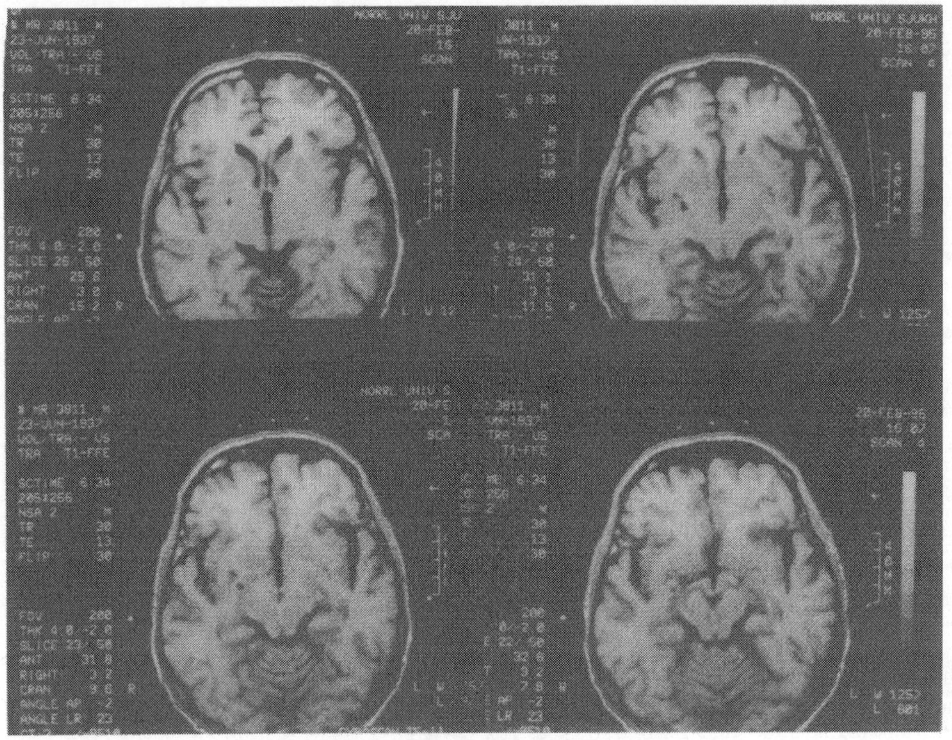

Fig. 2. Stereotactic 2 mm-thick axial MRI scans showing a 6 months-old RF lesion in the right pallidum. The lesion lies 22 mm lateral to the midline of the third ventricle at the most posteroventral edge of the right pallidum and encroaches on the dorsal amygdala, just lateral to the optic tract. (A putaminal lacune is visualized anterior and lateral to the pallidal lesion)

Table 2. *The Nature and Incidence of Long-Term Complications in Percent of Patients Operated Upon, and in Percent of Total Surgical Procedures*

Long-term complications	Number of side-effects	Incidence in % of patients	Incidence in % of surgical procedures
Fatigue and sleepiness	2	1.44	1.31
Worsening of memory	4	2.89	2.63
Depression	1	0.72	0.65
Aphonia	1	0.72	0.65
Dysarthria*	3	2.17	1.97
Visual field scotoma	1	0.72	0.65
Slight facial paresis*	1	0.72	0.65
Slight paresis of leg*	1	0.72	0.65
Delayed stroke	2	1.44	1.31
Total	14*	10.14	9.21

* Since one patient could have more than one long-term complication (*), the total number of patients (*) with long-term complications is inferior to the total sum of complications.

The long-term complications, noted in 14 patients (10.14% of patients, 9.21% of pallidotomies), are shown in Table 2: two patients complained for up to 1.5 years after surgery of increased need for sleep and continuous feeling of tiredness; there were no signs of depression in these patients. In four patients there was a long standing slight to moderate worsening of short term memory, noticeable by the patient him- or herself and/or by the patient's relatives. Two of these patients had already, before their left-side pallidotomy, a slight short term memory impairment, which worsened after surgery. The two other patients, who were operated on in the right pallidum, did not have a reported or noticeable memory impairment before surgery. One patient suffered long standing depression that needed psychiatric treatment. One patient with advanced dysphonia preoperatively was aphonic after surgery, and three patients had slight dysarthria. Only one patient had visual field scotoma after pallidotomy. One patient had a long standing slight dysarthria, and slight facial and leg paresis after surgery. Finally, delayed stroke appeared in two patients: in one patient, the stroke occurred 12 days after the second, bilateral pallidal lesion, and the ischaemic area extended into the internal capsule just posterior and ventral to the medially located pallidotomy lesion (Fig. 3).

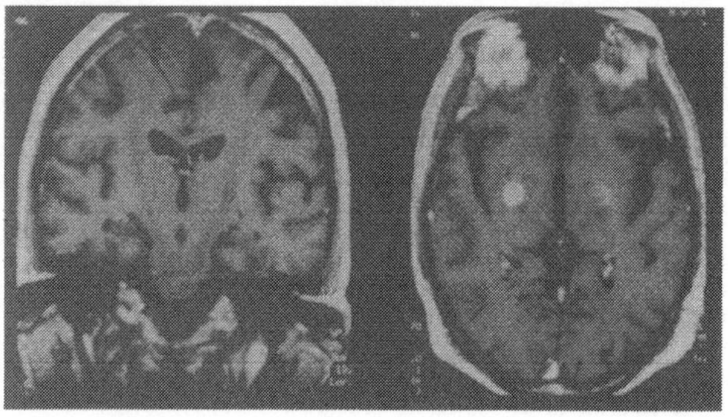

Fig. 3. Coronal and axial MRI scans performed 13 days after a second left-sided pallidotomy. Arrows indicate an infarction in the internal capsule, just posterior and ventral to the left-sided pallidotomy lesion

Discussion

Our experience in 152 consecutive pallidotomies showed that this surgical procedure is quite safe. There was no mortality and the morbidity, albeit present, was mild. Patients recovered well from the procedure and were discharged home usually one to two days after surgery. However five patients had to be re-admitted again within 1–3 weeks from surgery because of delayed complications. In two patients haematoma occurred at the third and seventh day, respectively, after pallidotomy. Both patients recovered completely without surgery, and one of them who is a farmer confessed later that he was feeling so well after his pallidotomy that he did some heavy lifting three days after surgery. Both patients asked for a new pallidotomy on the other side at the 6 months follow up! One patient was re-admitted for epileptic fits occurring 4 days after surgery, and two patients had stroke on the same side as their pallidotomy, 12 days and 3 weeks after surgery, respectively. The other listed complications neither prolonged the postoperative stay in hospital of the patients, nor did they require new hospitalization, with the exception of the patient with severe depression who had to be admitted to the psychiatric department.

The risks of PVP may be divided in two types: risks inherent to stereotactic surgery as such, and risks that can be attributed to the anatomical area of the brain targetted and eventually RF lesioned. Among the authors' complications, the subcortical haematomas and meningitis cannot be considered specific to pallidotomy. The same may apply to delayed stroke. On the other extreme, visual field scotoma is indeed a complication specific to pallidotomy, since the optic tract lies very close to the ventral medial border of the posteroventral pallidum. However, in this series the incidence was extremely low (0.65%) compared to the 14% incidence of the first report on PVP in 1992 [23].

Most of the other complications listed in this series of patients might have occurred had the patients undergone thalamotomy instead of pallidotomy. For 30 years, thalamotomy had been the dominant stereotactic procedure for patients with PD. Therefore, it was of interest to compare the complications of PVP to those reported by some authors following thalamotomy [4, 9, 15, 31, 33, 36]. For complications such as dysarthria and paresis, that appeared in our patients, their incidence, and especially their severity, seemed to be lower than for thalamotomy. These complications might have been avoided if the pallidal lesion did not lie so medial as to encroach on the internal capsule. In this respect, strict medial pallidotomy, especially if the medial pallidotomy is made more anteriorly as advocated by some [26], may carry increased risks as had already been shown by Bertrand in 1958 [2]. The authors believe that posteroventral pallidotomy should aim at the junction of the medial and lateral pallidum and should encompass both lateral and medial aspects of the pallidum at its most posterior and ventral level. Aphonia occurred in one patient who had severe dysphonia preoperatively; perhaps preoperative severe dysphonia should contraindicate pallidotomy.

The four patients with more or less permanent cognitive impairment were old and in three of them there was some evidence of slight memory deficit before surgery. Interestingly, the two patients with pallidotomy on the non-dominant brain had also some cognitive impairment following surgery. In agreement with others [1, 11, 17], the authors consider that patients with memory problems should not undergo pallidotomy, on either side of the brain. Epileptic fits have been reported after thalamotomy, especially when positive contrast ventriculography was used [9]. In the present series of patients, no ventriculography was used and in one of the two patients with epileptic fits it was believed that the convulsions were due to the pallidal lesion extending slightly into the dorsal amygdala ventrally. Both patients were free of epilepsy and without auticonvulsive medication within three months after surgery.

It is beyond doubt that provided that there is a careful targetting procedure and meticulous macrostimulation for assessment of the physiological target at surgery, pallidotomy does indeed carry less risks for the patients than thalamotomy. Furthermore, when complications occur, their severity is clearly less than after thalamotomy. Increased postural instability, sensory impairment, hemiplegia, dysphasia or unsteadiness upon walking, all of which are complications known to occur following thalamotomy [4, 15, 31, 33, 36] were not found in this series. It is also important to notice that pallidotomy-patients are generally older than thalamotomy-patients, and they suffer from a more advanced PD, since they do not only have tremor but often exhibit the full myriad of Parkinsonian symptoms including symptoms due to long-standing L-dopa treatment. The likelihood that these patients would therefore suffer more complications than the thalamotomy-patients cannot be sustained by this assessment.

The authors elected to assess patients operated on at two different centers in two different countries. Both centres use stereotactic systems that had been designed initially for functional stereotactic procedures and that have been historically used or are still in use by their designers and many others in a large number of thalamotomies and pallidotomies. Even though the number of patients operated on in each centre was not the same, the two stereotactic centres do use rather uniform techniques for target imaging, physiological intraoperative assessment of target area and incremental radiofrequency coagulation procedure. Therefore, the complications ought to be attributed to the procedure itself rather than reflect circumstances due to the surgery being performed in this or that centre. Nevertheless the distribution of the complications differed somewhat between the two centres: While both centres reported one patient with haematoma complication, the two delayed strokes and the depression occurred in patients of one of the centres and the two patients with epileptic fits and one patient with scotoma were operated on in the other. Although the incidence of complications were different in the two centres due to the uneven number of patients operated on, there was a definite correlation in both places between some of the complications and the anatomical location of the lesions within the pallidum: MRI or CT study showed that those patients who had either transient or permanent dysarthria and paresis had the lesion too medial and encroaching on the internal capsule. In one of the patients with epileptic fits MRI showed that the lesion had definitely irritated the dorsal amygdala.

In comparing the authors' complications with those reported by others following pallidotomy, two facts may be stated. One is that most reported series on pallidotomy are still too small and some of them do not address specifically the issue of complications of this surgery. The other fact is that the use of microelectrode recording and microstimulation during pallidotomy may contribute to an increase in the risks of severe complications [25].

Laitinen *et al.* in their first paper on CT-guided pallidotomy in 1992 reported 14% scotomata [23]. In further studies, the incidence decreased to virtually nil [22]. In the meantime, the imaging technique was refined, with axial and coronal MRI instead of CT for target definition and coordinate calculation. In addition, the stimulation and coagulation techniques were slightly modified [21, 22, 24]. In this present series, scotoma occurred only in one patient (0.65%). This patient was operated on in June 1992 with CT-directed target coordinates and with the old ventral to dorsal stimulation and coagulation technique. In patients operated on after 1993, MRI was the dominant target-imaging technique, and the stimulation and incremental coagulation were no longer conducted from a ventral to dorsal direction but from a dorsal to ventral direction in the posteroventral pallidum [22, 24].

Other stereotactic surgeons who started to perform pallidotomy benefited from the experience of Laitinen and the incidence of scotoma has now decreased so much that it is no longer a problem in performing pallidotomy. Some state that it was the use of a microelectrode technique during pallidotomy that decreased the risk of scotoma to virtually nil [26, 27]. In the authors' opinion, this may not be the case since neither they nor Laitinen use microelectrodes and their very low scotoma incidence compares favourably with others. Furthermore, it has been shown yet not that the microelectrode technique improved the results or decreased the complications of either thalamotomy [16] or pallidotomy [6, 19].

The complications of modern pallidotomy have been systematically analysed only in a few reports in a limited number of patients [10–12]. The classical paper of Svennilson and the Leksell group from 1960 [35] remains outstanding and unsurpassed in its careful and detailed description of the complications of PVP. In their series there were no complications of scotoma but the cognitive side-effects and the complications resulting from damage to the internal capsule were far more common than in the present series. It may be conduded that PVP today benefits from a much better imaging technique than was the case in the Fifties and Sixties. If performed with careful assessment of the target area with impedance monitoring and electrical stimulation, and if the most medial edge of the globus pallidus is avoided by the RF lesion, the modern posterior-ventral pallidotomy can be considered as a very safe operation for cognitively alert patients with advanced Parkinson's disease.

References

1. Alterman R, Kelly P, Beric A, Eidelberg D, Fazzini E, Perrine K, Sterio D (1996) Selection criteria for posteroventral pallidotomy. Acta Neurochir (Wien) 138: 636
2. Bertrand C (1958) A pneumotaxic technique for producing localized cerebral lesions and its use in the treatment of Parkinson's disease. J Neurosurg 15: 251–264
3. Bosch A, Schuurman R, Speelman H (1996) Posteroventral pallidotomy in movement disorders. Acta Neurochir (Wien) 138: 635–636
4. Bravo G, Parera C, Seiquer G (1966) Neurological side-effects in a series of operations on the basal ganglia. J Neurosurg 24: 640–647
5. Burchiel KJ, Favre J, Taha J (1966) Pallidotomy for Parkinson's disease: surgical technique and results. J Neurosurg 84: 336A
6. De Lotbinière ACJ (1996) Microelectrode recording: essential for the optimal placement of radiofrequency pallidotomy? Acta Neurochir (Wien) 138: 636
7. Dogali M, Fazzini E, Kolodny E, Eidelberg D, Sterio D, Devinski O, Beric A (1995) Stereotactic ventral pallidotomy for Parkinson's disease. Neurology 45: 753–761
8. Fazzini E, Dogali M, Eidelberg D, Beric A, Sterio G, Perrine K, Kolodny E (1996) Three-year follow up following unilateral pallidotomy in Parkinson's disease. Neurology 46: A200
9. Fox MW, Ahlskog JE, Kelly PJ (1991) Stereotactic ventrolateralis thalamotomy for medically refractory tremor in post-levodopa era Parkinson's disease patients. J Neurosurg 75: 723–730
10. Galvéz-Jiménez N, Lozano AM, Duff J, Trépanier L, Saint-Cyr JA, Lang AE (1996) Bilateral pallidotomy: pronounced amelioration of incapacitating levodopa-induced dyskinesias but accompanying cognitive decline. Mov Disord 11 [Suppl 1]: 242
11. Ghika J, Favre J, Frankhauser H, Regli F (1996) Neurological and neuropsychological complications of bilateral contemporaneous pallidotomy in Parkinson's disease. Neurology 46: A417
12. Green J, Vitek JL, Baron M, Bakey RAE, DeLong MR (1996) Neuropsychological sequelae of pallidotomy for treatment of Parkinson's disease: one year pilot findings. Neurology 46: A200
13. Hariz MI (1991) Clinical study on the accuracy of the Laitinen's non-invasive CT-guidance system in functional stereotaxis. Stereotact Funct Neurosurg 56: 109–128
14. Iacono RP, Shima F, Lonser RR, Kuniyoshi S, Maeda G, Yamada S (1995) The results, indications and physiology of posteroventral pallidotomy for patients with Parkinson's disease. Neurosurgery 36: 1118–1127
15. Jancovic J, Cardoso F, Grossman RG, Hamilton WJ (1995) Outcome after stereotactic thalamotomy for parkinsonian, essential, and other types of tremor. Neurosurgery 37: 680–687
16. Jones MW, Tasker RR (1990) The relationship of documented destruction of specific cell types to complications and effectiveness in thalamotomy for tremor in Parkinson's disease. Stereotact Funct Neurosurg 54 + 55: 207–211
17. Kelly PJ (1995) Pallidotomy in Parkinson's disease (editorial comment). Neurosurgery 36: 1154–1157
18. Kishore A, Turnbull I, de la Fuente-Fernandez R, Schulzer M, Calne DB, Snow BJ (1996) Ventral pallidotomy improves motor signs and dyskinesias in Parkinson's disease. Mov Disord 11 [Suppl 1]: 240
19. Kondziolka D, Bonaroti EA, Lunsford LD (1996) Pallidotomy for Parkinson's disease. Contemp Neurosurg 18(6): 1–7
20. Laitinen LV (1988) The Laitinen system. In: Lunsford LD (ed) Modern stereotactic neurosurgery. Nijhoff, Boston, pp 99–116
21. Laitinen LV (1994) Ventroposterolateral pallidotomy. Stereotact Funct Neurosurg 62: 41–52
22. Laitinen LV (1995) Pallidotomy for Parkinson's disease. Neurosurg Clin North Am 6: 105–112
23. Laitinen LV, Bergenheim AT, Hariz MI (1992) Leksell's posteroventral pallidotomy in the treatment of Parkinson's disease. J Neurosurg 76: 53–61
24. Laitinen LV, Hariz MI (1996) Movement disorders. In: Youmans JR (ed) Neurological surgery, 4th Edition. Saunders, Philadelphia, pp 3575–3609
25. Linazasoro G, Guridi J, Gorospe A, Ramos E, Mozo A, Obeso JA (1996) Posteroventral pallidotomy in Parkinson's disease. Clinical results in 27 patients. Mov Disord 11 [Suppl 1]: 240
26. Lozano A, Hutchison W, Kiss Z, Tasker R, Davis K, Dostrovsky J (1996) Methods for microelectrode-guided posteroventral pallidotomy. J Neurosurg 84: 194–202
27. Lozano AM, Lang AE, Galvez-Jimenez N, Miyasaki J, Duff J, Hutchison WD, Dostrovsky JO (1995) Effect of GPi pallidotomy on motor function in Parkinson's disease. Lancet 346: 1383–1387
28. Lunsford LD, Leksell D (1988) The Leksell system. In: Lunsford LD (ed) Modern stereotactic neurosurgery. Nijhoff, Boston, pp 27–46
29. Meyer CHA (1996) Pallidotomy for Parkinson's disease promptly improves a wide range of voluntary activities – especially gait and trunk movements. Acta Neurochir (Wien) 138: 635
30. Quinn N (1994) Reversal of Parkinson's akinesia by pallidotomy. Lancet 343: 1095–1096
31. Selby G (1967) Stereotactic surgery for the relief of Parkinson's disease. Part 2. An analysis of the results in a series of 303 patients (413 operations). J Neurol Sci 5: 343–375
32. Spiegelmann R, Chasin S (1996) Posteroventral pallidotomy: experience with 100 cases. Acta Neurochir (Wien) 138: 644
33. Struppler A, Jakob C, Lipinski H-G, Stimmer H (1996) Changes in muscle tone and control of force following stereotactic lesions on motor thalamus level. Mov Disord 11 [Suppl 1]: 241
34. Sutton JP, Coulwell W, Lew MF, Mallory L, Grafton S, DeGiorgio C, Welsh M, Apuzzo MLJ, Ahmadi J, Waters CH (1995) Ventroposterior medial pallidotomy in patients with advanced Parkinson's disease. Neurosurgery 36: 1112–1117
35. Svennilson E, Torvik A, Lowe R, Leksell L (1960) Treatment of Parkinsonism by stereotactic thermolesions in the pallidal region. Acta Psychiatr Neurol Scand 35: 358–377

36. Van Manen J (1969) Postural instability after ventrolateral thalamic lesions. In: Gillingham FJ, Donaldson IML (eds) Third symposium on Parkinson's disease. Livingstone, London, pp 237–241
37. Vitek JL, Hashimoto T, Baron M, Kaneoke Y, Turner R, Bakay R, DeLong MR (1994) Pallidotomy in Parkinson's disease: Correlation of lesion location to clinical outcome. Mov Disord 9: 477–478

Correspondence: Marwan I. Hariz, M.D., Ph.D., Department of Neurosurgery, University Hospital, S-901 85 Umeå, Sweden.

Acta Neurochir (1997) [Suppl] 68: 49–53

Deep Brain Stimulation and Thalamotomy for Tremor Compared

R. R. Tasker[1], M. Munz[1], F. S. C. K. Junn[1], Z. H. T. Kiss[1], K. Davis[1], J. O. Dostrovsky[2], and A. M. Lozano[1]

Department of [1]Surgery and [2]Physiology, University of Toronto, Division of Neurosurgery, The Toronto Hospital, Toronto, Canada

Summary

Deep brain stimulation (DBS) and thalamotomy are both capable of abolishing tremor. However, no technique is perfect and if thalamotomy proves inadequate so that tremor recurs, presumably because of suboptimal lesion location, the only option is to repeat the thalamotomy. With DBS all that has been necessary to date is to change the parameters of stimulation. Similarly with complications such as the "cerebellar" ones and paraesthesiae. If these occur after thalamotomy one can only wait and hope that they will subside and they do not always do so. With DBS, changing the parameters in the authors' patients has so far been successful in eliminating them.

DBS, like thalamotomy is very effective for controlling tremor in Parkinson's disease (PD) and essential tremor (ET) and for improving dexterity in ET, but both techniques are less useful for the control of dopa dyskinesia, Parkinsonian rigidity, or impaired dexterity in PD, though DBS may be better than thalamotomy for the latter condition. On the other hand, both DBS and thalamotomy are very effective in improving dexterity in PD and ET may depend upon the fact that in PD bradykinesia is a major component, whereas in ET only the tremor is. The advantages of DBS over thalamotomy have to be weighed against the peculiar risks of DBS and of course, its cost.

Keywords: Deep brain stimulation (DBS); thalamotomy; Parkinson's disease; microthalamotomy; cerebellar tremor.

Introduction

From the earliest days of surgery for Parkinson's disease (PD), it has been known that acute electrical stimulation at certain brain sites arrests tremor for the duration of the stimulation [9]. Siegfried and Rea [7] have pointed out, that, influenced by this striking phenomenon, Bechtereva *et al.*, Mundinger *et al.*, Brice and McLellan and Mazars and his associates all explored the possibility of using chronic stimulation instead of lesionmaking to control movement disorders. It was not until the 1980's, however, that concentrated efforts were made to use this modality of treatment by Siegfried and his colleagues [6, 7], Benabid [1, 2] and his group and many others.

The authors themselves implanted two patients in 1985, one with PD in whom an adequate lesion could not be made because of incipient dysarthria, and one with multiple sclerosis (MS) who had had a thalamotomy on the other side of the brain. However, equipment available to them at that time consisted only of a radiofrequency-coupled monopolar Medtronic PISCES electrode and they did not pursue deep brain stimulation (DBS) for tremor until there was access to more suitable equipment after 1993.

The purpose of this paper is not to present the results of DBS, but rather to compare the results of 20 DBS implantations with those of 35 thalamotomies for tremor in the same hands and during the same time-frame.

Methods

Technique

The authors' stereotactic technique for thalamotomy for tremor using the Leksell G frame, computerized tomography (CT), or magnetic resonance imaging (MRI), microelectrode recording and microstimulation has been described elsewhere [9, 10]. DBS differs from thalamotomy only in that a DBS electrode is inserted at the site where a lesion would normally be made. Table 1 lists the equipment used in 20 cases all performed by one of the authors (RRT). The electrodes used consist of 4 stimulating rings spread over a 1.0 cm length of electrode and these were inserted so that the centre of the array was located at what normally would be the thalamotomy lesion site.

For comparison, all patients undergoing a total of 35 thalamotomies were selected, all performed by the same surgeon (RRT) for tremor between 1990 and 1995. If one of these patients had undergone a previous thalamotomy the data from that procedure were also included in the study regardless of how long ago the operation took place. Procedures that were abandoned or repeated because of tremor recurrence on the same side were not considered separately.

Table 1. *DBS Equipment Used*

2	Neuromed time: Radiofrequency-coupled stimulator
10	Medtronic X-trel: Radiofrequency-coupled stimulator
8	Medtronic ITREL: Totally programmable battery powered stimulator

Table 2. *Follow-up Years, No. Procedures*

	DBS N = 20	Thalamotomy N = 35
<1/4	5	10
1/4–1/2	3	2
1/2–1	8	6
1–5	4	11
>5[a]	0	6

[a] Includes previous procedures on 1990–95 cases.
Abandoned and same side repeats excluded.
Bilateral procedures counted as 2 procedures.
Same side DBS/thalamotomy counted as 2 procedures.

Table 3. *Age and Sex at Surgery, No. Procedures*

		DBS N = 20	Thalamotomy N = 35
20–30 yr	M	0	0
	F	1	2
30–40	M	1	2
	F	0	1
40–50	M	4	2
	F	1	6
50–60	M	1	8
	F	2	2
60–70	M	7	4
	F	0	6
70–80	M	1	1
	F	2	1

Evaluation

All patients were evaluated semiquantitatively by one of the authors (RRT) preoperatively and at intervals postoperatively using an identical protocol in which maximum tremor was graded on a 0 (normal) to 5 scale at each body joint. Rigidity was similarly graded 0–5 while the patient patted as quickly as possible with the opposite hand. Dexterity for performing handwriting, repetitive finger-thumb touching, finger-nose touching, wrist rotation, patting, handwriting and, in the case of essential (ET) and cerebellar tremor (CT), drinking were also graded 0–5.

Follow-up

Patients were included in the study in whom adequate postoperative data were available over at least 3 months as listed in Table 2. Table 3 lists the age and sex of patients treated, Table 4 the indications, and Table 5 the side and type of surgery. One patient with PD who had previously undergone an unsuccessful left thalamotomy underwent simultaneous bilateral DBS implantation and one patient with ET underwent bilateral staged DBS. Four patients, 3 with PD, 1 with CT underwent both DBS and thalamotomy on opposite sides of the brain while 2 patients with PD underwent pallidotomy on the first, DBS on the second side of the brain, the pallidotomies having been done in an attempt to manage bradykinesia and dopa dyskinesia.

Table 4. *Indications for Surgery, No. Procedures*[a]

	DBS N = 20	Thalamotomy N = 35
Parkinson's disease	13	23
Essential tremor	3	2
Cerebellar tremor including MS	4	10

[a] Abandoned and same side repeats excluded.

Table 5. *Side of Surgery, No. Procedures*

	DBS $N = 20$	Thalamotomy $N = 35$
R	7	8
L	9	19
Both	2 (4 operations)	4 (8 operations)
Repeated	0	2R 6L
Abandoned, repeated	1	1
Abandoned	0	2

DBS, thalamotomy same side 1.
Opposite 4.
DBS, pallidotomy opposite 2.

Results

Microthalamotomy Effect

The phenomenon of " microthalamotomy" was seen in 12 of the 20 DBS patients, still persisting in one patient at the latest follow-up of 8 months. This confirms how sensitive the appropriate site in thalamus is for tremor control when the mere introduction of an electrode approximately 1 mm in diameter is sufficient to control tremor at least temporarily; on the other hand the microthalamotomy effect interferes with testing the DBS in the early postoperative period.

Effect on Tremor

PD and ET

Because of the small number of patients, tremor data were pooled for PD and ET as shown in Table 7.

Table 6. *Microthalamotomy Effect*

None	8
Present	12–1 wk–9 mos
Occasionally permanent	

Table 7. *PD-ET Tremor % Procedures*

	16 DBS	22 Thalamotomy
Abolished or insignificant	62.5	63.7
Slight	31.3	13.6
Significant or total recurrence	6.3	22.7
Repeated procedures in above series	0	27.3%

The incidence of total or virtually total (only trivial tremor occasionally being noted on the side contralateral to the surgery) abolition by DBS and thalamotomy were the same (62.5% and 63.7% respectively). This was achieved with thalamotomy, however, only after 27.3% of operations had been repeated after initial failure; no DBS had to be repeated because of tremor recurrence at the time of writing. This is a high incidence of repetition, 15% being this groups' usual rate over a long period (unpublished data) and reflects experience in two PD, both operated upon on both sides, in whom it proved almost impossible to abolish tremor using the usual operative strategies; experience with 4 "patient sides" in such a small series presenting this problem is unusual and distorts the data. A 15% thalamotomy repetition rate still contrasts sharply with the DBS experience.

Other Features of PD

Table 8 compares the relative effects of DBS and thalamotomy on rigidity, dexterity and writing in patients with PD and on dexterity and drinking in patients with ET. The effects of the two operations on rigidity appeared similar. In some DBS patients, striking abolition of rigidity occurred as soon as the DBS was activated, in much the same way as tremor was; in others the effect appeared minimal. This presumably reflects the site of electrode placement, it generally being agreed that thalamotomy lesions and therefore, presumably, DBS insertions must be more rostral in order to control rigidity than for tremor [5]. Similarly, there appeared little difference in the effects of DBS and thalamotomy on Parkinsonian writing, neither being very effective.

Table 8. *PD-ET Surgery – Rigidity and Dexterity % Procedures*

		DBS		Thalamotomy	
		PD	ET	PD	ET
Reduced rigidity	25–50%	10		14.3	
	>50%	50	—	64.3	—
Improved dexterity	25–50%	18		14.3	50
	>50%	64	100	14.3	50
Improved writing	25–50%	30		14.3	50
	>50%	20	100	7.1	50
Improved drinking	24–50%				50
	>50%	—	100	—	50

Table 9. *Dopa Dyskinesia, No. Procedures*

	DBS N = 13	Thalamotomy N = 21
Not present	8	9
Reduced or abolished	1 (20%)	6 (50%)
Not affected	4 (80%)	6 (50%)

Curiously, DBS appeared more effective in improving manual dexterity in PD than thalamotomy was. Whether this simply reflects the superiority of one technique over the other or whether it is also due to the fact that thalamotomy may induce iatrogenic ataxia [3, 11] is uncertain.

Dopa Dyskinesia

Table 9 shows an insignificant difference between DBS and thalamotomy in the relief of dopa dyskinesia in patients for whom data were available and follow-up adequate: – in both cases far below the degree of relief achieved by pallidotomy [4].

CT

Four patients with cerebellar tremor (CT) (3 with cerebellar degeneration of unknown etiology, 1 with MS) underwent DBS. 10 (5 with MS, 3 with cerebellar degeneration of unknown etiology, 1 with post-stroke and 1 with post-traumatic tremor) underwent thalamotomy as shown in Table 10. Despite the excellent early relief of tremor achieved in these patients by DBS, dexterous tasks were not dramatically better performed postoperatively and results were not any more satisfactory than with thalamotomy.

Table 10. *Cerebellar Tremor, No. Procedures*

	DBS		
	Excellent	Good–fair	Failed
Tremor	3	1	0
Dexterity	0	4	0
Writing	0	0	4
Drinking	0	2	2

Follow-up 5, 6, 12, 17 months.

	Thalamotomy		
	Excellent	Good–fair	Failed
Tremor	0	2	4
Dexterity	0	0	6
Writing	0	1	5
Drinking	1	1	4

Follow-up 2, 2, 4, 8, 18, 27 months.

Table 11. *Residual Tremor after DBS and Thalamotomy in Same Patient, 3 with Parkinson's Disease, 1 with Cerebellar Tremor*

No. procedures		
	DBS	Thalamotomy
None or insignificant	2	2
Slight	2	1
Moderate	1	
Recurrent		1

DBS and Thalamotomy in the Same Patient

Table 11 compares the results of DBS and thalamotomy in the same 3 patients with Parkinson's disease and in one with CT of unknown etiology reflecting the same trends as the whole group of patients with PD and ET.

Complications

Table 12 lists the complications peculiar to DBS and Table 13 those common to both procedures. Voltage escalation to control "breakthrough" tremor has been modest and has not thus far presented difficulties. One patient undergoing thalamotomy for ET suffered an intracerebral haematoma requiring craniotomy for evacuation with eventual recovery, including return of tremor. One patient with CT suffered a brief transient ischaemic attack consisting of upper limb monoparesis on the side of the body ipsilateral to the side of the thalamus being explored. The procedure was aborted,

Table 12.

% Complications - 20 DBS	
Extrusion	5
Pain, swelling at receiver	15
Voltage escalation	40
Antenna movement	5
Initial nausea, faintness	10

Table 13. *% Complications*

	20 DBS	35 Thalamotomy
Intracerebral haematoma		2.9(t)
Oedema–hemiparesis	5 same	
Ipsilateral TIA	5 patient (t)	
Emotional lability		2.9(t)
Aggravated central pain		2.9(p)
Hand ataxia	10(t)	2.9(t) 14.2(p)
Dysarthria	5(t)	5.7(t) 2.9(p)
Gait disturbance	5(t) 5(p)[a]	2.9(t) 5.7(p)
Paraesthesiae	4.5(t)	5.7(t) 11.4(p)
Parkinsonian crisis	5(t)	5.7(t)

(t) = transient or reversible, (p) = permanent, slight sequelae.
[a] Appeared 3 months postoperatively, questionably a complication of surgery.

no underlying cause could be found and the procedure was repeated uneventfully a week later. Unfortunately, this patient then developed severe postoperative cerebral oedema with disabling hemi-apraxia, paresis and dysphasia, which required 6 weeks to recover. She later went on to extrude, without infection, first, her X-trel which was removed, and then her DBS electrode which was reinserted into the subgaleal plane.

In general, the non-implant-related complications of DBS and thalamotomy are similar. Both procedures are equally likely to induce postoperative haemorrhage and both induce the so-called "cerebellar" complications of dysarthria, ataxia and gait disturbance [3, 11]. With DBS, however, altering the parameters of stimulation has thus far in the authors' experience always eliminated these problems whereas in some thalamotomy patients they constitute permanent disabilities.

Discussion

These results appear comparable to the much larger experience of Benabid and his group [2] who has reported his outcome data with 80 patients with PD, 20 with ET, 4 with MS and 13 with miscellaneous movement disorders. Because of a different evaluation technique, direct comparison of numbers cannot be made. They noted, at latest follow-up, that 88% of their PD and ET patients scored 3 or 4 on a 5 point scale for the upper limbs but that ET tended to recur during the follow-up period in 18.5% of patients. The authors have noted the same thing after thalamotomy for ET [8] whereas it is generally agreed that PD tremor rarely recurs if it has remained absent for 3 months after thalamotomy. Benabid et al found tremor to be the only Parkinsonian feature other than pain that benefitted from DBS whereas in the Toronto hospital experience there were some patients whose rigidity improved dramatically with stimulation and both procedures produced a modest degree of improvement in dopa dyskinesia. Benabid's group found the same less satisfactory results with MS and other dyskinesias as in the present series. They experienced a 2.6% incidence of superficial infection requiring removal of equipment and a 31.6% incidence of minor complications reversible by adjusting the parameters of stimulation. Their optimum frequencies for tremor control (130 Hz) are similar to the authors (130–185 Hz).

Conclusions

DBS and thalamotomy are both capable of abolishing tremor. DBS, like thalamotomy is very effective for controlling tremor in PD and ET and for improving dexterity in ET, but both techniques are less useful for the control of dopa dyskinesia, Parkinsonian rigidity, or impaired dexterity in PD, though DBS may be better than thalamotomy for the latter condition. The advantages of DBS over thalamotomy have to be weighed against the peculiar risks of DBS and of course, its cost.

References

1. Benabid AL, Pollak P, Louveau A, *et al* (1987) Combined (thalamotomy and stimulation) surgery of the VIM thalamic nucleus for bilateral Parkinson's disease. Appl Neurophysiol 50: 344–346
2. Benabid AL, Pollak P, Gao D, Hoffman D, Limousin P, Gay E, Payen I, Benazzouz A (1996) Chronic electrical stimulation of the ventralis intermedius nucleus of the thalamus as a treatment for movement disorders. J Neurosurg 84: 203–214
3. Hariz MI (1990) Correlation between clinical outcome and size and site of the lesion in computed tomography guided thalamotomy and pallidotomy. Stereotact Funct Neurosurg 54–55: 172–185
4. Lozano AM, Lang AE, Galvez-Jiminez N, *et al* (1995) GPi pallidotomy improves motor function in patients with Parkinson's disease. Lancet 346: 1383–1386
5. Narabayashi H (1988) Lessons from stereotaxic surgery using microelectrode techniques in understanding Parkinsonism. Mt Sinai J Med 55: 50–57
6. Siegfried J, Pamir MC (1985) Electrical stimulation in humans of the sensory thalamic nuclei and effects on dyskinesias and spasticity. In: Struppler A, Weindl A (eds) Clinical aspects of sensory motor integration. Springer, Berlin Heidelberg New York Tokyo, pp 283–288
7. Siegfried J, Rea GL (1988) Deep brain stimulation for the treatment'of motor disorders. In: Lunsford LD (ed) Modern stereotactic surgery. Martinus Nijhoff, Boston, pp 409–412
8. Shahzadi S, Tasker RR, Lozano A (1995) Thalamotomy for essential and cerebellar tremor. Stereotact Funct Neurosurg 65: 11–17
9. Tasker RR (1995) The use of microelectrodes in the human brain. In: B, Desmedt JE (eds) Pain and the brain: From nociception to cognition. Bromm Advances in pain research and therapy, vol 22. Raven, New York, pp 143–174
10. Tasker RR, Yamashiro K, Lenz FA, Dostrovsky JO (1988) Thalamotomy in Parkinson's disease: microelectrode techniques In: Lunsford D (ed) Modern stereotactic surgery. Martinus Nijhoff, Boston, pp 297–313
11. Yasui N, Narabayashi H, Kondo T, Ohye C (1976/77) Slight cerebellar signs in stereotactic thalamotomy and subthalamotomy for Parkinsonism. Appl Neurophysiol 39: 315–320

Correspondence: Ronald R. Tasker, M.D., 399 Bathurst St., 2–431 McL., Toronto, ONM5T 2S8, Canada.

Acta Neurochir (1997) [Suppl] 68: 54–60

Treatment of Deafferentation Pain by Chronic Stimulation of the Motor Cortex: Report of a Series of 20 Cases

J. P. Nguyen[1,2], Y. Keravel [1], A. Feve[1], T. Uchiyama[1], P. Cesaro[1,2], C. Le Guerinel[1], and B. Pollin[3]

[1] Département des Neurosciences, CHU Henri Mondor, Créteil, [2]INSERM U421, 8, rue du Général Sarrail, Faculté de Médecine, Créteil, and [3] Laboratoire de Physiologie de la Manducation, Université Denis Diderot, Paris, France

Summary

Twenty patients with deafferentation pain were treated by chronic stimulation of the motor cortex. The central fissure was localized using stereotactic MRI and the motor cortex was mapped using intra-operative somatosensory evoked potentials. Seven patients with trigeminal neuropathic pain experienced definite pain relief varying between 40 and 100%. Ten patients had central pain secondary to central nervous system lesions. A satisfactory long-lasting pain control (pain relief > 40%) was obtained in five of them (50% of cases). One patient with pain from peripheral nerve injury obtained more than 80% pain relief. Two patients had pain from spinal cord lesions. One did not respond but the other obtained an excellent long-term result.

The location of the effective stimulation plots was in agreement with the somatotopic maps of the primary motor cortex. One patient developed a small extradural haematoma which resolved spontaneously. None of the patients developed seizure activity. This study confirms the potential value of motor cortex stimulation in the treatment of certain forms of intractable pain, especially in cases with trigeminal neuropathic pain.

Keywords: Deafferentation pain; intra-operative somatosensory evoked potentials; chronic stimulation..

Introduction

So-called thalamic pain, related to a central lesion, is difficult to control medically [10]. Chronic stimulation of the posterior ventral nucleus of the thalamus, proposed in the 1970s [2], also proved to be disappointing, as it relieved only about one third of patients [9]. In 1991, Tsubokawa *et al.* [10] reported an improvement in the management of this type of pain by chronic stimulation of the motor cortex. The study by Meyerson *et al.* [3] showed that deafferentation pain of the face could also be improved by this technique. In contrast, patients presenting with thalamic pain in this series were not improved. The somatotopic arrangement of the motor cortex suggests that the stimulation sites to treat thalamic pain, generally affecting an entire hemibody, are different from those used to treat pain involving only the face.

The authors used stereotactic MRI in a series of 20 patients in order to define the ideal stimulation site in relation to the central sulcus and the somatotopic arrangement of the motor cortex for treatment of thalamic pain and deafferentation pain of the face.

Patients and Methods

Patients

Twenty patients presenting with refractory deafferentation pain were treated by chronic stimulation of the motor cortex between May 1993 and June 1995 (Table 1).

Ten patients suffered from central pain secondary to a cerebral lesion: deep ischaemic accident (thalamic or capsulothalamic) in 4 cases (cases 5, 6, 7 and 9), ischaemic accident involving the parietal lobe in 1 case (case 8), haematoma of the basal ganglia in 3 cases (cases 2, 3 and 4), deep post-traumatic cerebral lesions in 1 case (case 10) and thalamic abscess in 1 case (case 1).

Seven patients suffered from deafferentation pain of a hemiface. Three cases (cases 15, 16 and 17) suffered from painful anaesthesia of the face secondary to thermocoagulation of the trigeminal ganglion. In 2 cases (cases 11 and 13), this pain corresponded to the sequelae of an operation to the paranasal sinuses. In 1 case (case 12), pain appeared following trauma to the base of the skull. In case 14, the pain was related to a lesion of the trigeminal nerve in the cerebellopontine angle after several operations for recurrent acoustic neuroma.

Two patients experienced pain secondary to a post-traumatic spinal cord lesion: paraplegia in 1 case (case 19) and quadriplegia in the other (case 20). Both patients suffered from diffuse pain situated below the level of the lesion and deep visceral pain.

In patient 18, the pain was secondary to peripheral lesions involving the sciatic nerve, following resection of a neurofibrosarcoma in the context of Von Recklinghausen disease. All patients suffered from constant, severe pain, consisting of superficial burning pain,

Table 1. *Clinical Data and Results of Motor Cortex Stimulation*

Case	Sex	Age	Diagnosis	History (years)	Follow-up (months)	Results* (25 months)
1	F	35	thalamic abscess	7	22	good
2	M	50	basal ganglia haematoma	5	30	satisfactory → failure
3	M	65	basal ganglia haematoma	7	32	satisfactory
4	M	52	basal ganglia haematoma	4	25	good → satisfactory
5	M	68	thalamic infarct	7	18	satisfactory → failure
6	M	47	thalamic infarct	5	22	failure
7	F	58	thalamic infarct	5	28	satisfactory
8	F	47	parietal lobe infarct	6	14	excellent
9	M	70	thalamic infarct	5	30	good
10	M	59	deep post-trauma lesions	6	29	failure
11	F	75	trigeminal neuropathic pain	8	31	excellent
12	M	55	trigeminal neuropathic pain	5	17	good → satisfactory
13	F	60	trigeminal neuropathic pain	7	31	excellent
14	F	43	trigeminal neuropathic pain	8	39	excellent
15	F	59	trigeminal neuropathic pain	6	35	satisfactory
16	M	67	trigeminal neuropathic pain	15	27	satisfactory
17	F	77	trigeminal neuropathic pain	10	18	excellent → good
18	F	21	peripheral lesion	4	14	excellent
19	M	39	paraplegia	5	18	failure
20	M	35	tetraplegia	7	22	excellent

* Excellent, 80–100% reduction; good, 60–80% reduction; satisfactory, 40–60% reduction; failure, <40% reduction of pain on visual analogue scale.

more or less associated with deep feelings of constriction. 13 patients also suffered spontaneous episodes of pain: 4 cases of facial pain, 7 of thalamic pain and 2 of pain secondary to a spinal cord lesion. Eleven patients suffered from pain triggered by contact hyperpathia, allodynia and hyperaesthesia); 3 with facial pain and 8 cases with thalamic pain.

All patients were examined by a neurologist specialized in the management of chronic pain and by a psychiatrist. The pain intensity was scored by a visual analogue scale graduated from 0 to 100. Informed consent was obtained from the patient and family in every case. All patients suffered from chronic deafferentation pain, present for an average of 6.6 years (range: 4 to 15 years) and refractory to medical treatment (analgesics, anticonvulsants and antidepressants). At the preoperative evaluation, all patients had a score of between 70 and 100 on the visual analogue scale (mean score: 90.3). None of the patients had normal everyday activity. Three patients (cases 3, 10 and 11) had previously undergone unsuccessful stimulation of the VPM nucleus of the thalamus. Patient 18 had been treated initially by morphine, with a very incomplete result, followed by DREZOtomy, with partial pain relief which lasted only one month.

Surgical Procedure

In each patient, the central sulcus was located under stereotactic conditions (Leksell frame), based on MRI. The operation was performed under local anaesthesia. The exact site of the stereotactic target was verified by lateral teleradiography. A Resume 4-plot electrode (Medtronic, Minneapolis, USA) was introduced extradurally via a standard burr hole for the first patients and via a small craniotomy for the others. Somaesthetic evoked potentials (SEP) were recorded from the 4 contacts of the electrode after stimulation of the median, trigeminal or posterior tibial nerves, depending on the topography of the painful territory. In accordance with the technique and results reported by Wood [12], the contact situated over the sensory cortex recorded a negative wave, called (N20), 20 millimicrons after the stimulation, while the contact situated over the motor cortex recorded a positive wave, (P20). The position of the central sulcus could therefore be confirmed electrophysiologically when an inversion of this wave was observed between 2 adjacent contacts. The position of the electrode was considered to be definitive when the anatomical data (stereotactic localization) and physiological data (SEP) were concordant. Bipolar stimulation (0.6–3.5 milliamperes, 0.1 millimicrons, 30–40 Hertz) was then applied, using the contact or contacts situated over the motor cortex. Ideally, the patient described an almost immediate reduction of pain. Intraoperative stimulation never induced any paraesthesia.

Installation of the stimulator (ITREL 2, Medtronic) was performed about one week after the operation. Several trial stimulations were performed during this interval, using a connector brought out percutaneously.

Stimulation Parameters

In the majority of cases, patients were stimulated for 3-hour periods (including during the night), separated by intervals without stimulation also lasting 3 hours. Bipolar stimulation was performed with the negative pole situated over the motor cortex, as close as possible to the central sulcus. On average, the chronic stimulation parameters were as follows; frequency: 40.8 Hertz (25–55 Hz), duration: 90 microseconds (60–180 ms), amplitude: 2.4 volts (1.3–4 V). In view of the impedance of the system (mean: 1082.3 Ohms, range: 375 to 1993 Ohms), the mean intensity of stimulation was 2.75 milliamperes (0.8–6.7 mA).

Evaluation of the Results

The pain intensity was evaluated by a visual analogue scale during the test-stimulation period, and then every 3 months. The result was classified into 4 categories: 1) Excellent (80 to 100% pain reduction), 2) Good (60 to 79% improvement), 3) Satisfactory (40 to 59% improvement) and 4) Failure (< 40% improvement).

In order to establish correlations between the clinical result and the site of stimulation, the position of the electrodes was plotted in relation to the central sulcus on diagrams for the various patients. To allow combined analysis of the data, the central sulcus was represented graphically by a straight line drawn between its superior and inferior extremities. The superior point of the central sulcus was quite easy to determine on MRI. The inferior extremity of the central sulcus, situated at a variable distance from the lateral sulcus, is also fairly easy to recognize anatomically, but is not always quite so easy on MRI. It was found much easier and more reproducible to take, as the lower limit of the central sulcus, the midpoint of the superior insular line which constitutes a classical landmark, validated in particular by the anatomical and arteriographic studies conducted by Szikla [7]. Diagrams on which the position of the electrodes was identical in the various patients were obtained by standardizing these data. It was considered that a reliable mapping, including central sulcus landmarks and the position of the various stimulation plots, was obtained in 16 of the 20 patients.

Results

Results on Pain

Fifteen patients (75% of cases) were significantly improved (pain reduction of between 40 and 100%) in the long-term (mean follow-up: 25.1 months, range: 14 to 39 months). The result was considered to be good or excellent in 10 cases (50% of cases).

Twelve patients obtained a clear improvement of their pain during the intra-operative stimulation test. In the majority of these cases, this improvement was spontaneously maintained for an interval varying between 24 and 48 hours (post-effect).

All patients with deafferentation pain of the face were improved. The result was considered to be excellent or good in 4 cases (57% of cases) and satisfactory in 3 cases (43% of cases). All of the patients who obtained a good or excellent result resumed normal everyday activities, and virtually no longer required any analgesic medication. The result deteriorated over time in patients 12 and 17.

Of the 10 patients presenting with central pain, 3 obtained an excellent or good improvement and 2 obtained a satisfactory improvement. Patients 1 and 8 resumed an almost normal everyday life and 3 patients (cases 1, 8 and 9) markedly reduced their analgesic medication. In 3 patients (cases 2, 4 and 5), the initial improvement was better than the long-term improvement. In addition to constant background pain, patient 9 had also presented with major paroxysmal pain which totally disappeared during periods of stimulation. Patient 5 experienced a marked accentuation of pain when he mobilized the proximal part of the upper limb homolateral to the painful syndrome. This pain was markedly improved, allowing a certain degree of resumption of the main everyday activities.

One (case 20) of the 2 patients presenting with pain secondary to spinal cord lesions obtained an excellent result. This patient essentially experienced deep visceral pain which totally resolved. Diffuse pain situated in territories below the lesion was also improved. An excellent result was obtained in the patient with peripheral pain (case 18).

In the patients with facial pain, the improvement affected continuous pain as well as paroxysmal episodes and evoked pain. Continuous pain was improved in only 4 of the 10 patients with thalamic pain. Conversely, paroxysmal episodes were improved in 6 out of 7 cases and evoked pain was improved in 6 out of 8 cases.

A marked post-effect, with improvement of pain persisting for several hours or even several days after stopping the stimulator, was observed by the 1st month in the majority of cases. It was consequently not always easy to adjust the stimulator during the postoperative period, due to the persistent improvement of many patients following intraoperative stimulation. The duration of the post-effect decreased to 2 or 3 hours after the 1st or 2nd month. Due to this persistent effect, the follow-up visits were performed on the basis of a day-only admission, which allowed the performance of one or several modifications of the stimulation parameters, as required.

Adverse Effects

In 3 patients, stimulation at an intensity higher than 3 mA induced dysaesthesia appearing right from the start of stimulation and resolving after stopping the stimulator. Dysaesthesia affected the little finger in patient No. 3, and the hemiface in patients 12 and 15. In patient 6, the high intensity stimulation (6.6 mA) of the dominant hemisphere induced speech disorders which resolved as soon as the intensity was reduced. In 16 patients, in whom the stimulation did not induce any clinical phenomena, the efficacy of stimulation on pain was evaluated under double-blind conditions, in which the patient and one of the examiners did not

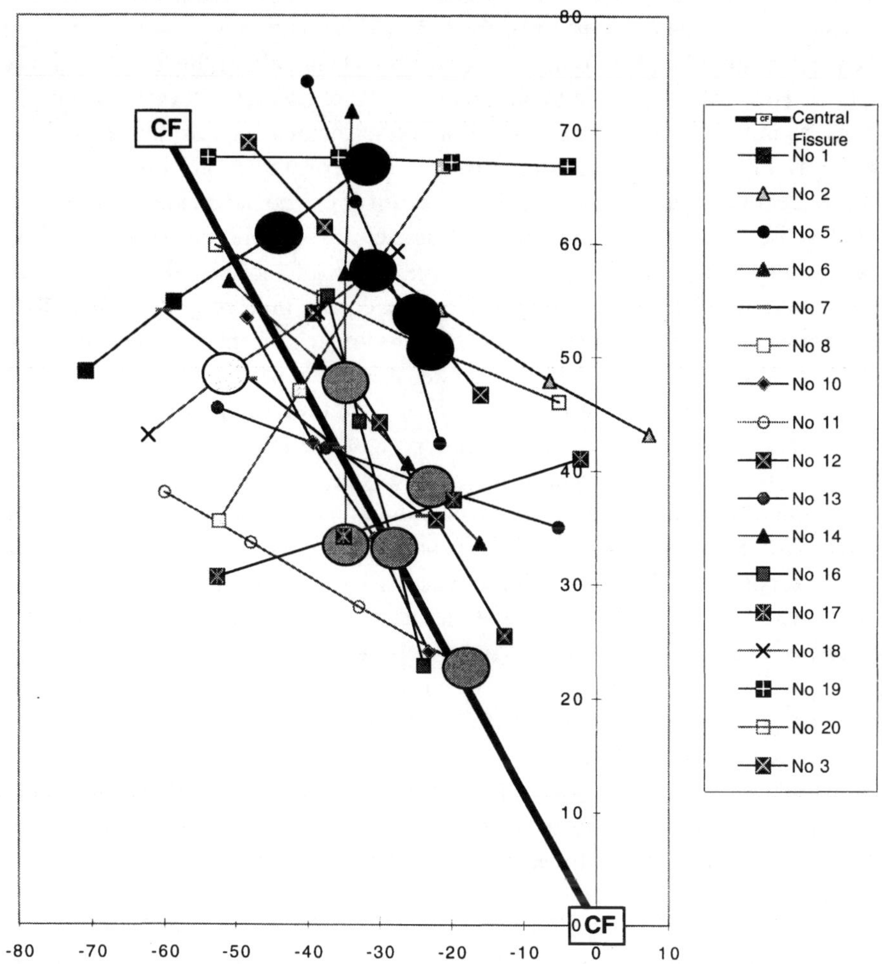

Fig. 1. Schematic lateral representation of central fissure (*CF*) and location of 4 polar stimulating plots in 16 patients. X axis corresponds to the level of the superior insular line (SIL) and Y axis is perpendicular to SIL at the level of it midpoint. The effective stimulation plots are circled. Light grey: trigeminal neuropathic pain. Dark grey: central pain. Black: quadriplegic pain. White: peripheral pain. Most of the effective stimulations plots are situated over the motor cortex and are in agreement with the main somatotopic maps

know whether or not the stimulator was turned on. One patient developed a small extradural haematoma, detected on the postoperative CT scan, with no clinical manifestations, which subsequently resolved spontaneously.

Stimulation did not induce any motor activation phenomena or any episodes of epilepsy in any of the patients.

No technical problems related to the equipment and no infections were observed.

Correlations Between Results and Position of the Electrodes

The use of a 4-plot electrode allowed testing 4 different stimulation sites in each patient. Each stimulation plot was tested in each of our 20 patients (total of 80 plots). Stimulation did not induce any beneficial effects in 3 patients, regardless of the stimulation plot used. In 13 patients, the effective stimulation zone was found to be very isolated, as the patients were only relieved by stimulation of a precise plot, and trial stimulations of the other plots were totally ineffective. In 3 patients (cases 5, 14 and 20), this zone was found to be larger, as a practically equivalent clinical result was obtained in 2 adjacent plots. The position of the electrodes in the 6 patients with deafferentation pain of the face is shown on Fig. 1. These sites were grouped in the middle third of the sensorimotor region.

The positions of the electrodes of the 7 patients with central pain and the 2 patients with pain secondary to a spinal cord lesion are shown on Fig. 1. The stimulation sites which improved central pain (cases 1, 5 and 8) were grouped in the upper third of the precentral region.

Discussion

It is now generally accepted that stimulation of certain structures of the central nervous system can induce analgesia [8]. Several studies have demonstrated that stimulation of the nucleus ventralis posterolateralis of the thalamus can control some forms of so-called deafferentation pain related to peripheral nerve lesions or central lesions [1, 2]. However, this technique was found to be fairly disappointing in the treatment of central pain, which, on average, is only improved in about 30% of cases [9]. Deafferentation pain of the face has also been found to be difficult to control [1]. Tsubokawa [10] recently reported satisfactory improvement of pain related to a central lesion by chronic stimulation of the motor cortex. The results obtained in 11 patients were initially very satisfactory, as 73% of patients were improved during the postoperative period. However, persistent long-term improvement was obtained in only 45% of cases. Meyerson [3] reported a series of 10 patients treated according to Tsubokawa's technique. The 6 patients with deafferentation pain of the face were considerably improved in the long-term, while patients with pain related to a central lesion or peripheral neuropathic pain were not improved.

The technique described by Tsubokawa [8, 10, 11] is mainly based on identification of the central sulcus by analysis of intra-operative somaesthetic evoked potentials. The position of this sulcus is indicated by inversion of the potential recorded 20 ms after stimulation of the median nerve (potential N20–P20) [12]. In order to confirm that the electrode is actually situated in the motor cortex, Meyerson [3] tried to induce muscular contractions in the contralateral arm or hand by high intensity and low frequency cortical stimulation. Tsubokawa [8, 10, 11] obtained motor responses in the lower limb by stimulating the superior part of the gyrus.

Somatotopy of the Motor Cortex

According to Penfield's studies on the somatotopy of the motor cortex [4], the electrode should be positioned in the inferior zone of the mediolateral part of the motor cortex in order to treat pain localized to the face. The data in the literature concerning the representation of the upper limb are also fairly concordant [12]. This zone is situated in the superior part of the gyrus, just above that corresponding to the representation of the face. The data in the literature concerning the lower limb are more discordant [6, 13]. Classically, in man, the zone of representation of the lower limb is situated in the medial surface of the hemisphere [4]. It has been shown, in man, that this zone could extend largely onto the lateral face of the hemisphere [6, 13]. This could explain why Tsubokawa obtained improvements in pain of the lower limb by a stimulation of the lateral surface of the precentral cortex. The authors results would support this hypothesis, but appear to be in contradiction with the results reported by Peyron [5], who recommended that the electrode be inserted in the subdural space, in direct contact with the cortex of the medial surface of the hemisphere to treat pain involving the lower limb. The authors results are in agreement with the classical data concerning the representation of the upper limb and the face. Facial pain was improved by stimulation in the inferior part of the lateral surface of the precentral region and pain of the upper and lower limbs was improved by stimulation in the superior part of the precentral region. The good concordance between the effect of stimulation and somatotopic data appears to indicate that no major modification of the somatotopic arrangement was observed in these patients. However, such modifications appeared obvious in one of the patients presenting in this study with quadriplegia, in whom improvement of bilateral pain of the lower limbs by unilateral stimulation appeared to be a surprising result. This result needs to be confirmed in a larger series of cases.

The efficacy of stimulation on pain related to a peripheral nervous lesion has not been clearly established. One of the 2 cases in Meyerson's series [3] was not improved. The authors obtained an excellent result in one patient with pain of the lower limb related to a neoplastic lesion of the trunk of the sciatic nerve. In this patient, morphine was virtually ineffective and DREZotomy had only very transiently improved the pain.

Localization of the Motor Cortex

Anatomical localization of the central sulcus is more easily performed using MRI than CT scan. It was found that it was very important to confirm, by intra-operative x-rays, that the electrode was correctly situated in the previously selected position and that it had not changed position during the procedure. The use of intra-operative SEP proved to be particularly useful to confirm the position of the central sulcus [12]. The localizing value of the motor effects of cortical stimulation appeared to be less reliable, as many studies have shown that these effects can be obtained by stimulation applied anteriorly as well as posteriorly to the central sulcus [4, 13]. Furthermore, large zones of the pre- and post-central region are able to give identical motor responses after stimulation, especially in terms of their site [13]. Functional magnetic resonance imaging will probably be very useful as it appears capable of generating somatotopic maps of the primary motor cortex in individual subjects [6].

The clinical effects of stimulation on pain can also facilitate positioning of the electrode, as, in several cases in this series, intra-operative cortical stimulation induced an almost immediate improvement of pain, thereby validating the correct positioning of the electrode. Although very inconstant, this effect justifies performing the procedure under local anaesthesia and selection of patients able to reply coherently during the operation.

Complications

The risks of the technique are still incompletely known. Complications directly related to the operative procedure appear to be very rare. Detachment of the dura mater can predispose to the formation of an extradural haematoma, as in one patient. The use of a small craniotomy, rather than a simple burr hole would help to avoid this complication. The risk of inducing real epilepsy has to be considered. This complication has not been reported in any of the patients published in the literature [3, 5, 8, 10, 11]. However, great caution is required in relation to this potential complication and experimental studies are needed, as the long-term effects of chronic stimulation on the structure of the cortex are not known.

Mechanism of Action

The mechanism of action of chronic stimulation of the motor cortex is unknown. Tsubokawa proposed several hypotheses which have not yet been confirmed, in particular a long-term neuroplastic effect [8, 11]. Two aspects need to be discussed:

(i) The effect of stimulation on the cortex itself, which could vary as a function of the cortical layers submitted to stimulation. A relatively high stimulation frequency could also induce a tonic depolarization and cortical inactivation effect, which is known to inhibit thalamic relays [8]. Conversely, stimulation could excite certain pyramidal neurons. Experimental studies are required to analyse in more detail the physiological effects of this type of stimulation at the cellular level.

(ii) It may appear paradoxical that the stimulation plots placed over the motor cortex rather than over the parietal cortex exerted the more effective analgesic effect. This could be explained by an effect on the cortex itself (especially frontal cortex, intracortical connections, parietal cortex) and/or on subcortical structures (lateral and median thalamic relays or reticular nucleus) [5] or even a role of inhibitory pyramidal connections on spinal somaesthetic relays [8].

Conclusion

This pilot study is in line with the main series of the literature and confirms the potential value of chronic stimulation of the motor cortex in the treatment of certain forms of neurological pain refractory to other treatments. The anatomical localization of the central sulcus by MRI and optimization of the positioning of the stimulation plots appear to be essential both to improve the results of treatment and to allow a better understanding of the mechanism of the analgesic effects.

References

1. Hosobuchi Y, Adams JE, Rutkin B (1973) Chronic thalamic stimulation for the control of facial anesthesia dolorosa. Arch Neurol 29: 158–161
2. Mazars GJ (1975) Intermittent stimulation of nucleus ventralis posterolateralis for intractable pain. Surg Neurol 4: 93–95
3. Meyerson BA, Lindblom U, Linderoth B, Lind G, Herregodts P (1993) Motor cortex stimulation as treatment of trigeminal neuropathic pain. Acta Neurochir (Wien) 58: 150–153
4. Penfield W, Boldrey E (1938) Somatic motor and sensory representation in the cerebral cortex of man as studied by electrical stimulation. Brain 15: 389–443
5. Peyron R, Garcia-Larrea L, Deiber MP, Cinotti L, Convers P, Sindou M, Mauguiere F, Laurent B (1995) Electrical stimulation of precentral cortical area in the treatment of central pain: electrophysiological and PET study. Pain 62: 275–286
6. Rao SM, Binder JR, Hammeke TA, Bandettini PA, Bobholz JA, Frost JA, Myklebust BM, Jacobson RD, Hyde JS (1995) Somatotopic mapping of the human primary motor cortex with functional magnetic resonance imaging. Neurology 45: 919–924
7. Szikla G, Bouvier G, Hori T, Petrov V (1977) Angiography of the human brain cortex. Springer, Berlin Heidelberg New York
8. Tsubokawa T (1995) Motor cortex stimulation for deafferentation pain relief in various clinical syndromes and its possible mechanism. In: Besson JM, Guilbaud G, Ollat H (eds) Forebrain areas involved in pain processing. Libbey, Eurotext, Paris, pp 261–276
9. Tsubokawa T, Katayama Y, Yamamoto T, Hirayama T (1985) Deafferentation pain and stimulation of thalamic sensory relay nucleus: clinical and experimental study. Appl Neurophysiol 48: 166–171
10. Tsubokawa T, Katayama Y, Yamamoto T, Hirayama T, Koyama S (1991) Chronic motor cortex stimulation for the

treatment of central pain. Acta Neurochir (Wien) 52: 137–139
11. Tsubokawa T, Katayama Y, Yamamoto T, Hirayama T, Koyama S (1993) Chronic motor cortex stimulation in patients with thalamic pain. J Neurosurg 78: 393–401
12. Wood CC, Spencer DD, Allison T, Mc Carthy G, Williamson PD, Goff WR (1988) Localization of human sensorimotor cortex during surgery by cortical surface recording of somatosensory evoked potentials. J Neurosurg 68: 99–111
13. Woolsey CN, Erickson TC, Gilson WE (1979) Localization in somatic sensory and motor areas of human cerebral cortex as determined by direct recording of evoked potentials and electrical stimulation. J Neurosurg 51: 476–506

Correspondence: Dr Jean Paul Nguyen, Service de Neurochirurgie, CHU Henri Mondor, 51 av. du Mal de Lattre de Tassigny, 94010 Créteil cedex, France.

Acta Neurochir (1997) [Suppl] 68: 61–63

Obsessive Compulsive Disorder and the Right Hemisphere: Topographic Analysis of Lesions After Anterior Capsulotomy Performed with Thermocoagulation

B. Lippitz[1], **P. Mindus**[2], **B. A. Meyerson**[1], **L. Kihlström**[1], and **Ch. Lindquist**[1]

Departments of [1]Neurosurgery and [2]Psychiatry, Karolinska Hospital and Institute, Stockholm, Sweden

Summary

Considerable but uncontrolled evidence suggests that stereotactic capsulotomy by means of thermolesions may provide symptomatic relief for patients with otherwise therapy refractory "malignant" obsessive compulsive disorder (OCD). Unlike in other functional stereotactic interventions, target localization for capsulotomy is based upon anatomical definition only. Few systematic attempts have been made to correlate the site and size of the capsular lesions with postoperative clinical outcome. Between 1976 and 1989 bilateral thermo-capsulotomy (TC) was performed in 22 OCD patients. In 19 patients complete quantitative pre- and postoperative psychiatric rating of OCD symptoms and long-term postoperative MRI studies were available. Cohorts of patients fulfilling criteria for good or poor outcome were contrasted, cases with intermediate treatment effect being excluded. Median postoperative MRI follow-up was 8.4 years (2.4–20.3 y). 9/19 patients fulfilled criteria for good postoperative outcome. In these patients all lesion sites overlapped covering a small area within the right anterior limb of the internal capsule. Lesions within the group of patients with poor outcome (n = 5) were located elsewhere, mostly further anterior in the internal capsule. Differences of lesion overlap between the two outcome groups were significant for the right side (Fisher's Exact Test: $p < 0.005$). Common topographic features of lesion sites within the *right* internal capsule were identified in OCD patients responding favourably to capsulotomy.

Keywords: OCD; anterior capsulotomy; thermolesion; postoperative control.

Introduction

Obsessive-compulsive disorder (OCD) is one of the most prevalent and chronic forms of mental disorders in the general population. Presently favoured neurobiological hypotheses of OCD assume that the disease is caused by or associated with an imbalance in the cortico-striatal-thalamo-cortical circuit [12]. A great number of patients relapse after pharmacological treatment or do not respond at all. About 20% experience a progressively disabling course and are refractory to psycho- and pharmacotherapy. Some of these patients are candidates for surgical anti-obsessive therapy.

A limited number of patients with a chronic deteriorating clinical course, intractable by all current non-surgical therapeutic options, have been operated with bilateral anterior thermo-capsulotomy. Only few systematic attempts have been made to correlate the anatomical location of these lesions to the individual postoperative clinical outcome [10].

The current retrospective study was designed to define the lesion sites in OCD patients treated with bilateral stereotactic thermo-capsulotomy. A geometric system for interindividual comparison of lesion parameters was developed based upon postoperative long-term MRI investigations. The preliminary results are reported.

Patients and Methods

Between 1976 and 1989 22 patients with otherwise therapy refractory OCD were treated with bilateral Thermo-Capsulotomy (TC) at the Karolinska Hospital Stockholm. The patients fulfilled the diagnostic criteria of the current DSM for OCD, their duration of illness exceeded 5 years causing severe subjective suffering and considerable reduction in psychosocial functioning. All non-operative treatment options had been tried systematically without appreciable effect [11]. The clinical morbidity was monitored prospectively using standardized psychiatric rating scales (CPRS-OC) as described earlier in detail [8–11]. Nineteen patients with complete pre- and postoperative psychiatric ratings and long-term postoperative MRI studies (male/female: 8/11) fulfilled all criteria for further evaluation. Their median age was 39 years (range 26.8–53.3 y; mean 40.3 y). All patients were right-handed.

Patients were assigned to two outcome categories based upon percent change over time in their CPRS-OC rating: Nine patients experienced more than 50% postoperative symptom relief and were classified as having a good clinical outcome and 5 patients showed no clinical change. Data pertaining to the two groups of patients fulfilling criteria for good or poor outcome were contrasted, cases with intermediate treatment effect being excluded for the current quantitative evaluation.

Operative Technique

The details of the stereotactical operative technique [5, 11] have been described before. In brief, the bilateral capsulotomy lesions were placed between the anterior and the middle thirds of the anterior limb of the internal capsule as defined on CT or MRI tomograms at the approximate level of the foramen of Monro [11]. The radiofrequency lesions were intended to be about 20 mm in height and 8 mm in width [5]. The basal portion of the capsule was to be included in the lesion. The coagulation electrode was aligned to the internal capsule's 25–30 degree angulation from the vertical plane [11].

Quantitative Anatomical MRI Evaluation

Median postoperative MRI follow-up was 8.4 years (range 2.4–20.3 y; mean: 8.5 y). All MRI studies were performed on a 1.5 Tesla Signa Advantage Unit (General Electric). In order to achieve optimal anatomical orientation, T2 proton weighted (pulse gated fast spin) echo sequences (TR 4000 ms and TE 35 + 80 ms) in the axial plane were selected. Slice thickness was 5 mm and interslice gap 2 mm. Field of view was 25 cm and matrix size 256 × 256 covering the whole brain. A well demarcated hyperintense signal change within the anterior limb of the internal capsule on proton weighted sequences was defined as a lesion. Images were reformatted on the MRI console with an equal angulation parallel to the AC-PC line as individually defined in all cases. The resulting reformatted slice thickness was 0.86 mm.

For quantitative interindividual comparison of lesion localization the following anatomical landmarks were selected: for definition of the stereotactic z-plane the anterior commissure, the foramen of Monro and the internal cerebral vein. The lesion extent within the internal capsule in the x- and y- planes was measured on a superimposed ruler in relation to the adjoining putamen: the part of the anterior limb of the internal capsule at the lateral edge of the putamen was assigned to constitute the 0 coordinate, the capsular part adjacent to the medial putaminal edge was defined as the 100 coordinate. A lesion's start- and endpoint on this virtual ruler was measured in every reformatted MR slice and expressed in discrete numbers allowing interindividual comparison. Right and left sided lesions were analyzed separately.

Results

Quantitative Analysis

Nine out of 19 patients fulfilled the criteria for good clinical postoperative outcome. All lesions in these patients overlapped covering a volume in the middle of the right anterior limb of the internal capsule at the level of the foramen of Monro (coordinates 38–64) and (4 mm above) on the plane with the internal cerebral vein (coordinates 48–50). By contrast, lesions within the group of patients with poor outcome were located elsewhere, mostly further anterior in the internal capsule. Differences of lesion overlap between the two outcome groups were significant for the right side (Fisher's Exact Test: $p < 0.005$). Left sided lesions showed no corresponding differences with regard to outcome.

The detailed neuropsychiatric results will be reported elsewhere.

Discussion

The present results demonstrate a correlation between outcome and capsulotomy lesion site, and provides some evidence for the right-sided lesion in the successfully treated patients. Nine out of these 19 otherwise therapy refractory patients manifested clinical improvement following the stereotactic intervention. The lesioned volume, common to all those patients with a favourable outcome, is located within the right-sided anterior limb of the internal capsule. By contrast, no such overlap could be demonstrated on the left side.

So far only a few systematic attempts have been made to correlate the anatomical location of the functional lesions to postoperative clinical outcome or side-effects [6, 10]. In an early MRI study without quantitative anatomical assessment Mindus *et al.* reported that MRI had failed to visualize distinct, bilateral lesions in two patients with unsarisfactory outcome after capsulotomy with the Gamma Knife, whereas all successfully treated patients had shown adequate lesions [10].

In the present study patients were subjected to a standardized operative technique, MRI protocol and quantitative psychiatric assessment, in order to reduce difficulties in the interindividual comparison. The problem of quantitative anatomical comparison was addressed by using standardized digitally reformatted MRI images in combination of anatomical landmarks and numerical measurements. Since lesion coordinates were expressed relative to common anatomical landmarks, MRI distortion was considered negligible for the current investigation. Remaining potential sources for inaccuracies are subjective judgments with regard to the lesion extent and the lack of sub-millimeter measurements on the MRI console.

The present data can contribute to a further optimization of the anatomical target identification for capsulotomy lesions. The study provides evidence for the relevance of right sided lesions in the successful stereotactic treatment of OCD. Likewise metabolic PET studies indicate the importance of right hemispheric structures in the aetiology and treatment of OCD: The basal ganglia and the orbitofrontal cortex are accepted as playing a crucial role [1–3]. PET studies of patients with obsessive-compulsive disorder exposed to individual symptom provoking stimuli demonstrated right caudate activation [7, 13] and right [7] and bilateral [13] orbitofrontal activation in the symptomatic state. Mc Guire *et al.* reported positive correlations between symptom intensity and rCBF in the lower portion of the right inferior frontal gyrus and caudate nucleus [7]. Several studies describe therapy dependent regional metabolic effects in OCD patients and demonstrate orbitofrontal hyperactivation on the right side before treatment [4, 14, 15]. Capsulotomy is supposed to interrupt thalamo-cortical projections within the anterior limb of the internal capsule [12] and may be assumed to interfere with the inappropriate activation of the orbitofrontal cortex associated with OCD.

The current results reflect the potential importance of a minimal lesioned volume defined by the mid-part of the right anterior limb of the internal capsule at the level of the foramen of Monro and the internal cerebral vein. The evaluation of more recently treated patients and of patients subjected to radiosurgical capsulotomy with the Gamma Knife will further help to optimize the target identification. A prospective study is planned with a unilateral right-sided capsulotomy target as defined by the current anatomical investigation in order to reproduce the topographical parameters.

References

1. Alexander GE, Crutcher MD, DeLong M (1990) Basal Ganglia-thalamocortical circuits: parallel substrates for motor, oculomotor, "prefrontal", and "limbic" functions. In: Uylings HBM, Van Eden CG, DeBruin JPC, Corner MA, Feenstra MGP (eds) Progress in brain research, vol 85. Elsevier, Amsterdam pp 119–146
2. Baxter L, Schwartz J, Mazziotta JC, Phelps ME, Pahl JJ, Guze BH, Fairbanks L (1988) Cerebral glucose metabolic rates in non-depressed patients with obsessive-compulsive disorder. Am J Psychiatry 145: 1560–1563
3. Baxter L, Schwartz JM, Bergmann KS Szuba MP, Guze BH, Mazziotta JC, Alazraki A, Selin CE, Ferng H-K, Munford P, Phelps ME (1992) Caudate glucose metabolic rate changes with both drug and behaviour therapy for obsessive-compulsive disorder. Arch Gen Psychiatry 49: 681–689
4. Benkelfat C, Nordhal TE, Scmple W (1990) Local cerebral glucose metabolic rates in obsessive-compulsive disorder. Arch Gen Psychiatry 47: 840–848
5. Bingley T, Leksell L, Meyerson BA, Rylander G (1972) Stereotactic capsulotomy in anxiety and obsessive-compulsive states. In: Laitinen LV, Livingston KE (eds) Surgical approaches in psychiatry. MTP, pp 159–164
6. Hay P, Sachdev P, Cumming S, Smith JS, Lee T, Kitchener P, Metheson J (1993) Treatment of obsessive-compulsive disorder by psychosurgery. Acta Psychiatr Scand 87: 197–207
7. McGuire PK, Bench CJ, Frith CD, Marks IM, Frackowiak RS, Dolan RJ (1994) Functional anatomy of obsessive-compulsive phenomena. Br J Psychiatry 164(4): 459–68
8. Meyerson BA (1996) Neurosurgical treatment of mental disorders. Introduction and indications. In: Gildenberg P, Tasker R (eds) Textbook of stereotactic and functional neurosurgery. In press
9. Mindus P, Rasmussen SA, Lindquist C (1994) Neurosurgical treatment for refractory obsessive-compulsive disorder: Implications for understanding frontal lobe function. J Neuropsych Clin Neurosci 6: 467–477
10. Mindus P, Bergström K, Levander SE, Noren G, Hindmarsh T, Thuomas KA (1987) Magnetic resonance images related to clinical outcome after psychosurgical intervention in severe anxiety disorder. J Neurol Neurosurg Psychiatry 50: 1288–1293
11. Mindus P, Meyerson BA (1995) Anterior capsulotomy for intractable anxiety disorders. In: Schmidek HH, Sweet WH (eds) Operative neurosurgical techniques. Indications, methods, and results, 3rd ed. Saunders, Philadelphia, pp 1443–1454
12. Modell JG, Mountz JM, Curtis GC, Greden JF (1989) Neurophysiologic dysfunction in basal ganglia/limbic striatal and thalamocortical circuits as a pathogenetic mechanism of obsessive-compulsive disorder. J Neuropsych 1(1): 27–36
13. Rauch SL, Jenike MA, Alpert NM, Baer L, Breiter HCR, Savage CR, Fishman AJ (1994) Regional cerebral blood flow measured during symptom provocation in obsessive-compulsive disorder using oxygen 15-labeled carbon dioxide and positron emission tomography. Arch Gen Psychiatry 51: 62–70
14. Simpson S, Baldwin B (1995) Neuropsychiatry and SPECT in an acute obsessive compulsive syndrome patient. Br J Psych 166(3): 390–392
15. Swedo SE, Pietrini P, Leonard HL, Schapiro MB, Rettew DC, Goldberger EL, Rappoport SI, Rappoport JL, Grady CL (1992) Cerebral glucose metabolism in childhood-onset obsessive compulsive disorder. Revisualization during pharmacotherapy. Arch Gen Psychiatry 49: 690–694

Correspondence: Bodo Lippitz, M.D, Department of Neurosurgery, Karolinska Hospital, Box 130, S-17176 Stockholm, Sweden.

Acta Neurochir (1997) [Suppl] 68: 64–69

Lesionectomy in Epileptogenic Temporal Lobe Lesions: Preoperative Seizure Course and Postoperative Outcome

M. Casazza, G. Avanzini, E. Ciceri, R. Spreafico, and **G. Broggi**

Istituto Nazionale Neurologico "C. Besta", Milano, Italy

Summary

A series of 54 patients operated on for temporal epileptogenic lesions is reported: 36 had slow growing tumours, 18 supratentorial cavernous angiomas. The patients were divided into two different groups according to the presence of seizures controlled (group 1) or not controlled (group 2) by antiepileptic drugs (AEDs).

All the patients underwent preoperative scalp EEG and magnetic resonance imaging (MRI). They were operated on by pure lesionectomy, associated with amygdalo-hippocampectomy in 8 cases of uncontrolled seizures. Postoperatively they underwent MRI examination which revealed an incomplete lesionectomy in 12 cases.

Patients were followed up after surgery for at least 2 years, 6 of them were reoperated on for the persistence (or regrowth) of the tumour. The results of epilepsy outcome are reported. These cases underline the importance of preoperative electroclinical study, in order to determine the relationship between lesion location and epileptic focus. If good concordance is present, a complete lesionectomy is enough to cure the patient. In other cases associated amygdalo-hippocampectomy leads to better results, while more complicated cases may need preoperative stereo-EEG studies.

Keywords: Epilepsy; temporal lobe lesion; lesionectomy; amygdalo-hippocampectomy.

Introduction

MRI leads to the preoperative identification of anatomic lesions in a very high percentage of patients with epilepsy, particularly with temporal lobe epilepsy (TLE). The identification of the morphologic change, responsible for seizures can help in localizing the epileptogenic zone, but the presence of a structural lesion in a patient with seizures does not allow a statement of cause and effect. These considerations are increased in the temporal lobe by the presence of such structures as the hippocampus which are often implicated in seizure generation [10]. It has also been suggested that a secondary mesiotemporal focus may develop independently from a distant lesion, which may also induce morphological changes in the hippocampus [12].

The most frequent histological types of epileptogenic temporal lesions are slow growing gliomas such as astrocytomas, gangliogliomas and dysembryoplastic tumours [19], but malignant degeneration in some of them has been reported [3]. Only biopsy or excision can lead to histological diagnosis so that traditional surgery is considered convenient by many authors for oncological reasons in all of these cases [14].

Arterio-venous malformations and cavernous angiomas are often observed in cases of epilepsy [8, 18]. In these patients the risk of spontaneous bleeding is not completely assessed [7, 18] but it is well documented by MRI [20] and has been related to epilepsy onset, persistence or deterioration [16]. All these considerations underline the importance of establishing a correct surgical and medical approach to radiologically evident lesions in patients with epilepsy, in order to give a prognostic indication for the various options in presurgical investigations and in surgical techniques [2, 5, 13]. The authors have reviewed critically their patients, who underwent lesionectomy in recent years, to determine a positive integrated approach to epileptic patients with temporal lesions.

Methods and Material

The patients of this study were selected from 1988 to 1994 from the surgical series of the authors' institute. They were operated on for temporal lobe lesions presenting with one or more epileptic seizures. Clinical data on preoperative epileptic seizures, with particular regard for symptomatology, were collected. The patients underwent preoperative scalp EEG: in 5 patients sphenoidal electrodes were successfully used to record seizures and in 3 of them foramen Hovale electrodes have also been employed. All patients were studied with pre- and postoperative MRI (Philips Gyroscan 0.5 Tesla, Philips Gyroscan ACS 1.5 Tesla). Standard examination included T1 weighted images (w.i.) sagittal and coronal sections, proton density and T2 w.i. (Spin Echo: TE 50, TR 2000; TE 100, TR 2000) axial and coronal sections. Contrast medium (gadolinium) was used only in selected cases.

Patients were divided into two groups: group 1 included those with sporadic or controlled seizures and group 2 was formed by patients with refractory seizures.

Forty-six patients underwent pure lesionectomy. In 5 cases they were reoperated on for the persistence of seizures associated with incomplete lesionectomy, and surgery was extended to amygdalo-hippocampectomy in 3 cases. One patient had further surgery for tumour regrowth.

In 8 patients lesionectomy was combined with the removal of amygdala and hippocampus. Follow-up lasted more than 2 years in all cases. Postoperative MRI and seizure outcome, using Engel classification [9], are considered.

Results

Mean age at seizure onset appears higher in patients with cavernomas (Table 1) than with tumours, while mean illness durations is much shorter only in cavernomas of group 1. The 14 patients of group 1 had only isolated preoperative seizures controlled by AEDs. Eight of them had a cavernous angioma, temporolateral in 7 cases and mesial in 1 case. Six had a slow growing tumour (4 low grade astrocytomas, 1 ganglioglioma, 1 teratoma), located temporo-laterally in 3 cases, mesially in 1 case, mesially and laterally in 1 case.

In these patients surgical approach was lesionectomy, complete in all cavernomas and in 6 tumours, incomplete in 2 tumours.

The mean follow-up is 5 ± 1.2 years. One patient with psychiatric disorders dropped out. Six patients with cavernomas are postoperatively in Engel class IA and one in class IC. Only one patient with a mesial cavernous angioma had a postoperative worsening of her seizures (class IV C), probably due to surgical complications: she had in fact a temporo-basal malacia.

Two patients with tumour are in class IA, but one of them relapsed 5 years postoperatively coincidentally with tumour regrowth. She has recently been reoperated on and no postoperative data are yet available.

One patient with incomplete lesionectomy of a mesial tumour is in class IC while another with a residual lateral tumour, which recurred postoperatively and required reoperation (performed elsewhere) and radiotherapy, is in class III B. Another patient from this group is in class IV C: she had a lateral teratoma pressing on mesial structures. After a complete lesionectomy she was seizure free for only one year. Seizures then recurred and are difficult to control.

Table 1

		Mean age at onset	Mean illness duration	Mean age at surgery
Cavernomas	group 1	30.1 ± 14.7	2.1 ± 2.6	32.1 ± 14.8
	group 2	28.9 ± 10.3	10.9 ± 8.7	39.6 ± 10.9
Tumours	group 1	21.9 ± 14.1	9.2 ± 8.2	31 ± 10.2
	group 2	18.4 ± 9.4	9.6 ± 6.1	28 ± 8.2

Table 2. *Preoperative Seizure Course (Group 2)*

	Cavernous angiomas	Tumours
Seizure frequency		
1–12/year	0/10	1/30
>1/month	7/10	8/30
>1/week	1/10	14/30
>1/day	2/10	7/30
Seizure semeiology		
Aura	8/10	27/30
Impairment of consciousness		
– preceded by aura	6/10	22/30
– not preceded by aura	2/10	3/30
Somatomotor phenomena	3/10	7/30
Secondary generalization	3/10	13/30

In group 2, 10 patients had cavernomas (7 lateral, 2 lateral and mesial, 1 mesial) and 30 had slow growing tumours (15 mesial, 12 lateral, 3 mesial and lateral): 11 were gangliogliomas, 7 low grade astrocytomas, 5 oligodendrogliomas, 2 calcific telangiectatic hamartomas, 2 ependymomas, 1 each oligoastrocytoma, neurinoma, epidermoid and dysembryo-neuroepithelioma. These patients had refractory seizures.

Preoperative seizure frequency and semeiology are reported in Table 2: while frequency is higher in tumours than in cavernomas, there are no differences in the semeiology of seizures, particulary with regard to the impairment of consciousness and effects of extratemporal diffusion (somato-motor phenomena and secondary generalization). Interictal EEG was normal in 3 patients, showed non-specific theta activity in 2 and slow (theta-delta) and epileptiform focal activity spatially concordant with the site of the lesion in 34 patients. In 4 of these this activity diffused contralaterally and in 3 it was associated with epileptiform contralateral asynchronous abnormalities. In one case, only contralateral sharp-waves were observed.

Table 3. *Postoperative Outcome (Group 2)*

Mean follow-up	4.6 ± 1.8 years		
	Class	No.	
Cavernous angiomas	I A	5	
	I D	2	(relapse only at drug withdrawal)
	II C	2	(1 with multiple angiomas, 1 with temporomesial angioma)
	IV B	1	(contralateral hippocampal atrophy)
Tumours	I A	14	(4 incomplete lesionectomies)
	I D	2	
	II B	2	
	II C	2	
	III A	2	
	IV A	1	
	IV B	6	
	IV C	1	

In sixteen patients seizures were recorded, in 12 cases from the scalp, in 5 also with sphenoidal electrodes and in 3 with foramen ovale electrodes. Four patients had multiple scalp recordings with sphenoidal and/or foramen ovale electrodes. In 15 patients seizures fitted with lesion site. In the only one case in which they did not the outcome was IV B. Patients with cavernomas were operated on by lesionectomy, which resulted in complete removal in all cases. In patients with tumours, lesionectomy was shown as complete on the postoperative MR control in 12 cases and incomplete in 10. Five of these patients therefore received further surgery and in 3 of them the lesionectomy was enlarged to amygdalo-hippocampectomy.

In 8 patients electroclinical data led to a different surgical approach, i.e. lesionectomy plus amygdalo-hippocampectomy.

Mean follow-up has lasted 4.6 ± 1.8 years. Postoperative seizure outcome is rather different in cavernomas and tumours (Table 3). Most patients with cavernous angioma are in class I (70%), 2 of them in class ID: they relapsed only on withdrawal of AEDs, seizures were promptly controlled by the resumption of their medication. The only patient in class IV B of this group had interictal epileptiform activity contralateral to the cavernoma and a mild hippocampal atrophy on that side. Seizures were not recorded and had no lateralizing signs.

Only 50% of the patients with tumours are in class I. Four of them had an incomplete lesionectomy, due to the extension of the lesion, but an amygdalo-hippocampectomy for electroclinical reasons (Figs. 1 and 2). Three patients, in whom the hippocampus was not involved in the lesion and seizures did not have mesiotemporal semeiology, were cured by the complete lesionectomy.

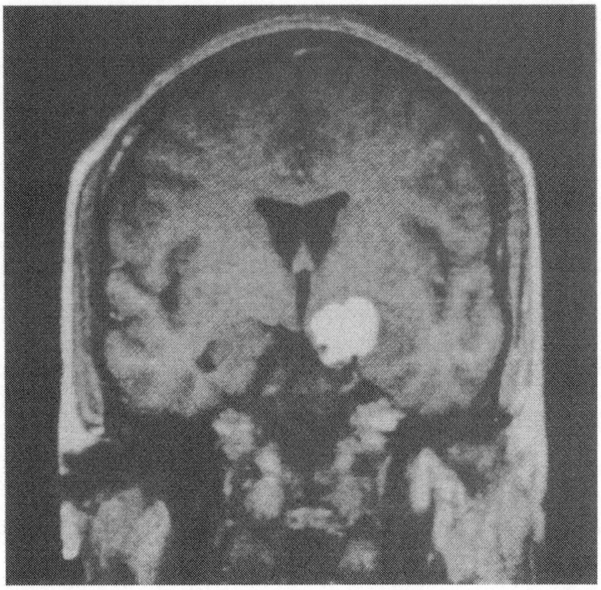

Fig. 1. MR coronal images with gadolinium (SE 600/20). Thirty-three-year old patient with refractory mesio-temporal seizures. The intensely enhancing lesion (ganglioglioma) involves the posterior part of the left amygdala and the anterior part of the hippocampus

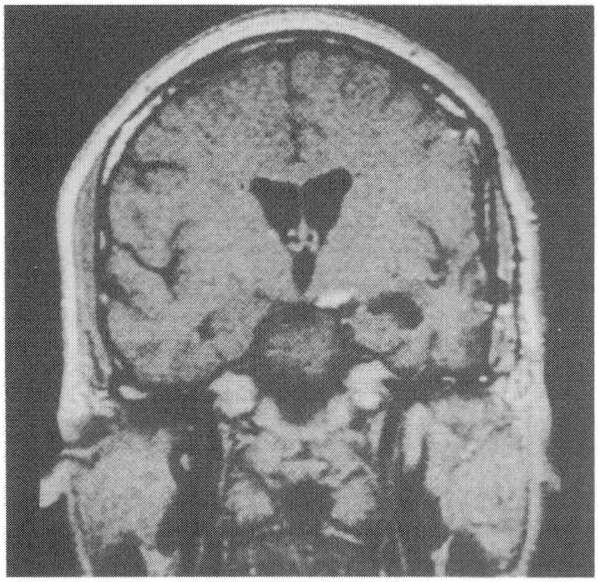

Fig. 2. MR coronal images with gadolinium (SE 600/20). In the postoperative follow-up the complete removal of the intra-axial lesion with partial amygdalo-hippocampectomy is well demonstrated. The patient is seizure free

Among those with peristence or worsening of sei-

Table 4. *Semeiology of Seizures and Outcome*

Outcome	Temporal aura	Extratemporal aura	Loss of contact preceded by aura	Loss of contact not preceded by aura	Somatomotor phenomena	Total
I A	16	1	12	2	3	19
I D	4	0	2	0	2	4
II B	2	0	2	0	0	2
II C	4	0	4	0	2	4
II A	2	0	2	0	0	2
IV A	0	0	0	1	0	1
IV B	4	1	4	2	3	7
IV C	0	1	1	0	1	1

Table 5. *Outcome of Patients with Recorded Seizures*

I A	7/16
I D	1/16
II B	2/16
II C	3/16
III A	1/16
IV B	2/16

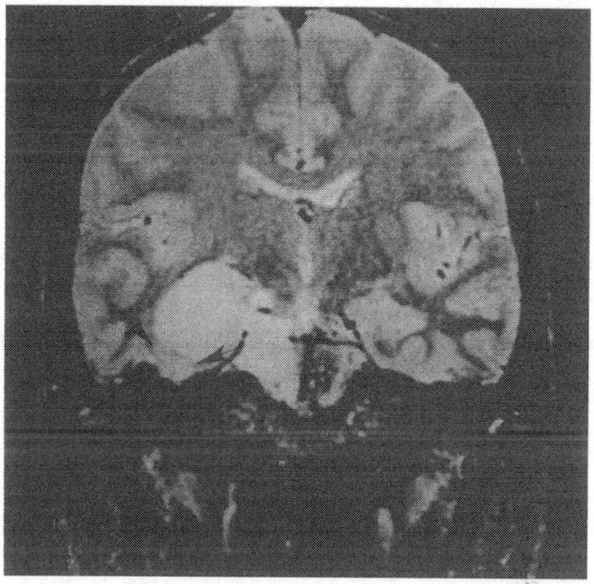

Fig. 3. MR coronal images (SE 2000/100). Twenty-one-year old patient with refractory seizures of possible mesio-temporal origin. A large, extra-axial hyperintense lesion is well demonstrated in the right ponto-cerebellar angle extending into the ambiens cistern. The middle temporal lobe structures are markedly compressed (arrows)

zures, extratemporal aura, loss of contact not preceded by localizing aura and somatomotor phenomena are more frequent than in patients of class I (Table 4). The recording of ictal EEG by itself is not enough to improve the outcome (Table 5). Only in one patient did recorded seizures not fit with tumour location. This patient is in class IV B, and had an operation for a temporo-lateral oligodendroglioma. Two other cases with lateral tumours and complete lesionectomy are in class IV B. In both cases there is no localizing effect from seizure semeiology.

In 5 patients seizures were compatible with the location of the lesion, but lesionectomy as demonstrated by postoperative MR imaging was incomplete. Two cases may have double pathology: in one the temporal lobe homolateral to the partially excised mesio-temporal astrocytoma has a complex malformative aspect, in another a temporo-lateral epidermoid probably induced a structural rearrangement of mesio-temporal structures. Even after complete removal of the tumour seizures were unchanged (Figs. 3 and 4).

Discussion

In slow growing hemispheric tumours epilepsy is present in 70% of cases [11] and seizures are often refractory to AEDs [1]. In addition, cavernous angiomas provoke epileptic seizures in almost 50% of cases [17].

MRI now fairly easily and precisely gives the size and location of these lesions but it does not provide information on their epileptogeneity [4, 6]. The temporal lobe has been studied widely for its involvement in seizures, mostly due to mesio-temporal structures [10]. It is therefore the most frequent target of non-lesional epilepsy surgery with encouraging results [3]. In the presence of a lesion and refractory epilepsy, the surgical approach is discussed: if seizures are triggered by the lesion, a pure lesionectomy can cure the patient, but the presence of a distant electric focus

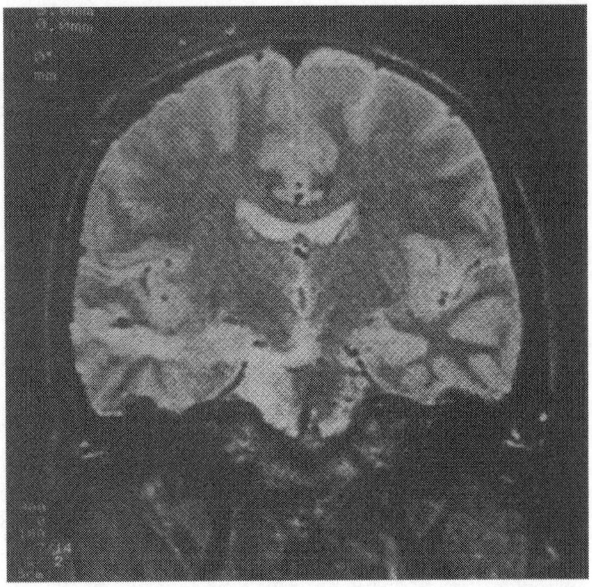

Fig. 4. MR coronal images (SE 2000/100). Postoperative follow-up shows the complete removal of the supra-tentorial part of the epidermoid. No postoperative seizure modifications

of non-concordant semeiology requires a tailoring of surgery of associated cortectomy [15, 19, 21]. Postoperative results confirm this approach: patients are cured in 95% of cases after a more extensive approach to the lesion, and 50% after pure lesionectomy in the series of Spencer [19]. Wyllie [21] also emphasises a better prognosis in the presence of a complete excision of an electrical focus, even if the lesionectomy itself is incomplete. Awad [1] however, reports a better control of seizures if lesionectomy is complete.

In the authors' series patients with sporadic seizures (group 1) and with refractory epilepsy (group 2) have been considered separately. In group 1, where lesionectomy is the treatment of choice, failure in control of seizures is due either to postoperative complications to incomplete lesionectomy or to tumour regrowth. In only one case did the presence of an extracerebral tumour (teratoma) lead probably to mesiotemporal compression and to postoperative seizures, e.g. a case of epidermoid in group 2, in whom a radiological structural rearrangement of those structures was also observed. In group 2 a complete lesionectomy, demonstrated by MRI, correlates with better results if seizures arise from the lesion, as shown by preoperative electroclinical studies. This is particularly true for mesio-temporal lesions. In the cases in which a residuum of the tumour does not involve the epileptic focus, patients may be seizure free postoperatively.

A careful electroclinical evaluation of seizures may suggest the combined approach of lesionectomy and amygdalo-hippocampectomy, even without deep electrodes or ECoG studies. Such an approach has led in the authors' series to good results. VideoEEG is an important tool, but sometimes may not be sufficient to distinguish a temporo-mesial from a lateral seizure onset. The clinical pattern of seizures can be even more important than ictal recording, while in more complicated and selected cases with non-localizing convulsive features, stereoEEG is the only means of identifying an epileptic focus.

In conclusion, the association of seizures and temporal lesions must be critically considered in order to establish the indications for surgery, distinguishing an oncological from an epileptologic approach. In the latter case preoperative studies should be directed to the demonstration of concordance between the lesion and seizures or its absence.

References

1. Awad IA, Rosenfeld J, Ahl J, Hahn JF, Lüders HO (1991) Intractable epilepsy and structural lesions of the brain; mapping, resection strategies, and seizure outcome. Epilepsia 32: 179–186
2. Berger SM, Ghatan S, Haglund MM, Dobbins Y, Ojemann GA (1993) Low grade gliomas associated with intractable epilepsy: seizures outcome utilizing electrocorticography during tumor resection. J Neurosurg 79: 62–69
3. Boon PA, Williamson PD, Fried I, Spencer DD, Novelly RA, Spencer SS, Mattson RH (1991) Intracranial, intraaxial, space-occupying lesions in patients with intractable partial seizures: an anatomoclinical, neuropsychological and surgical correlation. Epilepsia 32: 467–476
4. Bracchi M, Casazza M, Bradac GB, Avanzini G, Broggi G, Grisoli M (1994) Vascular anomalies in epilepsy. In: Shorvon AD *et al* (eds) Magnetic resonance scanning and epilepsy. NATO ASI Series. A 264. Plenum, New York, pp 191–193
5. Cascino GD (1990) Epilepsy and brain tumours: implications for treatment. Epilepsia 31 [Suppl 3]: 37–44
6. Cascino GD, Jack CR jr, Sharbrough FW, Kelly PY (1994) Non-malignant tumoral lesions. In: Shorvon AD *et al* (eds) Magnetic resonance scanning and epilepsy. NATO ASI Series, A 264. Plenum, New York, pp 185–189
7. Del Curling O jr, Kelly DL, Elster AD, Craven TE (1991) An analysis of the natural history of cavernous angiomas. J Neurosurg 75: 702–708
8. Dodick DN, Cascino GD, Meyer FB (1994) Vascular malformations and intractable epilepsy: outcome after surgical treatment. Mayo Clin Proc 69: 741–745
9. Engel J (1987) Outcome with respect to epileptic seizures. In: Engel J (ed) Surgical treatment of the epilepsies. Raven, New York, pp 553–571
10. Engel J (1989) Basic mechanisms of epilepsy. In: Plum F *et al* (eds) Seizures and epilepsy, vol 31. FA Davis Company, pp 71–111
11. Ettinger AB (1994) Structural causes of epilepsy. Neurol Clin 12 (1): 41–56

12. Fried I, Jung K, Spencer DD (1992) Hippocampal pathology in patients with intractable seizures and temporal lobe masses. J Neurosurg 76: 735–740
13. Fried I, Cascino GD (1993) Lesional surgery. In: Engel J (ed) Surgical treatment of the epilepsies, 2nd ed. Raven, New York, pp 501–509
14. Goldring S, Rich KM, Picker S (1986) Experience with gliomas in patients presenting with a chronic seizure disorder. In: Little JR (ed) Clincial neurosurgery, vol 33. Williams and Wilkins, Baltimore, pp 15–42
15. Kahane P, Munari C, Hoffmann D, Tassi L, Gallina P, Francione S, Di Leo M, Quarato P, Lo Russo G, Benabid AL (1994) Approche chirurgicale multimodale des angiomes caverneux épileptogènes. Epilepsies 6: 113–130
16. Kraemer DL, Awad IA (1994) Vascular malformations and epilepsy: clinical considerations and basic mechanisms. Epilepsia 35 [Suppl 6]: 30–43
17. Requena I, Arias M, Lopez-Ibor C, Pereiro I, Barba A, Alonso A, Monton E (1991) Cavernomas of the central nervous system: clinical and neuroimaging manifestations in 47 patients. J Neurol Neurosurg Psychiatry 54: 590–594
18. Robinson JR, Awad IA, Little JR (1991) Natural history of the cavernous angioma. J Neurosurg 75: 709–714
19. Spencer DD, Spencer SS, Mattson RH, Williamson PD (1984) Intracerebral masses in patients with intractable partial epilepsy. Neurology 34: 432–436
20. Vielvoye GJ, Pijl MEJ (1992) Magnetic resonance imaging of the so-called cerebral cryptic angiomas. Clin Neurol Neurosurg 94 [Suppl]: 171–175
21. Wyllie E, Lüders HO, Morris HN, Lesser RP, Dinner DS, Hahn J, Estes ML, Rothner AD, Erenberg G, Cruse R, Friedman D (1987) Clinical outcome after complete or partial cortical resection for intractable epilepsy. Neurology 37: 1634–1641

Correspondence: Marina Casazza, M.D., Istituto Nazionale Neurologico "C. Besta", via Celoria 11, 20133 Milano, Italia.

Acta Neurochir (1997) [Suppl] 68: 70–74

Low Grade Glioma in Intractable Epilepsy: Lesionectomy versus Epilepsy Surgery

D. Lombardi[1], **R. Marsh**[2], and **N. de Tribolet**[1]

[1] Department of Neurosurgery, University Hospital of Geneva, Geneva, Switzerland and [2]Department of Neurosurgery, Mayo Clinic, Rochester, USA

Summary

In approximately 30% of patients with intractable partial epilepsy, an intra-axial cerebral lesion is the aetiology of the seizure disorder. Lesions adjacent to mesiotemporal structures often result in secondary epileptogenicity in the same region.

The authors present 22 cases of low-grade gliomas associated with intractable epilepsy. In 15 cases the location was temporal (8 extrahippocampal and 7 with invasion of the amygdalo-hippocampus), 7 cases were extratemporal in eloquent areas. The eight extrahippocampal tumours were originally treated with lesionectomy. The seizure outcome was class 1 in only 4 cases, the remaining 4 were class 4 according to Engel's classification. The 4 cases with class 4 outcome required additional temporal lobectomy associated with amygdalo-hippocampectomy for seizure control. The 2 cases with associated hippocampal atrophy at MRI after lobectomy had outcome class 1. The 2 cases without hippocampal atrophy at MRI presented outcome class 2. The 7 cases with invasion of amygdala and hippocampus were treated with selective lesionectomy + amygdalo-hippocampectomy. In all these cases convergence of focal structural abnormality, ictal onset of epileptiform EEG abnormality and interictal epileptiform EEG abnormality provided powerful evidence of focal epileptogenicity. All these patients had a favourable epilepsy outcome (class 1–2). In the seven extratemporal cases the first step was lesionectomy. In 1 case located in the parietal region intraoperative mapping was required. 5 had class 1 outcome, one case had outcome class 2 and one case had an outcome class 4. The last patient required a second step operation with intraoperative strip and deep electrode monitoring that led subsequently to a frontal lobectomy. This patient is seizure free 2 years after surgery.

There was no perioperative mortality and post-operative morbidity was 3/22.

This study indicates that lesionectomy may be the first step procedure if the structural abnormality is localized to extra-temporal eloquent cortex and concordance is documented. Patients may subsequently be candidates for a cortical resection as a second step procedure if the lesionectomy does not provide an adequate reduction in seizure tendency.

Since MRI identified hippocampal atrophy was predictive in this study of an unsatisfactory seizure outcome after lesionectomy, MRI defined dual pathologies consisting of a temporal lesion plus hippocampal atrophy necessitate temporal lobectomy + amygdalo-hippocampectomy.

In patients with negative MRI findings of hippocampal atrophy and temporal lobe lesions, intraoperative electrocorticography and deep electrode monitoring are indicated for planning the surgical strategy.

Keywords: Partial epilepsy; lesionectomy; amygdalo-hippocampectomy; low-grade gliomas.

Introduction

In approximately 30% of patients with intractable partial epilepsy an intra-axial cerebral lesion is the aetiology of the seizure disorder [1–3]. The concordance of focal structural abnormality, ictal onset and inter-ictal epileptiform EEG abnormality and neuronal dysfunction in a given region of the brain provides powerful evidence of focal epileptogenicity [4, 5]. In instances where there is no such absolute concordance the neurosurgeon should be suspicious of possible mislocalization of epileptogenicity [6, 7]. The tumour exerts a pathological effect on nearby brain parenchyma rendering this region of the brain epileptogenic. The effect of a mass lesion on surrounding brain parenchyma may be mechanical, causing increased pressure and/or ischaemia or may be related to specific trophic factors derived from blood leakage or haemosiderosis [8, 9]. Lesions adjacent to mesiotemporal structures often result in secondary epileptogenicity in these structures. The incidence of mesio-temporal sclerosis and extra-hippocampal tumour in the temporal lobe has ranged from 8 to 22% [7]. In some cases the brain around the lesion is irreversibly kindled so as to remain epileptogenic despite lesion resection. This phenomenon appears to be greater in patients with temporal extra-hippocampal lesions.

Material and Methods

All the patients with the exception of the group with critical extra-temporal location of the tumour entered the seizure protocol including prolonged video-EEG monitoring, neuropsychological testing, MRI hippocampal volumetry and intraoperative deep electrodes monitoring and corticography. WADA test was administered in 8 cases.

Results

Twenty-two cases of low grade gliomas are presented associated with intractable epilepsy, classified as partial complex seizures. The mean age of the patients was 36 years (range 16–52) and the mean duration of intractable seizure disorder was 5.6 years (range 2–14). In 15 cases the location was temporal (8 extra-hippocampal and 7 with invasion of the amygdalo-hippocampus), 7 cases were extra-temporal in eloquent areas (Table 1). The eight temporal extra-hippocampal tumours were originally treated with lesionectomy (Fig. 1A). In 4 out of 8 cases intra-operative deep electrodes and corticography showed independent desynchronized epileptic activity in the amygdala and hippocampus. The seizure outcome was class 1 in only 4 cases, the remaining 4 in which deep electrodes were showing autonomous desynchronized activity were class 4 according to Engel's classification. The four cases with class 4 outcome required additional temporal lobectomy associated with amygdalo-hippocampectomy for seizure control. The 2 cases with associated hippocampal atrophy at MRI (Fig. 1B) after temporal lobectomy and amygdalo-hippocampectomy had outcome class 1. The 2 cases without hippocampal atrophy at MRI, after the same surgical procedure, presented outcomes class 2.

The 7 cases with invasion of amygdalo and hippocampus (Fig. 2A) were treated with a trans-Sylvian tumourectomy and selective amygdalo-hippocampectomy (Fig. 2B). In all these cases convergence of focal structural abnormality, ictal onset and inter-ictal epileptiform EEG abnormality confirmed epileptiform activity confined to the amygdala and hippocampus. Intra-operative deep electrode recordings and corticography provided powerful evidence of focal epileptogenicity. All these patients had a favourable epilepsy outcome (class 1–2).

Table 1. *Site of Cerebral Lesions and Relationship to Outcome of Seizure Activity after Microsurgical Lesionectomy*

Localization	Engel's class				Follow-up (months)
	I	II	III	IV	mean
Temporal, extrahippocampal	4	—	—	4	16
Hippocampal	5	2	—	—	18
Frontal	—	—	—	1	18
Parietal	1	—	—	—	28
Occipital	1	—	—	—	22
Fronto-parietal	2	—	—	—	35
Temporo-parietal	1	—	—	—	35
Parieto-occipital	—	1	—	—	37

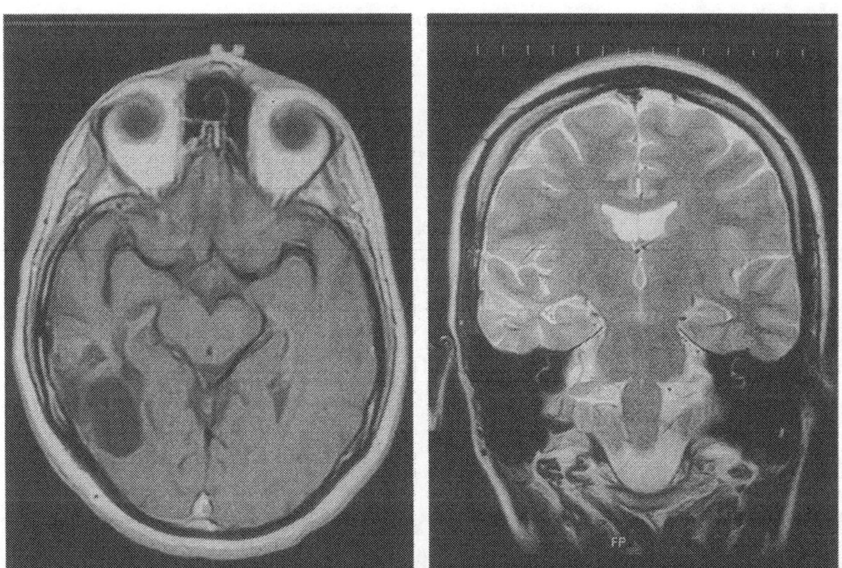

a b

Fig. 1. (a) Axial MRI after lesionectomy of a grade II temporal astrocytoma. The patient showed persistence of partial complex seizures after surgery. (b) Coronal T2 weighted MRI of the same patient shows left hippocampal atrophy in association with the surgically treated temporal lesion. The patient underwent as 2nd step surgery temporal lobectomy and amygdalo-hippocampectomy which allowed complete control of epilepsy

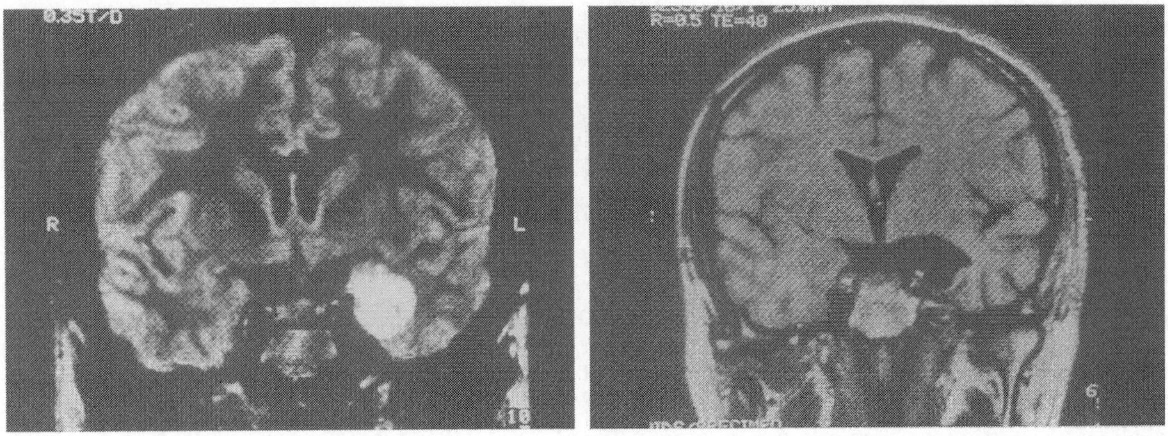

a b

Fig. 2. (a) Coronal MRI with gadolinium injection of a 21 years old man suffering from partial complex seizures since the age of 7. The enhancing lesion invading the left amygdala and hippocampus at histology was classified as ganglioglioma. (b) Coronal MRI with gadolinium injection after tumourectomy and selective amygdalo-hippocampectomy through a trans-Sylvian approach. This procedure allowed complete control of the epilepsy

In the seven extra-temporal cases (Fig. 3A) the first step was lesionectomy because of the location in eloquent areas (Fig. 3B). In 1 case located in the parietal region intraoperative mapping was required. Five patients had class 1 outcome, one case had class 2 and the other had class 4 outcome. The last patient required a second step operation with intraoperative deep electrodes and corticography which subsequently led to a frontal lobectomy. This patient is now seizure free 2 years after surgery.

The histological diagnosis was astrocytoma grade II in 8 cases, oligodendroglioma grade I in 3 cases and grade II in 2 cases, ganglioglioma in 6 cases and DNT (dysembryoblastic-neuroepithelial-tumour) in 3 cases. Hippocampal gliosis with cell loss associated with temporal tumour was documented at the histological examination in 4 cases. In these 4 cases desynchronized epileptiform activity was documented intraoperatively in the amygdala and hippocampus independently from the perilesional area. At the preoperative MRI volumetry only 2 out of 4 cases of hippocampal atrophy were confirmed from the quantitative study (Table 2).

Surface electrodes and deep electrodes implanted within the tumours did not show epileptiform activ-

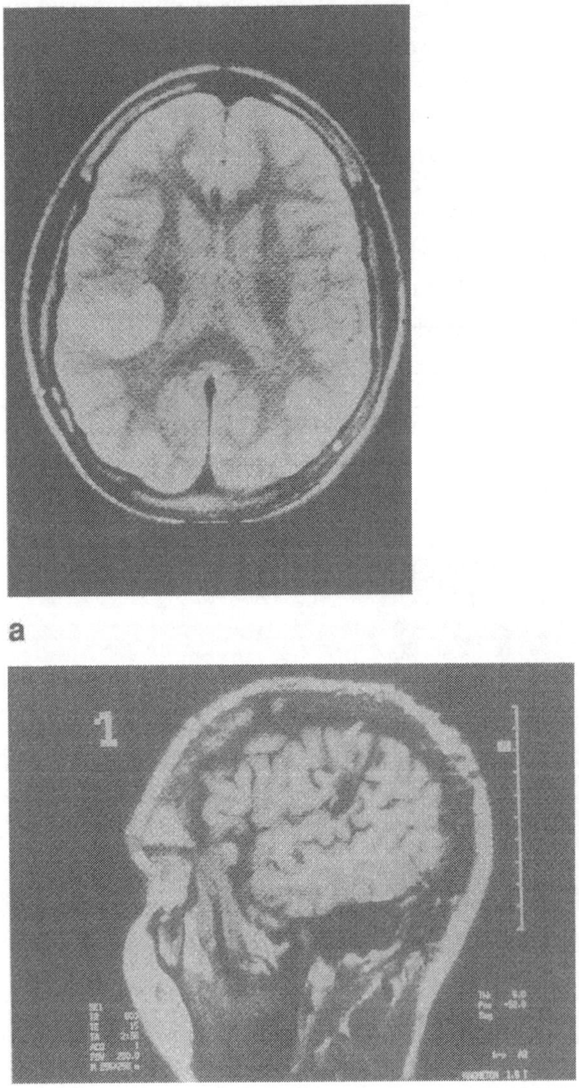

a

b

Fig. 3. (a) Axial T2 weighted MRI of a 16 years old boy suffering from partial complex seizures since the age of 14 years. The lesion, spontaneously hyperintense, localized in the supramarginal gyrus on histology was classified as astrocytoma grade II. (b) Sagittal MRI after gross total removal of the lesion through a trans-sulcal approach. The lesionectomy allowed complete control of the epilepsy

Table 2. *Correlation of Hippocampal Formation Atrophy and Surgical Outcome in Patients with Extra-Hippocampal Temporal Lobe Lesions and Partial Epilepsy*

Patients	Seizure	Hippocampic atrophy		Pathology	Outcome		Deep electrodes
		MRI volumetry	Histology		Lesionectomy	TL and AHE	
1	left	left	+	astrocytoma	IV	I	+
2	right	right	+	ganglioglioma	IV	I	+
3	right	no	+	oligodendroglioma	IV	II	+
4	right	no	–	astrocytoma	I	–	–
5	left	no	–	DNT	I	–	–
6	left	no	–	oligodendroglioma	I	–	–
7	right	no	–	astrocytoma	I	–	–
8	left	no	+	astrocytoma	IV	II	+

TL and *AHE* = temporal lobectomy and amygdalo-hippocampectomy.

ity with the exception of 3 out of 4 cases of DNT in which epileptiform activity, synchronized with the perilesional region, was observed. There was no perioperative mortality and surgical morbidity consisted of right transient hemiparesis in a patient with a left parietal oligodendroglioma, transient anomic aphasia in a patient with a left medial postero-temporal grade II astrocytoma and Kluwer-Bucy syndrome in a patient with an oligodendroglioma infiltrating the amygdalo-hippocampus.

Discussion

This study indicates that lesionectomy may be the first step procedure if the tumour is localized to extratemporal eloquent cortex especially when preoperative studies show concordance. Patients may subsequently be candidates for a cortical resection as a second step epilepsy procedure if the lesionectomy does not provide an adequate reduction in seizure tendency.

MRI identified hippocampal atrophy was predictive in this study of an unsatisfactory seizure outcome after lesionectomy in cases of dual pathology. All patients with documented MRI evidence of hippocampal pathology had an unfavourable outcome after resection of the extra-hippocampal lesion alone. The absence of MRI identified hippocampal atrophy however did not have the same prognostic importance. The authors conclude that MRI defined dual pathologies consisting of a temporal lesion and hippocampal atrophy necessitate temporal lobectomy and amygdalo-hippocampectomy. In patients with intractable epilepsy with negative MRI findings of hippocampal atrophy and presenting with a temporal lobe tumour, preoperative prolonged video-EEG and intraoperative deep electrodes recordings with corticography are indicated for planning the surgical strategy.

When electrodes implanted in the amygdala and hippocampus record a desynchronized independent activity from the perilesional region the authors recommend the combination of an amygdalo-hippocampectomy and temporal lobectomy with the lesionectomy. This should be performed even in the absence of a structural abnormality of the mesial temporal structures visualized by MRI hippocampal volumetry. Indeed, there is no information in the literature about how long it would take for a functional anomaly of the hippocampus to became morphologically visible at MRI. Four out of eight extra-hippocampal temporal tumours showed autonomous desynchronized activity in the amygdala and hippocampus and this was predictive of poor epilepsy control with lesionectomy only.

The opposite phenomenon of hippocampal tumour provoking autonomous desynchronized activity in the cortical surface of the temporal lobe did not occur in this series. It is more likely for a tumour at the surface of the temporal lobe to "kindle" the mesiotemporal structures than for a tumour of the hippocampus to "kindle" the temporal cortex. This is confirmed by the good results obtained with the simple tumour removal through a trans-sylvian tumourectomy and amygdalo-hippocampectomy in cases of hippocampal tumours.

The same 4 cases which showed during the intraoperative deep electrodes recording desynchronized activity of the amygdala and hippocampus from the perilesional region presented at the histological study gliosis with cell loss, but in only two cases this was visible at the preoperative MRI volumetry as

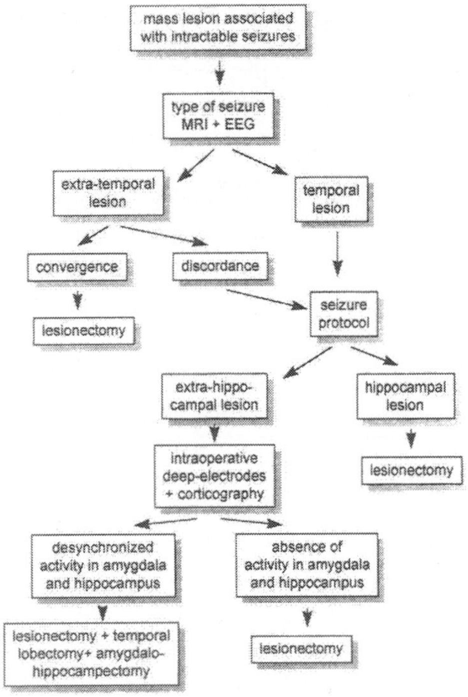

Fig. 4. Surgical strategy in mass lesions associated with intractable seizures

hippocampal asymmetry. Deep electrodes recording in this series was superior in predictive value than MRI volumetry and correlated better with anatomo-pathological findings (Fig. 4).

DNT, finally, represent from the functional and anatomical point of view, a different class of tumours. The presence of intervening functional neuronal tissue causes these tumours not to be electrically silent but to present intrinsic epileptic activity.

References

1. Awad I, Rosenfeld J, Ahl J, *et al* (1991) Intractable epilepsy and structural lesions of the brain: Mapping, resection strategies, and seizure outcome. Epilepsia 32: 179–186
2. Berger M, Ghatan S, Haglund M, *et al* (1993) Low-grade gliomas associated with intractable epilepsy: Seizure outcome utilizing electrocorticography during tumor resection. J Neurosurg 79: 62–69
3. Cascino G, Kelly P, Marsh W, *et al* (1990) Stereotactic resection of intra-axial cerebral lesions in partial epilepsy. Mayo Clin Proc 65: 1053–1060
4. Cascino G, Kelly P, Sharbrough R, *et al* (1992) Long-term follow-up of stereotactic lesionectomy in partial epilepsy. Epilepsia 33: 639–644
5. Fish D, Andermann F, Olivier A (1991) Complex partial seizures and small posterior temporal or extratemporal structural lesions: Surgical management. Neurology 41: 1781–1784
6. Fried I, Cascino G (1993) Lesional surgery. In: Engel J Jr (ed) Surgical treatment of the epilepsies 2. Raven P, New York, pp 501–509
7. Fried I, Kim JH, Spencer DD (1992) Hippocampal pathology in patients with intractable seizures and temporal lobe masses. J Neurosurg 76: 735–740
8. Kirkpatrick P, Honavar M, Janota I, *et al* (1993) Control of temporal lobe epilepsy following en bloc resection of low-grade tumors. J Neurosurg 78: 19–25
9. Penfield W, Jasper H (1954) Epilepsy and the functional anatomy of the human brain. Little Brown, Boston

Correspondence: Daniela Lombardi, M.D., Department of Neurosurgery, University Hospital of Geneva, 24 rue Micheli du Crest, 1211 Geneva, Switzerland.

Acta Neurochir (1997) [Suppl] 68: 75–80

Incorporation of Ultrasonic Imaging in an Optically Coupled Frameless Stereotactic System

H. Hirschberg and **G. Unsgaard**

Departments of Neurosurgery, The National Hospital Oslo and The Regional Hospital Trondheim, Norway

Summary

Frameless stereotactic interactive tracking systems relate a point in the surgical field to a corresponding point on the patients MR or CT scans in multiple planes. A basic weakness with these systems is that they cannot compensate for movement of target points due to brain shift caused by CSF drainage or lesion removal. Real time images can be obtained using ultrasonic techniques but the poor quality and definition and the ill-defined scan plane make interpretation difficult and reduce the usefulness of this modality. The authors have combined these two modalities by mounting light emitting diodes (LEDs) on the ultrasonic probe, thus allowing a "virtual tip" to be developed in the centre of the ultrasonic beam, and tracked via an optically coupled frameless stereotactic system (Radionics, OTS). This has allowed a direct correlation between pre-operative MR and the per-operative ultrasonic images using reformatted MR images. Ultrasound images are obtained through a separate skull opening and the image plane is determined by the position of the virtual tip. The ultrasonic and MR images are presented side by side for visual comparison. Minimally invasive tumour resection or haematoma removal could be carried out under ultrasonic guidance with direct interactive relation to the preoperative MR scans. Alternatively interactive image directed surgical procedures can be up-dated in real time by dynamic ultrasonic images taken in clearly defined scan planes.

Keywords: Image directed surgery; ultrasonic imaging.

Introduction

Interactive image directed stereotactic systems, (neuronavigation, frameless stereotaxy), rely on transformation of the imaging digital data to the stereotactic operative field space. Various technologies have been adapted to implement this goal, using both framebased and frameless stereotactic systems. Most of the frameless systems developed employ some sort of pointing device either coupled mechanically in the form of an articulate arm [4–6, 15] or via sonic [1, 2, 13], optical [3, 16] or magnetic [11] transmission.

The authors have employed a system, where light emitting diodes (LEDs) mounted on various surgical instruments, have been used as an armless pointing device and which, mounted on the surgical microscope, has allowed the focal plane of the microscope to be correlated with the relevant CT/MR scan (OTS, Radionics Inc Burlington, Mass, USA) [7].

Any mechanical shift in the brain during surgery will not be reported by these systems since they use "historical" data sets as images. On the other hand ultrasonic imaging techniques give real time information but their lack of definition and poorly defined scan planes make their interpretation difficult. The authors have combined these two modalities by mounting two -three LEDs on the ultrasonic probe allowing a virtual tip to be developed in the centre of the ultrasonic beam. MR images indicating the position of the virtual tip were displayed along with the corresponding ultrasonic image. This greatly increased the value of the information obtained from the ultrasonic scans. They present here their preliminary experience with this system.

Materials and Methods

The optical digitizer employed in this study uses three linear television cameras to define a volume in three dimensional space (IGT Boulder Col.). The position of up to 15 infrared light emitting diodes can be determined in this three dimensional volume and each one independently tracked. The size of the defined three dimensional volume and the accuracy of the system is dependent on the distances from the array to the operative field. Light emitting diodes have been attached to bipolar forceps, to a frame mounted on the operating table to compensate for movement of the table during surgery, on a frame mounted on the surgical microscope and two or three LEDs on a 7 Mhz ultrasonic probe (B&K Medical Copenhagen Denmark).

Coordinates generated by the digitizer are transferred to a Hewlett-Packard workstation running specialised software (RSA OTS

1,1 Burlington Mass). Axial, coronal and sagittal images are displayed or the images can be reformatted in the plane of the probe. The ultrasonic images were displayed on a separate monitor where the images could be rotated to correspond to the format of the MR scans.

Patients all had intra-axial tumours and were not previously operated. Phantom studies were performed on a gelatine filled box with MR visible targets embedded inside and registration fiducials on the surface.

Image Acquisition

MR scans were performed on a Sieman's Impact MR scanner, using the Turbo-flash mode The produced slices are contiguous and are approximately 2.2 mm in thickness and consist of 64 scans. All scanning was done in the axial plane. A remountable non-invasive stereo-adapter was used to carry 6 MR visible markers and to immobilise the patient's head during the 7 minutes required to perform volumetric scan [8, 10, 14]. The use of a remountable guide allows great flexibility in the scheduling of the operative procedure. The phantom was scanned in an identical manner but using surface fiducials.

Image Registration

The fiducial points were identified and marked on the display. Four fiducials are necessary for the registration process and they are selected to give a good distribution around the volume of the head and the surgical field. On the day of the operation the stereo-adapter was remounted in an identical fashion to that used during the MR scanning procedure and the patient's head immobilised in a conventional manner using the Mayfield 3 point fixation system. The fiducial markers are small plastic doughnuts permanently filled with MR contrast and show up as two points on the scans regardless of the directional orientation. Each fiducial is identified on the corresponding axial scan, then the tip of the probe placed in the central hole of the selected fiducial and the coordinate recorded. The remountable guide is then removed and the burr hole for the ultrasonic probe and a separate skin flap and craniotomy opening can now be planned using the system and a special probe with a variable distance between the probe tip and the two mounted LEDs which allows simulated penetration of the brain identical to the ultrasonic virtual tip. The configuration of the stereotactic ultrasonic probe is shown in two planes in Fig. 1.

Studies were first performed on a ultrasonic compatible gelatin phantom where MR and ultrasound visible targets were imbedded. After scanning the phantom was registered in the OTS via 4 surface fiducials. Fig. 2 shows the three MR views of the scans determined by the virtual tip of the ultrasonic probe and the corresponding ultrasonic image. The ultrasonic image is in a similar plane to the axial MR. The MR "map" greatly simplifies the interpretation of the ultrasonic images. The degree of target shift could also be approximated in this model.

Five patients were also operated on using this combined modality. Fig. 3 shows a set of images from a patient with a cystic glioma. A small separate burr hole (10 mm) was made for the ultrasonic probe and the tumour was sonicated at a different angle to the operative trajectory to allow the ultrasonic visualisation of the surgical instruments used (Fig. 1). The tumour was removed through a separate craniotomy opening (30 mm). A cortical incision of approximately 10 mm was used and a silicon catheter was first placed from the cortical surface to the tumour with the OTS navigation system. This

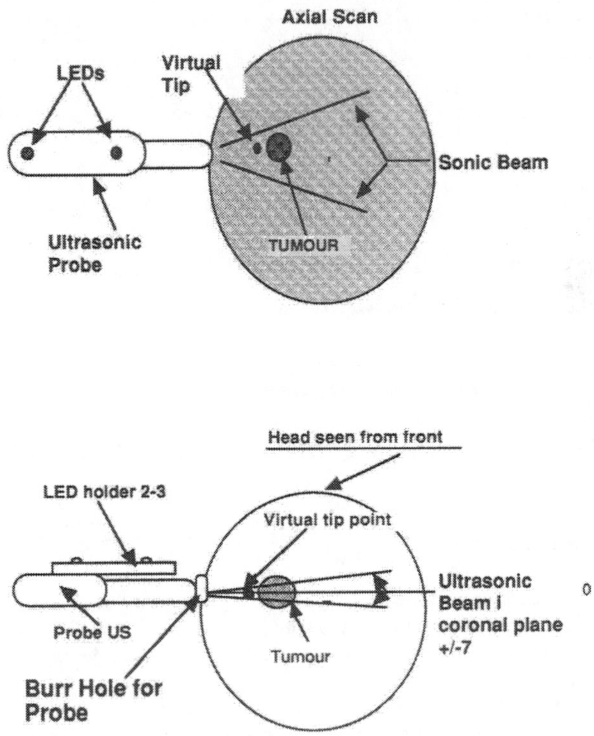

Fig. 1. The configuration of the stereotactic ultrasonic probe and its relationship to the skull in two planes. The beam is 60 degrees in width in the horizontal plane (axial) and 15 degrees in the vertical plane. The virtual tip can be either at a fixed (2 LEDs, 135 mm) or variable (3 LEDs) distance from the probe tip. The ultrasonic picture will now correlate with the MRI scans

allowed immediate identification of the operative trajectory with minimal damage to brain tissue. The tumour was removed with the ultrasonic aspirator under ultrasonic guidance. Local brain shift in this case was about 20 mm due to cyst drainage although tumour shift was less owing to its proximity to the falc cerebri as seen on the images. Similar techniques were used in the other cases, three of which were glioblastoma and one cerebral metastasis. The addition of ultrasonic derived information was valuable in all of the cases.

Discussion

Modern interactive image directed systems offer the neurosurgeons a new degree of precision and cost effectiveness. Most of the systems available today have an accuracy in the mm range determined using phantoms or other forms for models. During actual surgery, however, the degree of precision is greatly reduced due to movement of the brain compared to its position during initial scanning and patient registration with an intact skull. System accuracy of greater than 2 mm is therefore not really useful in open surgery since the large errors caused by brain shift are much greater

a

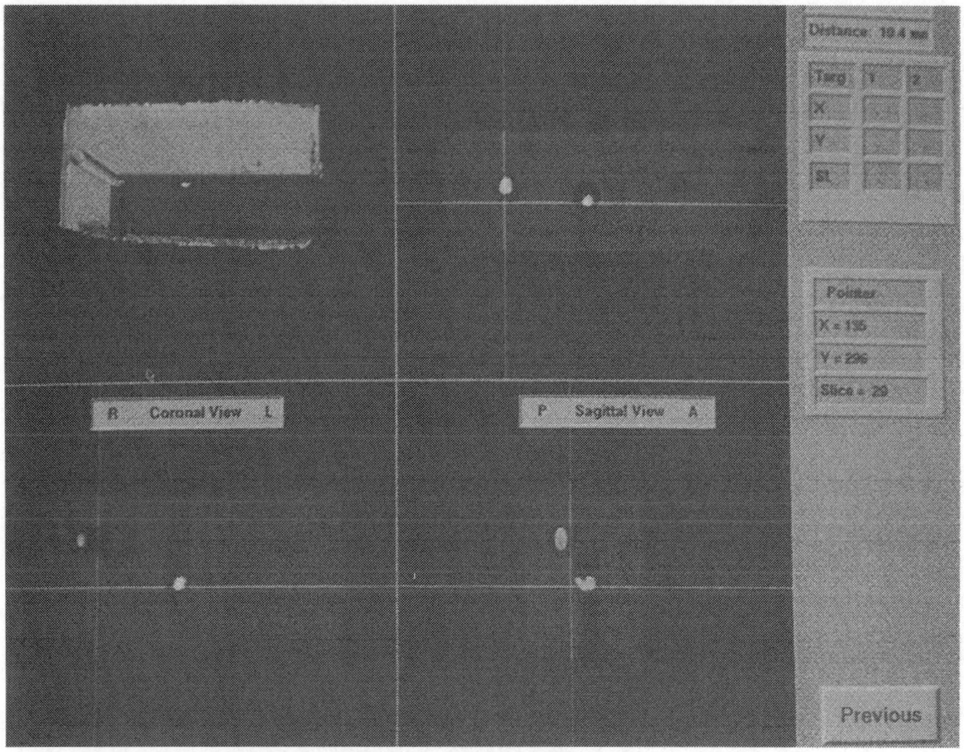

b

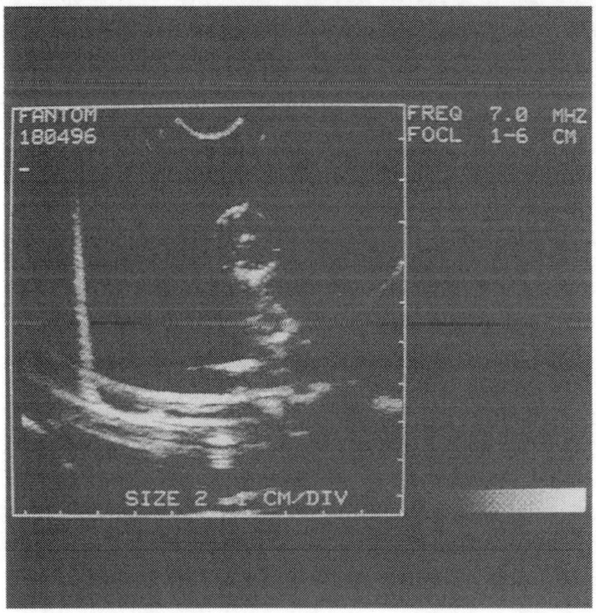

Fig. 2. MR and ultrasonic images of a gelatin phantom. The phantom consisted of a plastic rectangular box filled with hardened gelatine. Hollow tubes (10 mm diameter) containing vitamin capsules were imbedded in the gelatin in various planes. The phantom was scanned in the axial plane and registered in the OTS via 4 surface fiducials. (a) Shows the reformatted MR images in all three planes corresponding to the "virtual tip" in the ultrasonic beam as indicated by the cross hairs. (b) Shows the axial ultrasonic image of the target at this level. The tube wall and the MR target are clearly identified from the reflection artifacts

than this value. Various solutions to this problem have been proposed such as small craniotomies, adjusting patient position or by marking the boundary of the tumour with stereotactically placed catheters or dye injection. The authors have employed the latter technique with the injection of isotonic methylene blue in 6 to 8 tracks around the periphery of the tumour determined by the contrast ring in MR scans. The dye was injected using image directed guidance before resection of the tumour was started employing a special probe and OTS equipment. The tumour was then resected until the dye became visible. In two cases using this technique large infiltration of macrophages was noted in the histological specimens. This could be caused either by rapid migration of macrophage infiltration due to the dye itself or increased staining of

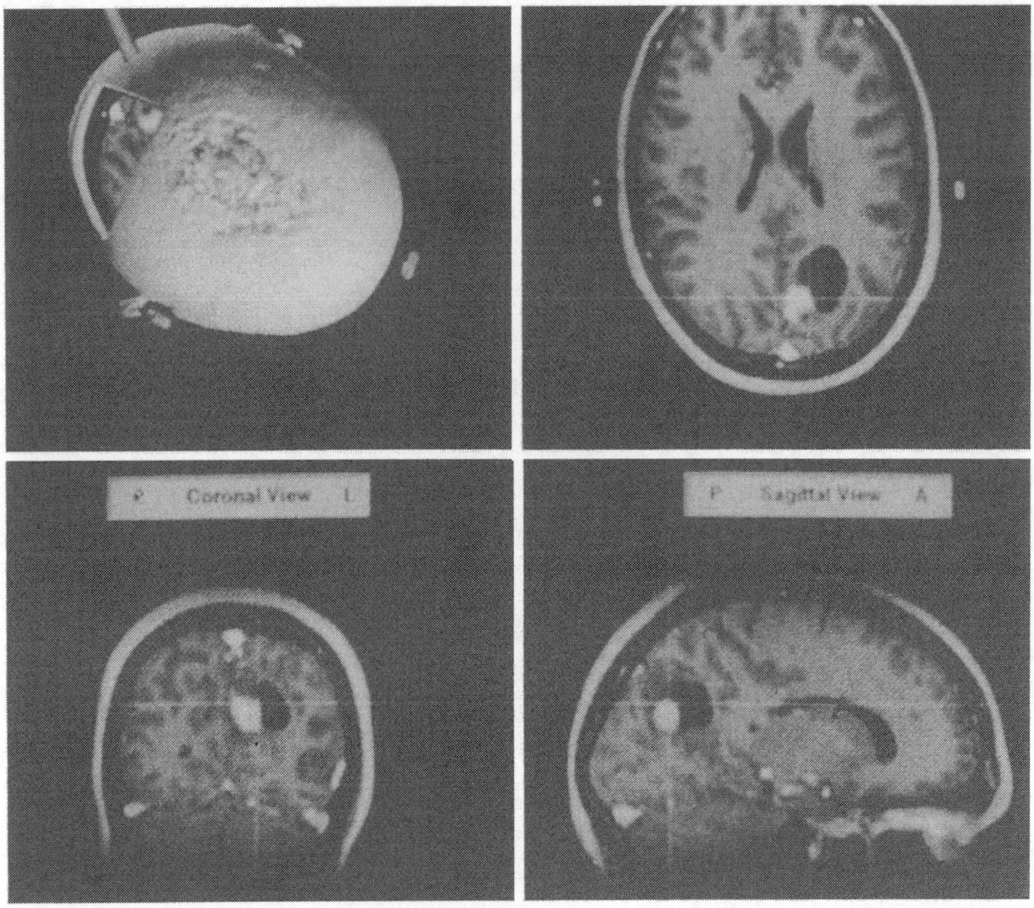

a

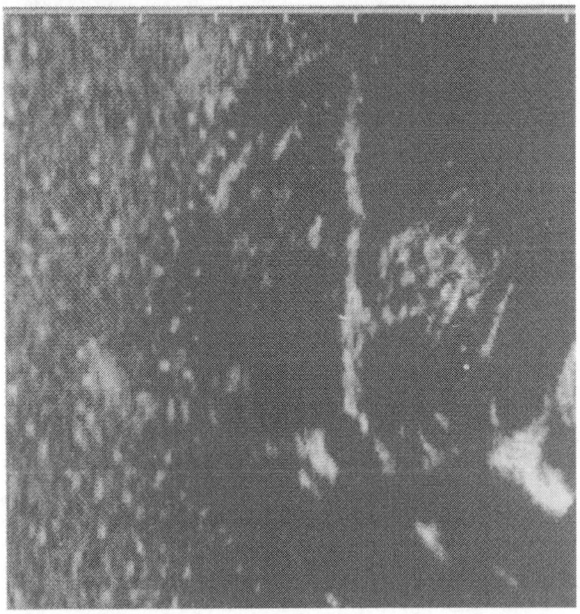

b

Fig. 3. (a) Reformatted MR scans of a patient harbouring a cystic glioma. The virtual tip is shown at the superior lateral border of the tumour. (b) Corresponding ultrasonic image sonicated through a separate burr hole clearly shows the tumour and the falc cerebri. The image was obtained after puncture of the cyst which caused significant local shift. The tumour was removed through a small craniotomy and cortical opening with ultrasonic guidance

macrophages which are usually found within gliomas by the dye making them more visible.

These techniques are only approximate and require multiple injection tracks into the brain or tumour. Cystic tumours are especially difficult if the cyst is punctured and drained at an early stage in the operation causing significant shifts.

Direct image registration based on anatomic surface

marking is another technique which theoretically, to a certain degree, could compensate for brain shift. This technique, however, is still in an experimental stage and no commercial systems based on it are available at the present moment.

Intraoperative imaging using ultrasonic techniques can provide real time information concerning the position of structures and surgical instruments in the brain [9, 12]. It can also follow changes caused by manipulations of the brain. Ultrasonic imaging, however, is often difficult to interpret due to its poor resolution, lack of contrast and difficulty in defining the scan planes at which the images are produced. A high order of echogenicity is necessary for reasonable resolution of structures in the brain.

Even the simple method presented here of developing a so-called virtual tip in the ultrasonic beam (centred close to the pathology of interest) and then using the ultrasonic probe as a stereotactic pointing device keyed to MR images has shown itself to be quite helpful. As presently implemented the ultrasonic beam should be in the plane of the axial images to allow direct correlation. Work is in progress to reformat the MR-images in the plane of the beam in almost real time so that a direct visual correlation between ultrasonic and reformatted MR-images can be obtained at any scan angle. Sweeping through the image volume of interest with the probe, would, since the corresponding MR slices are known and can be used as a three dimensional "map", also allow the generation of three-dimensional ultrasonic images to be built up rapidly. The addition of a frame grabber in the computer will also allow the presentation of the ultrasonic image directly on the same display which is now used for displaying the MR views.

Some neurosurgical procedures can be carried out quite effectively under ultrasonic guidance alone, for example aspiration of brain abscesses and removal of intracranial haematomas. These can be performed using a minimally invasive technique requiring only a small opening in the cortex. The addition of navigation information via an interactive image guidance system greatly increases the accuracy of such a procedure and even the simple matter of placing burr holes or bone flaps to allow optimum visualisation and sonication of pathology is greatly simplified. It has also been suggested that by using advanced computer technology it should be possible to employ directly the knowledge obtained from ultrasonic images of shifting normal structures to "distort the MR image in such a way that they are brought up to date. This technique, though, will require powerful computers and high resolution ultrasonics to make it feasible.

The introduction of both pre-operative and per-operative imaging techniques have proven highly valuable to the neurosurgeon. On the other hand they can be unnecessarily distracting in the OR. One most not lose sight of the fact that surgery is still primarily guided by direct visualisation of the brain and its pathology. Image guidance system merely give an occasional update and cannot in their present form replace the skills and experience necessary for successful neurosurgery.

References

1. Barnett GH, Kormos DW, Steiner CP, Piraino D, Weisenberger J, Hajjar F, Wood C, McNally J (1993) Frameless stereotaxy using a sonic digitizing wand. Development and adaptation to the Picker ViStar Medical Imaging System. In: Maciunas RJ (ed) Interactive image-guided neurosurgery. AANS, Park Ridge, pp 113–119
2. Barnett GH, Kormos DW, Steiner CP, Weisenberger J (1993) Use of a frameless, armless stereotactic wand for brain tumor localization with 2-D and 3-D neuroimaging. Neurosurgery 33: 674–678
3. Bucholz RD, Smith KR (1993) A comparision of sonic digitizers versus light emitting diode-based location. In: Maciunas RJ (ed) Interactive image-guided neurosurgery. AANS, Park Ridge, pp 179–200
4. Galloway RL Jr, Maciunas RJ (1993) An articulated arm for neurosurgical use. In: Maciunas RJ (ed) Interactive imaged-guided surgery. AANS, Park Ridge, pp 159–168
5. Golfinos JC, Fitzpatrick BC, *et al* (1995) Clinical use of a frameless stereotactic arm: Results of 325 cases. J Neurosurg 83: 197–205
6. Guthrie BL, Kaplan R, Florek D (1992) Stereotactic neurosurgical operating arm system. Stereotact Funct Neurosurg 58: 144–145
7. Hirschberg H (1996) Implementation of a stereotactic microscope using an optically coupled tracking system. Stereotact Funct Neurosurg in press
8. Hirschberg H (1997) Interactive image directed neurosurgery: Patient registration employing the Laitinen stereo adaptor. Minim Invasive Neurosurg in press
9. Koivukangas J, Louhisalmi Y, *et al* (1993) Ultrasound controlled neuronavigator-guided brain surgery. J Neurosurg 79: 36–42
10. Laitinen LV, Liliequist B, *et al* (1985) An adapter for computed tomography-guided stereotaxis. Surg Neurol 23: 559–66
11. Manwaring KH (1993) Intraoperative microendoscopy. In: Maciunas RJ (ed) Interactive image-guided surgery. AANS, Park Ridge, pp 217–232
12. Oikarinen J, Alakuijala J, *et al* (1993) The Oulu neuronavigator system: Intraoperative ultrasonography in the verification of neurosurgical localization and visualization. In: Maciunas RJ (ed) Interactive image-guided neurosurgery. AANS, Park Ridge, pp 223–246
13. Roberts DW, Strohbehn JW, *et al* (1986) A frameless stereo-

taxic integration of computerized tomographic imaging and the operating microscope. J Neurosurg 65: 545–549
14. Takizawa T (1993) Neurosurgical navigation using a non-invasive stereotadapter. Surg Neur 40: 1–6
15. Watanabe E, Mayanagi Y, *et al* (1991) Open surgery assisted by the neuronavigator, a stereotactic, articulated, sensitive arm. Neurosurgery 28: 792–800
16. Zamorano L, Nolte LP, *et al* (1994) Interactive intraoperative localization using an infrared-based system. Stereotact Funct Neurosurg 63: 84–88

Correspondence: Henry Hirschberg, M.D., Ph.D., Department of Neurosurgery, Riks Hospital, N-0027 Oslo, Norway.

Acta Neurochir (1997) [Suppl] 68: 81–84

Magnetoencephalography (MEG) in Epilepsy Surgery

N. Forss

Brain Research Unit, Low Temperature Laboratory, Helsinki University of Technology, Espoo, Finland

Summary

Whole-scalp MEG has proved to be a suitable tool for pre-operative evaluation of patients suffering from drug-resistant focal epilepsy. MEG recordings are non-invasive and safe for the subject, and no demanding preparations of the patient are needed before measurement. The MEG recordings may reveal several epileptic foci, and the order of activation can be resolved in millisecond scale. In addition, epileptic cortex can be localized with respect to important functional areas, such as sensorimotor or visual cortices, and these areas can be visualized in a same brain reconstruction. This helps in patient selection and planning of the operation. Moreover, prior MEG localization of epileptic foci and functionally important areas aids in placing the intracranial electrodes to right places, when needed.

Keywords: Magnetoencephalography; localization; epilepsy.

Introduction

Brain surgery has become increasingly important in the treatment of patients suffering from focal, drug resistance epilepsy. Preoperative evaluation of suitable candidates is of crucial importance for the success of the surgery. New imaging techniques are continuously searched for to reduce the need of time consuming and demanding invasive recordings, which are not totally without risk for the patient. With good spatial and excellent temporal resolution, magnetoencephalography (MEG) is one of the new promising non-invasive methods in locating epileptogenic cortex.

Methods

During any brain function at least thousands of pyramidal cells in the cerebral cortex are activated almost simultaneously. The apical dendrites of these cells lie parallel to each other and perpendicular to the cortical surface, which is thus also the main direction of the intracellular currents. These synchronized intracellular currents of the pyramidal cells are the source of cerebral magnetic fields, which can be measured non-invasively outside the head with very sensitive magnetometers. This method is called magnetoencephalography (MEG).

In electric recordings, skull and scalp distort the electric potentials recorded on the scalp which makes the exact localisation of active areas very difficult. These structures, however, are practically transparent to magnetic fields, and therefore they do not disturb MEG measurements. MEG measures tangential currents which arise from fissural activity; radial currents are magnetically silent outside of the head. Usually several cortical areas are simultaneously activated and therefore MEG's selectivity to tangential currents is an advantage in practical work, because it makes the interpretation of the data more simple. MEG detects mainly cortical activity, but the depth from which activity can be detected depends on the strength of the source. Sources of evoked fields are usually a few centimetres below the surface of the skull, but very strong activity, such as epileptic spikes, can be recorded also from deeper structures.

The whole-scalp Neuromag-122^{TM} magnetometer of the Helsinki University of Technology houses 122 superconducting SQUID sensors in liquid helium. The helmet shaped bottom of the magnetometer covers the whole scalp and therefore allows detection of simultaneous activity of several sources all over the cortex. The measurements are performed in a magnetically shielded room to reduce the effect of environmental noise (Fig. 1).

The exact location of the head with respect to the sensors is found by measuring the magnetic signals produced by currents in three head position indicator coils placed at known sites on the scalp. The locations of the coils with respect to anatomical landmarks on the head are determined with a 3-D digitizer to allow alignment of the MEG and MRI coordinate systems. For further technical details of the MEG/MR integration, see [3]. The spatial resolution of MEG for cortical sources is a few millimeters under favourable conditions, and the temporal resolution is better than a millisecond, which makes it possible to follow the extremely fast spatio-temporal changes in brain activity.

When a large group of neurons act in synchrony, the resulting net current can be approximated by a current dipole. The equivalent current dipole (ECD) that best accounts for the measured signals can be calculated on the basis of the measured magnetic field distribution. As a result the dipole's location in three-dimensional space, its orientation and strength may be obtained. The ECDs can then be superimposed on the subject's MRI to show the source location with respect to anatomical structures. Although the areas activated in association with epileptic seizures are usually large, the ECD locations represent centre of gravity of epileptic activity.

Already from the early 1980s, sharp localization of irritative MEG activity has been succesfully performed [1, 5]. In MEG recordings,

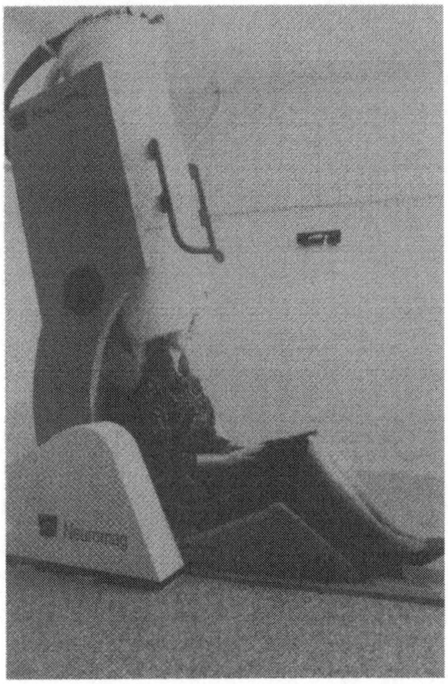

Fig. 1. Whole-scalp Neuromag-122™ neuromagnetometer. The measurements are performed in a magnetically shielded room

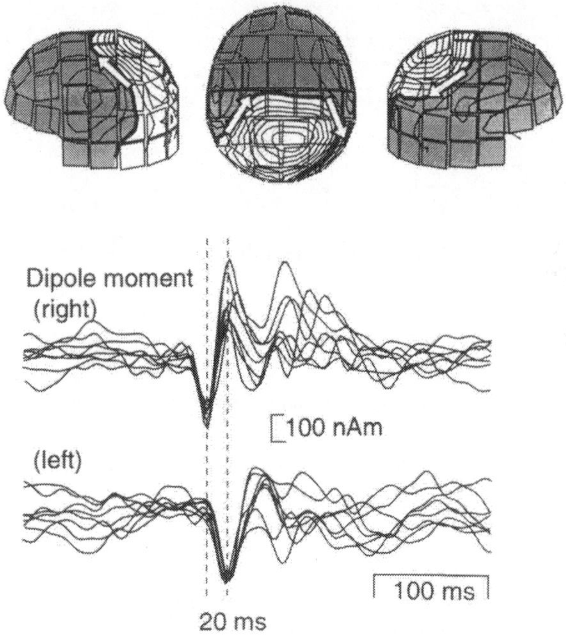

Fig. 2. Top: Magnetic field patterns of Patient 1 during a single time moment of one spike. The sensor array is viewed from left, top, and right. The shadowed areas indicate magnetic flux out of the head. The white arrows show the sites and orientations of the two dipoles required to account for the field pattern. Bottom: Dipole moments of the two dipoles as a function of time. Each trace corresponds to one unaveraged spike. (Modified from [4])

the epileptic focus can be localized with respect to functional landmarks [8, 9]. At present, multichannel MEG instruments covering whole scalp are available, and a number of epileptic patients have been studied with MEG as part of their preoperative evaluation.

Patient Examples

Patient 1 [4] demonstrates MEG's ability to separate the primary and secondary epileptic foci. The patient is a 18-years old female who had suffered from epilepsy over 11 years. Scalp EEG showed interictal activity over the right hemisphere in the centroparietal region. In videotelemetry the right-sided epileptic activity was occasionally associated with smaller amplitude spikes in the left parietal region.

MEG measurements revealed two epileptic foci, one in the right and the other in the left hemisphere. The activity in the left hemisphere was constantly delayed by 20 ms compared with the right (Fig. 2). The epileptic foci were located about 1 cm posterior to SI hand area in both hemispheres, and the epileptic activity was probably conducted from right to left hemisphere via callosal connections. No independent epileptic activity was observed in the left hemisphere, suggesting that removal of the right-sided focus would be sufficient.

Patient 2 [2] is a 38-year-old man, who has suffered from epilepsy since teenage. The seizures begin with an odd feeling or pain in the left gums, after which develop left-sided facial twitches. CT and PET were normal. In MRI the right hippocampus was thinner than the left. Several EEG and videotelemetry recordings showed either a left temporobasal or a right midtemporal focus. Despite all these studies the epileptic focus was not reliably identified.

Figure 3 shows the patient's MEG traces during a self-triggered seizure with left hemifacial convulsions. At the beginning of the seizure, spikes started to emerge more frequently and became polyphasic in morphology in the right frontoparietal channels. About 6 s after the beginning of the discharges the seizure spread to the left. The seizure continued for about 14 s and ended abruptly. The following activity was clearly dampened, and the interictal spikes, frequently seen at the beginning of the measurement, reemerged only after 65 s from the end of the seizure.

Sources of somatosensory evoked fields to median nerve stimulation and auditory evoked fields to tone beeps served as functional landmarks. Sources of both

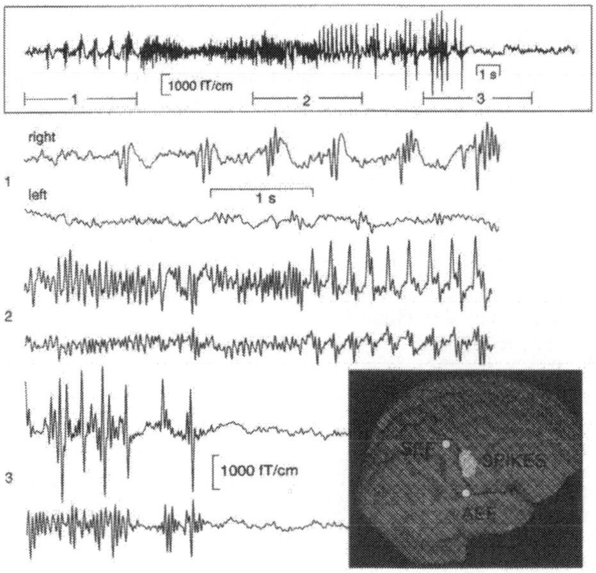

Fig. 3. Epileptic discharge in Patient 2. The curve at the top shows the whole seizure recorded from the the channel over right fronto-temporal region. In the lower part selected periods (1, 2, and 3) are expanded, and corresponding signals from the left side are shown for comparison. Bottom right: Locations of dipoles for ictal and interictal spikes (grey cluster) and for auditory (AEF) and somatosensory (SEF) evoked fields (white spheres) superimposed on the patient's MRI surface rendering. The Rolandic and Sylvian fissures are highlighted. (Modified from [2])

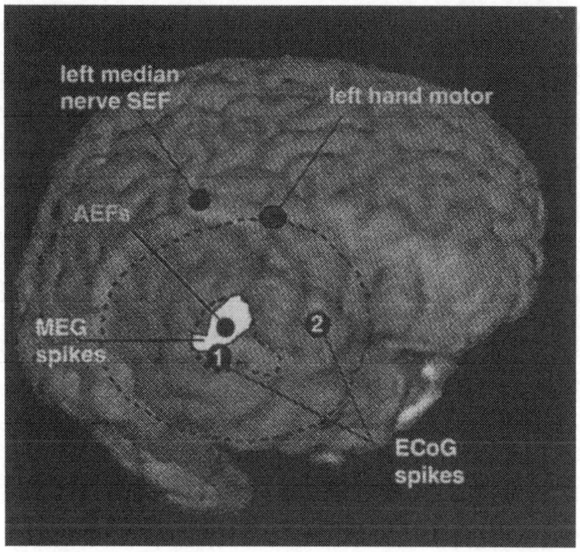

Fig. 4. A cortical surface map of the Patient 3's functional brain anatomy. Preoperative MEG localization of the primary auditory cortex (AEFs) and hand area of the left primary somatosensory cortex (SEF) is indicated by black spots and spike generator area by white area. Peroperative cortical stimulation elicited left hand motor movements (grey spot), and ECoG revealed spikes over a smaller (dashed line, #1) and a larger (dashed line, #2) areas in the temporal lobe. The MEG source agreed completely with smaller area of ECoG; multiple subpial transsection on the intrasylvian planum temporale and the adjoining angular gyrus abolished all epileptic activity. (Modified from [7])

ictal and interictal spikes clustered anterior and lateral to the hand area of the SI, indicating that discharges originated in the face representation area of the right primary motor cortex. The left-sided activation followed the right-sided signals with a constant delay of 22 ms, suggesting a secondary focus in the left frontal area.

Patient 3 [7] is an 8-years old girl who suffers from Landau-Kleffner syndrome. In this syndrome the patients may lose their ability to understand speech after normal initial development, and their EEG often show epileptic spikes. Continuous epileptic spiking in the cortical auditory areas may prevent the patient from proper analysis of auditory stimuli [6]. The ability to use language may be improved if epileptic activity can be dampened.

Figure 4 summarizes the preoperational MEG data and peroperational electrocorticography and electric stimulation data of this child. EcoG picked up epileptic activity from two regions, smaller and larger ones around the supratemporal auditory cortex. The smaller area agreed well with MEG source area, and therefore it was first trans-sected. That procedure managed to stop all the epileptic activity, and no further resections were needed.

Combination of MEG and PET

Positron emission tomography (PET) is widely accepted as a reliable tool for preoperative evaluation of epileptic patients. Combination of PET's spatial accuracy with MEG's excellent temporal resolution might significantly improve the value of preoperative evaluation. In the present ongoing study in co-operation with Turku University Hospital, 10 temporal lobe epilepsy patients, who were candidates for surgical treatment, have been studied with whole-head MEG and PET. In 7 out of 10 patients, the PET and MEG results were in good agreement. In two patients MEG suggested bilateral foci whereas the PET findings suggested a unilateral one. However, even in these two patients the epileptic activity in MEG was clearly stronger in the hemisphere showing significant blood flow changes in PET.

Other Applications of MEG in Neurosurgery

Because of large inter-individual variation in the patterns of cortical sulci, it is difficult to define locations of important functional areas on the basis of anatomy alone. The task is even more difficult if a brain tumour or other lesion has altered the brain structure. With MEG it is possible to reliably and non-invasively locate certain functional areas such as the sensorimotor strip, and to visualize that area with respect to the brain. Recordings of somatosensory evoked magnetic fields agreed with electrocorticographic (ECoG) data in determining the course of the central sulcus [8].

Conclusion

Whole-scalp MEG has proved to be a suitable tool for preoperative evaluation of patients suffering from drug-resistant focal epilepsy. MEG recordings are non-invasive and safe for the subject, and no demanding preparations of the patient are needed before measurement. The MEG recordings may reveal several epileptic foci, and the order of activation can be resolved in millisecond scale. In addition, epileptic cortex can be localized with respect to important functional areas, such as sensorimotor or visual cortices, and these areas can be visualized in a same brain reconstruction. This helps in patient selection and planning of the operation. Moreover, prior MEG localization of epileptic foci and functionally important areas aids in placing the intracranial electrodes to the right place, when needed.

Acknowledgements

These studies were financially supported by the Academy of Finland and by the Sigrid Jusélius Foundation. I thank Prof. Riitta Hari for comments on the manuscript.

References

1. Barth D, Sutherling W, Engel JJ, Beatty J (1982) Neuromagnetic localization of epileptiform spike activity in the human brain. Science 218: 891–894
2. Forss N, Mäkelä JP, Keränen T, Hari R (1991) Trigeminally triggered epileptic hemifacial convulsions. NeuroReport 2: 918–920
3. Hämäläinen M, Hari R, Ilmoniemi R, Knuutila J, Lounasmaa OV (1993) Magnetoencephalography – theory, instrumentation, and applications to noninvasive studies of the working human brain. Rev Mod Phys 65: 413–497
4. Hari R, Ahonen A, Forss N, Granström ML, Hämäläinen M, Kajola M, Knuutila J, Lounasmaa OV, Mäkelä JP, Paetau R, Salmelin R, Simola J (1993) Parietal epileptic mirror focus detected with a whole-head neuromagnetometer. NeuroReport 5: 45–48
5. Modena I, Ricci GB, Barbanera S, Leoni R, Romani GL, Carelli P (1982) Biomagnetic measurements of spontaneous brain activity in epileptic patients. Electroenceph Clin Neurophys 54: 622–628
6. Paetau R, Kajola M, Korman M, Hämäläinen M, Granström ML, Hari R (1991) Landau-Kleffner syndrome: epileptic activity in the auditory cortex. NeuroReport 2: 201–204
7. Paetau R, Appelqvist K, Blomstedt G, Gaily G, Granström ML, Jousmäki V, Lindahl E, Salonen O (1996) Magnetoencephalography (MEG) helps in surgical treatment of acquired epileptic aphasia. In preparation
8. Sutherling W, Crandall P, Darcey T, Becker D, Levesque M, Barth D (1988) The magnetic and electric fields agree with intracranial localizations of somatosensory cortex. Neurology 38: 1705–1714
9. Tiihonen J, Hari R, Kajola M, Nousiainen U, Vapalahti M (1990) Localization of epileptic foci using a large-area magnetometer and functional brain anatomy. Ann Neurol 27: 283–290

Correspondence: N. Forss, M.D., Brain Research Unit, Low Temperature Laboratory, Helsinki University of Technology, Otakaari 3A, FIN-2150 Espoo, Finland.

Acta Neurochir (1997) [Suppl] 68: 85–89

Integration of Functional Brain Mapping in Image-Guided Neurosurgery

A. R. Rezai[1], **A. Y. Mogilner**[1], **J. Cappell**[2], **M. Hund**[2], **R. R. Llinás**[2], and **P. J. Kelly**[1]

Departments of [1]Neurosurgery and [2]Physiology and Neuroscience, New York University Medical Center, New York, NY, USA

Summary

Magnetoencephalographic (MEG) brain mapping was performed in 90 patients with lesions associated with eloquent sensorimotor cortex. The MEG-derived sensorimotor mapping information was utilised for risk analysis and planning. Subsequently, these patients underwent either stereotactic volumetric resection, stereotactic biopsy or non-surgical management of their lesions.

In seventeen patients, the MEG sensorimotor localization was integrated into an operative stereotactic database (consisting of CT, MRI and digital angiography) to be used in an interactive fashion during computer-assisted stereotactic volumetric resection procedures. The spatial relationship between the MEG derived functional anatomy, the structural/radiological anatomy and the pathology could then be viewed simultaneously, thereby affording a safer trajectory and approach. In addition, the real-time availability of functional mapping information in an interactive fashion helped reduce surgical risk and minimise functional morbidity. All of these patients had resection of their lesions with no change in their neurological status.

In conclusion, MEG is a non-invasive, accurate, and reproducible method for pre-operative assessment of patients with lesions associated with eloquent sensory and motor cortex. The interactive use of MEG functional mapping in the operating room can allow for a safer approach and resection of these eloquent cortex lesions.

Keywords: Magnetoencephalography; brain mapping; stereotactic neurosurgery; image-guided neurosurgery.

Introduction

Resection of brain lesions in the vicinity of eloquent cortex, such as sensorimotor or speech cortices, is a formidable task. Accurate preoperative and intraoperative localization of functional cortex is paramount for planning surgical resection with minimum morbidity. Sole reliance on anatomical criteria to localise functional cortex can result in inaccurate identification of cortical areas [20], which may contribute to post-operative morbidity. Traditionally, direct cortical mapping has been used intraoperatively to establish the relationship between eloquent cortex and the lesion. Recent advances in functional imaging have provided clinicians with a variety of non-invasive methods of mapping functional cortex pre-operatively. Magnetoencephalography (MEG) is a noninvasive functional imaging modality that has been demonstrated to localise accurately sensorimotor cortex in normal individuals. The authors are routinely employing MEG for preoperative mapping, and have developed a technique integrating MEG functional imaging data with stereotactic neurosurgery.

Methods

Patient Population

From 1994 to 1996, 90 patients, all of whom harboured lesions in the vicinity of sensorimotor cortex as seen on initial MRI and CT scans, underwent preoperative MEG mapping. Forty-two females and 48 males were studied, ranging in age from 9 to 60 years. There were 65 tumours and 25 arteriovenous malformations studied.

As a test of the reproducibility and precision of MEG mapping, thirty normal adult controls underwent high-resolution MRI scanning and repeated MEG sensorimotor mapping.

MEG Mapping

MEG mapping was performed using a MAGNES 37 channel or dual 37 channel MEG system (Biomagnetic Technologies, Inc. San Diego, CA) located at the Center for Neuromagnetism at NYU Medical Center. At the start of the recording, the three reference points (the left and right preauricular regions and the nasion) defining the MEG head-based coordinate system, as well as two additional reference points on the forehead, were identified using a stylus-type transmitting wand [5, 7, 14, 20]. Somatosensory cortical localization was performed using repetitive tactile stimulation (air-puff or buzzer stimulation) of the digits of the hand, the lips, the face and the toes [9, 14, 15, 25]. Motor mapping was done using a button paradigm involving alternating flexion and extension of the third finger or first toe in response to a visual cue. The evoked responses were averaged and localised into the three dimensional space of the head-based coordinate system using a single dipole model [9, 14, 15, 25, 28].

Immediately following the MEG procedure, the aforementioned MEG reference points were marked with MRI visible Vitamin E markers, and a high-resolution MRI was performed for each patient. The MEG data were then overlaid onto the MRI data both in two dimensions (axial, coronal and sagittal planes) as well as onto three-dimensional reconstructions of the MRI images, thus providing a clear visualization of the location of sensorimotor cortex with respect to the lesion.

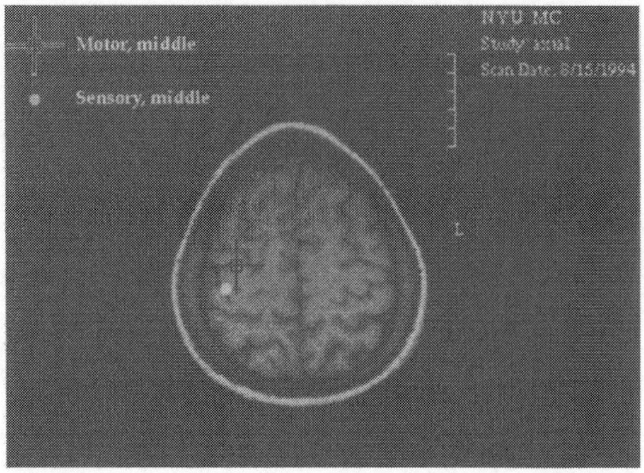

Fig. 1. Normative MEG data: MEG localization of sensorimotor cortex in a normal (28 year old right-handed female) adult. Sensory and motor evoked magnetic fields were recorded in response to tactile stimulation of and motor activity of the left middle finger, respectively. The equivalent magnetic source dipoles were mapped onto MRI scans. These dipoles localise the precentral motor cortex, the postcentral sensory cortex and the central sulcus

Intraoperative Integration

Seventeen patients had their MEG results incorporated into the COMPASS (COMPASS international, Rochester, MN) neurosurgical stereotactic database. This database includes CT, MR, and digital subtraction angiography information and is routinely used for computer-assisted stereotactic volumetric resections [11, 12]. A mathematical vector transformation procedure [20] was used to transform the MEG dipole locations into the corresponding stereotactic coordinates. These transformed MEG dipole sources could then be visualised in an interactive fashion via heads-up display on the operating microscope or on video monitors in the operating room. Additionally, standard intraoperative electrocorticographic monitoring of somatosensory and motor evoked potentials was performed for all patients.

Results

Repeated MEG measurements in the control group revealed highly precise and reproducible mapping of sensorimotor cortex. A typical localization is shown in Fig. 1. The central sulcus can thus be easily identified based on the functional data.

In the 90 patients studied, MEG provided definitive information as to the proximity of the lesion to sensorimotor cortex. This information was then used in the subsequent management of these patients, specifically influencing the decision whether to proceed with lesion resection, biopsy or non-operative management. Figure 2 displays the MRI scans of a patient with a right frontal lobe lesion along with the overlaid MEG motor and sensory sources. Whereas the location of central sulcus may not be obvious based on the MRI alone, the MEG localises the motor cortex to be at the posterior margin of the lesion, and the location of the central sulcus is clearly identifiable.

Interactive MEG guidance provides continuous orientation and localization with respect to the tumour and the surrounding functional and structural anatomy. An example of an interactive MEG-guided computer-assisted volumetric resection is shown in figure 3. In Fig. 3a, a bony trephine with the underlying cortex and tumour is shown in a three-dimensional MRI reconstruction. Cross-sectional representations of the tumour as well as MEG sensorimotor sources at those levels are displayed in this volumetric reconstruction. Figure 3b demonstrates a representative cross-section as it would appear intraoperatively on a monitor or on a heads-up display. None of the patients undergoing this procedure had any permanent neurologic sequelae subsequent to the surgery.

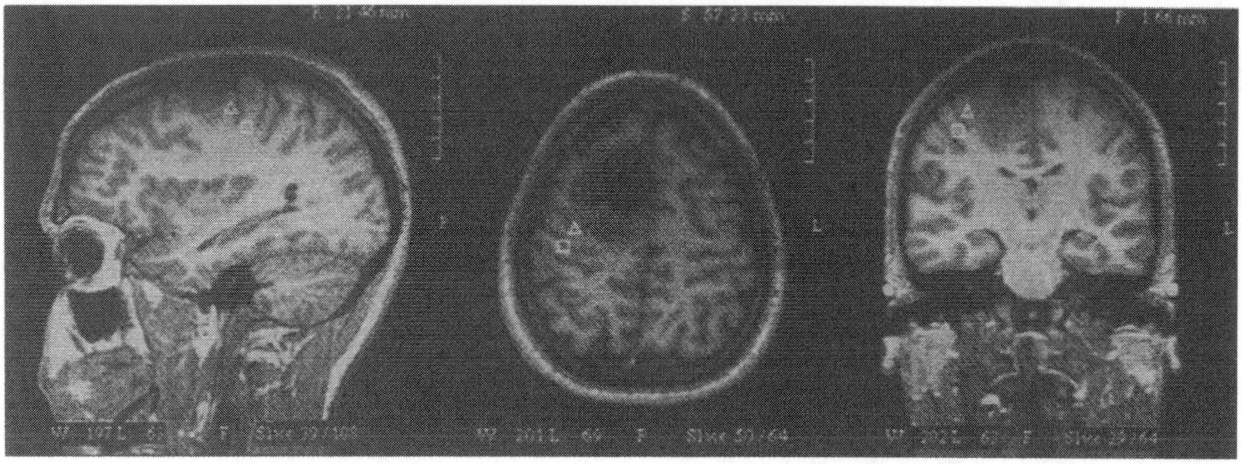

a b c

Fig. 2. (a–c) Patient data: Localization of sensorimotor cortex in an adult with a right frontal lesion. The patient is a 24 year old left-handed male who presented with a 2 year history of focal as well as generalised seizures. Neurological testing revealed no deficits. Imaging studies demonstrated a large, irregularly shaped hypodense lesion in the right frontal lobe. Preoperative MEG mapping was performed revealing index finger motor (triangle) and thumb sensory (square) dipole sources. These sources are shown projected onto sagittal (a), axial (b), and coronal (c) MRI images. On the basis of MEG localization of the central sulcus, the tumour was determined to be immediately anterior and adjacent to, but not involving, the motor cortex

Discussion

Traditionally, preoperative localization of eloquent cortices has been accomplished using structural/anatomical criteria from imaging data (e.g. CT and MRI), as well as via stereotactic atlases based on surface landmarks [2, 21, 26]. There is evidence to suggest, however, that sole reliance upon these methods is inadequate. Large mass lesions have been demonstrated to distort the normal brain anatomy, and cerebral oedema may obscure the usual radiographic gyral/sulcal pattern [2, 4, 10, 18, 21, 23, 24]. Moreover, intraoperative mapping via direct cortical stimulation has demonstrated variability in the functional architecture of the brain [1, 8, 17, 27]. Additionally, human cortical plasticity, i.e. the dynamic reorganization of sensory and motor maps, has been demonstrated following both transient and permanent injuries/alterations in both the central and peripheral nervous system [3, 13, 14, 19, 23].

Functional brain imaging techniques such as PET, fMRI, and MEG, are increasingly being employed in clinical settings [4, 6, 7, 14, 15, 18, 24, 27], each technique having its own particular advantages. PET and fMRI, which reflect metabolic changes, have a long integration time which may be beneficial for higher level activities such as language and complex motor paradigms. Moreover, these modalities can simultaneously detect concurrent activity at multiple sites which can be useful for mapping a distributed brain function. PET, however, is limited by its low temporal resolution (minutes), as well as by its invasive nature, necessitating intravenous injections of radiolabelled substances. Functional MRI is particularly advantageous since it is available at many clinical centres, necessitating only an upgrade to already available conventional MRI equipment [16, 22]. The temporal resolution of functional MRI, however, is currently on the order of seconds, and that of PET in the order of minutes, and thus not suitable for mapping such activity as epileptogenic foci.

Magnetoencephalography (MEG) is entirely non-invasive, and has the additional advantages of high spatial (millimeter) and temporal (millisecond) resolution. Numerous studies have demonstrated the accurate and reproducible localization of sensorimotor cortex using MEG [6, 7, 14, 15, 18, 25]. The authors have been using MEG at their institution for pre-operative mapping and surgical planning since 1993, and to date have performed pre-operative mapping and risk analysis in 90 patients.

The interactive use of MEG information intra-operatively provides a number of benefits. Specifically, it allows for smaller craniotomies and safer approach planning. Furthermore, continuous visualization of anatomy, functional anatomy and pathology allows for more aggressive yet safer resections.

Future applications of this technology include the

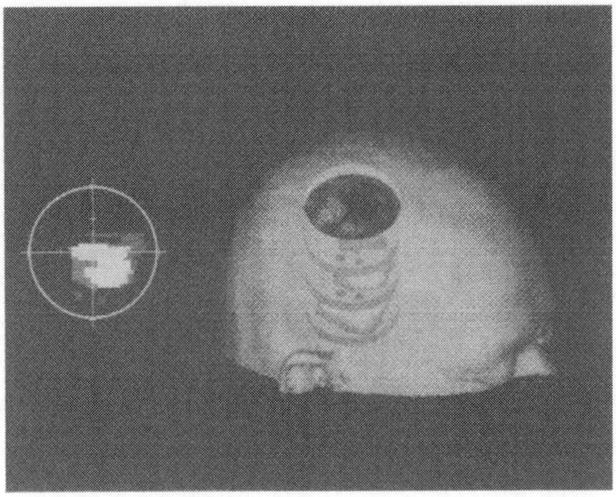

Fig. 3. Interactive MEG Guidance and computer-assisted volumetric resection. Right: A three-dimensional MRI reconstruction of the patient's head is shown. Volumetric cross-sectional levels (1 mm thick) through the tumour are depicted underneath an intraoperative photograph of the tumour and surrounding brain tissue. The MEG source dipoles for motor and sensory cortex are shown on the relevant cross sections as grey circles. Left: A representative sample of the cross sectional data as it appears in the COMPASS stereotactic database. This corresponds to the middle section (right figure part). The circle represents the 1.5 inch diameter bony trephine. The cross-sectional tumour volume derived from the contrast-enhanced CT and T1 MRI with contrast is depicted in white and grey, respectively. The location of the MEG motor and sensory dipoles in stereotactic space are seen as grey squares

integration of MEG data into other image-guided frame-based and frameless systems. Additionally, integrating a variety of different functional imaging modalities into such systems may provide complementary information not obtainable via one modality alone. Thus, the management of lesions associated with eloquent cortex should continue to become safer and more efficacious as these technologies continue to develop.

References

1. Berger MS, Kincaid J, Ojemann GA, *et al* (1989) Brain mapping technique to maximize resection, safety, and seizure control in children with brain tumours. Neurosurgery 25: 786–792
2. Bucholz RD (1993) The central sulcus and surgical planning. AJNR 14: 926–927
3. Cohen L, Pascual-Leone A, Hallet M (1993) Plasticity of cortical motor output organization following deafferentation, cerebral lesion, and skill acquisition. In (eds) Advances in neurology: Electrical and magnetic stimulation of the brain and the spinal cord. Raven, New York, pp 187–201
4. Fried I, Nenov V, Ojemann SG, *et al* (1995) Functional MR and PET imaging of rolandic and visual cortices for neurosurgical planning. J Neurosurg 83: 854–861
5. Gallen CC, Schwartz B, Bucholz RD, *et al* (1995) Presurgical localization of functional cortex using magnetic source imaging. J Neurosurg 82: 988–994
6. Gallen CC, Schwartz B, Reike K (1994) Intrasubject reliability and validity of somatosensory source localization using a large array biomagnetometer. Electroencephalogr Clin Neurophys 90: 145–156
7. Gallen CC, Sobel DF, Waltz T, *et al* (1993) Non-invasive presurgical neuromagnetic mapping of the somatosensory cortex. Neurosurgery 33: 260–268
8. Goldring S, Aras E, Weber PC (1970) Comparative study of sensory input to motor cortex in animals and man. Electroencephalogr Clin Neurophys 29: 537–550
9. Hämalainen H, Kekoni J, Sams M, et al (1990) Human Somatosensory Evoked potentials to mechanical pulses and vibration: Contributions of S1 and S2 somatosensory cortices to P50 and P100 components. Electroencephalogr Clin Neurophys 75: 13–21
10. Iwasaki S, Nakagawa H, Fukusumi A (1991) Identification of pre- and post central gyri on CT and MRI images on the basis of the medullary pattern of cerebral white matter. Radiology 179: 207–213
11. Kelly PJ (1991) Stereotactic resection: General principles. In: Kelly PJ (eds) Tumour stereotaxis. Saunders, Philadelphia pp 292–295
12. Kelly PJ (1991) Tumour stereotaxis. Saunders, Philadelphia
13. Lewine JD, Astur RS, Davis LE, *et al* (1994) Cortical organization in adulthood is modified by neonatal infarct: A case study. Radiology 190: 93–96
14. Mogilner A, Grossman JA, Ribary U, *et al* (1993) Somatosensory cortical plasticity in adult humans revealed by magnetoencephalography. Proc Natl Acad Sci USA 90: 3593–3597
15. Mogilner A, Nomura M, Ribary U, *et al* (1994) Neuromagnetic studies of the lip area of primary somatosensory cortex in humans: evidence for an oscillotopic organization. Exp Br Res 99: 137–147
16. Mueller WM, Yetkin Z, Hammeke T, *et al* (1996) Functional magnetic resonance imaging mapping of the motor cortex in patients with cerebral tumours. Neurosurgery 39: 515–512
17. Ojemann GA (1979) Individual variability in cortical localization of language. J Neurosurg 50: 164–169
18. Orrison WW, Rose DF, Hart BL, *et al* (1992) Noninvasive preoperative cortical localization by magnetic source imaging. Am J Neurorad 13: 1124–1128
19. Ramachandran VS, Rogers-Ramachandran D, Stewart M (1992) Perceptual correlates of massive cortical reorganization. Science 258: 1159–1160
20. Rezai AR, Hund M, Kronberg E, *et al* (1996) The interactive use of magnetoencephalography in stereotactic image-guided neurosurgery. Neurosurgery 39: 92–102
21. Roland PE, Zilles K (1994) Brain atlases – a new research tool. Trends Neurosci 17: 458–467
22. Sanders JA, Lewine JD, Orrison WW (1996) Comparison of primary motor cortex localization using functional magnetic resonance imaging and magnetoencephalography. Human Brain Mapping 4: 47–57
23. Seitz RJ, Yanxiong H, Knorr U, *et al* (1995) Large-scale plasticity of the human motor cortex. Clin Neurosci Neuropath 6: 742–744
24. Sobel DF, Gallen CC, Schwartz BJ, *et al* (1993) Central sulcus localization in humans: comparison of MR anatomic and magnetoencephalograhphic functional methods. Am J Neuroradiol 14: 915–927
25. Suk J, Ribary U, Cappell J, *et al* (1993) Anatomical localization revealed by MEG recording of the human somatosensory system. Electroencephalogr Clini Neurophys 78: 185–196

26. Talairach J, Tournoux P (1993) Referentially oriented cerebral MRI anatomy. Atlas of stereotactic anatomical correlation for grey and white matter. Thieme, Stuttgart
27. Wise R, Hadar U, Howard D, *et al* (1991) Language activation studies with positron emission tomography. In: Symposium. Exploring brain functional anatomy with positron tomography. Wiley, Chichester, pp 218–234
28. Yamamoto T, Williamson SJ, Kaufman L, *et al* (1988) Magnetic localization of neuronal activity in the human brain. Proc Natl Acad Sci USA 85: 8732–8736

Correspondence: A. R. Rezai, M.D., Department of Neurosurgery, New York University Medical Center, New York, NY 10016, USA.

Acta Neurochir (1997) [Suppl] 68: 90–92

Significant Reduction of Seizure Incidence and Increase of Benzodiazepine Receptor Density after Interstitial Radiosurgery in Low-Grade Gliomas

P. C. Warnke, A. Berlis, A. Weyerbrock, and **C. B. Ostertag**

Abteilung Stereotaktische Neurochirurgie, Neurozentrum, Freiburg, Federal Republic of Germany

Summary

Epilepsy is the leading symptom in low grade gliomas. In order to evaluate the effect of interstitial radiosurgery on seizure incidence the authors retrospectively analysed the outcome of 80 patients with temporal grade II astrocytomas and a history of epilepsy. Patients were treated by 125-iodine temporary implants using 60 Gy as reference dose. The dose rate was 9.6 ± 1.6 cGy/h. Median follow-up was 4.1 years. In 20 patients benzodiazepine receptor imaging was performed using single photon emission computed tomography and iomazenil. Treatment with carbamazepine alone led to a significant reduction in seizure incidence with 28% of patients being seizure-free ($p < 0.05$). Interstitial radiosurgery led to a further reduction of seizures rendering 40% of patients seizure-free after 3 months. After 6 months only 21% of patients still had seizures that were refractory to medical treatment ($p < 0.01$). SPECT imaging revealed that all tumours had a significant reduction of benzodiazepine receptors which also applied to the surrounding brain. After interstitial radiosurgery of tumours, receptor density increased in brain adjacent to the tumour (0.68 to 0.94 ratio ipsi to contralateral brain, $p < 0.01$) coincident with significant tumour shrinkage. Thus, in epileptogenic temporal low grade gliomas, interstitial radiosurgery not only reduced the tumour burden but also effectively treated the concomitant epilepsy, resulting in 79% of patients being seizure-free after combined treatment by radiosurgery and anticonvulsive medication.

These results compare favourably to the outcome after resection in lesional epilepsy raising the issue of radiosurgery as a less invasive alternative to open epilepsy surgery.

Keywords: Low grade glioma; epilepsy; interstitial radiosurgery; benzodiazepine receptors.

Introduction

Epileptic seizures are the most common presenting symptom in low grade gliomas before the neuroradiological evaluation reveals a space occupying lesion. In these benign gliomas with a slow – though age related – tendency to grow, symptomatic epilepsy may be the leading and primary symptom for a long time before other neurological deficits evolve. Therefore treatment of symptomatic epilepsy of low grade gliomas is of significant relevance in these patients who otherwise remain functional for a long period. As the tumour itself can be treated effectively by interstitial radiosurgery [7] the question arises as to whether interstitial radiosurgery might also have a positive effect on the concomitant epilepsy. To evaluate the effect of interstitial radiosurgery on seizure incidence the authors examined retrospectively a group of 80 patients with temporal low grade gliomas who presented with epileptic seizures. The last 20 patients of this group were also evaluated by pre- and post-radiosurgery SPECT imaging of central benzodiazepine receptors in the tumour and adjacent brain. The objective of the study was to establish the effect of interstitial radiosurgery on seizure incidence in temporal low grade gliomas.

Material and Methods

80 patients treated between 1986 and 1995 were used for retrospective evaluation of their seizure history. All patients were diagnosed as having astrocytomas grade II of either the right ($N = 34$) or left ($N = 46$) temporal lobe. Diagnosis was established by serial stereotactic biopsy. Epileptic seizures were classified according to the International Classification of the Epilepsy Liga. Anticonvulsant medication was recorded as well as the seizure incidence and, if available, serial screening of serum levels of anticonvulsive drugs.

Patients were treated by interstitial radiosurgery using temporary implants with iodine-125. The reference dose to the tumour margin was 60 Gy and the effective dose rate was 9.6 ± 1.6 cGy/h for all tumours. Mean patient age was 31.6 ± 6.2 years. 48 patients were male, 32 were females. Median follow-up was 4.1 years.

In 20 patients pre- and 3 months post-radiosurgery SPECT studies were performed using iodine-123 labelled iomazenil, a specific ligand to benzodiazepine receptors [1]. Mean activity applied was 110 MBq. Examinations were performed using a single head SPECT system (Siemens orbiter) with a full width half maximum spatial resolution of 8 × 8 mm. Imaging was performed 10 minutes and 2 hours after i.v.injection. Images were obtained with 64 views over 360 degrees to create a 64 × 64 matrix. A Shepp-Logan-Hanning filter was used for image reconstruction.

Statistical analysis was performed as univariate analysis concerning seizure incidence pre- and post-radiosurgery and seizure incidence pre- and post-anticonvulsant medication. The iomazenil binding pre- and post-radiosurgery was also quantitatively evaluated and analysed using both two-way ANOVA and the chi-square test.

Results

Out of the 80 patients who were enrolled into the study 72 presented with seizures which required medical treatment before the initiation of radiosurgery. The most widely used drug in this population cohort was carbamazepine which in 28% of all patients completely abolished seizure activity. Out of the 80 patients 58 received carbamazepine as the primary and only treatment. 12 patients received phenytoin as primary treatment and 10 patients were treated with phenobarbital. The longitudinal analysis of seizure incidence before and after radiosurgical treatment is outlined in Fig. 1. Immediately after explantation of the radioactive source, which took place after a median time lag of 26.2 days, there was a nonsignificant increase in seizure incidence. This increase was attributed to spherical blood-brain barrier breakdown due to the rapid formation of a radionecrotic centre inside the tumour and the concomitant perifocal oedema. Three months after interstitial radiosurgery a significant reduction in seizure incidence without any change in medication was seen, with another 40% of patients being seizure-free. Six months after radiosurgery another significant reduction occurred resulting in only 21% of the total patient population still having seizures. Further follow-up after 12 and 24 months showed no further significant reduction in seizure incidence. Thus, overall, around 20% of the patients with temporal low grade astrocytomas still had seizures after radiosurgery.

The effect of interstitial stereotactic radiosurgery on benzodiazepine receptor expression before and six months after treatment is shown in Fig. 2. All tumours showed significant reduction of benzodiazepine receptor expression compared with contralateral mirror-imaged brain areas. After radiosurgery a small but non-significant increase of benzodiazepine receptor expression could be seen in the tumour itself. The brain adjacent to the tumour which also showed a significant reduction of benzodiazepine receptors before radiosurgery showed a significant increase in ligand binding after radiosurgery, with a concomitant shrinking of the area of low receptor density.

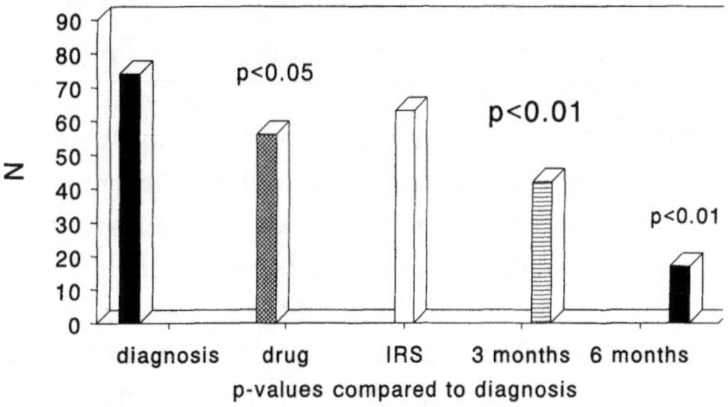

Fig. 1. Longitudinal incidence of seizures in temporal astrocytomas grade II before and after interstitial radiosurgery. The y-axis shows the actual number of patients with seizures. The x-axis depicts the time points at which seizure incidence was evaluated

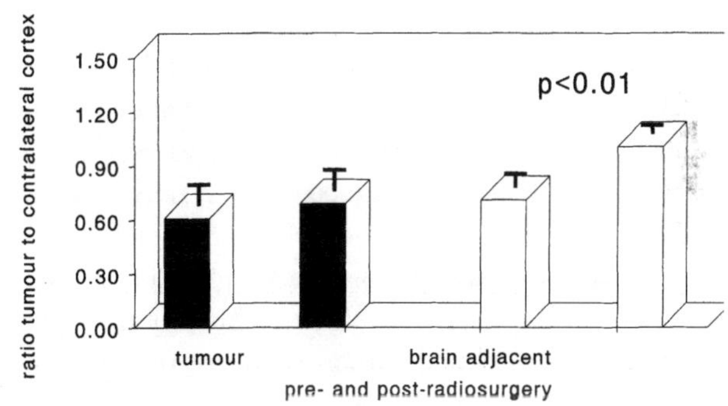

Fig. 2. Imaging of central benzodiazepine receptors in temporal astrocytomas grade II and surrounding brain before and after radiosurgery (6 months). Whereas within the tumour there was no significant effect of interstitial radiosurgery on receptor binding, there was a significant increase in the brain adjacent to the tumour

Discussion

Though limited by the retrospective nature of this study, it could be shown that in epilepsy-prone temporal lobe grade II astrocytomas treated by interstitial radiosurgery a significant reduction of seizure incidence could be achieved. A decrease in seizure incidence using low dose rate implants with a mean dose rate of 9.6 cGy/h and a tumour reference dose of 60 Gy occurs earliest, 3 months after radiosurgery concomitant with tumour shrinking. A further decrease in seizure incidence could be seen six months after interstitial radiosurgery whereas longer follow-up did not show any further reduction in seizure activity. Although all patients were also on anticonvulsive medication, drug treatment contributed only a little to the overall decrease in seizure incidence as carbamazepine treatment alone resulted in a mere 28% of patients being seizure-free whereas interstitial radiosurgery significantly improved outcome by reducing the percentage of patients still having seizures six months after radiosurgery to only 21%. Thus the main contribution towards relief from epilepsy in temporal low grade astrocytomas came from the radiosurgical procedure itself. Earlier reports with much lower numbers of patients have hinted already at the beneficial effect of interstitial radiosurgery on symptomatic epilepsy in low grade gliomas [10] and experimental as well as clinical work has shown the efficacy of radiosurgery using linear accelerators on epileptic foci [2, 3, 5]. However, the mechanism by which seizure incidence is reduced or seizures are abolished remains unknown. In analogy to surgical resection of epileptic foci, one could speculate that the creation of radionecrosis and the necrotizing of the epileptic focus may be responsible for the effect of interstitial radiosurgery on the patient's epilepsy [4]. Furthermore, as the authors could show by SPECT imaging, the shrinking of the tumour volume as induced by interstitial radiosurgery leads to a re-expression of central benzodiazepine receptors in the brain adjacent to the tumour especially in the overlying cortex. This might be the result of a re-established normal ion homeostasis in the extracellular space which was previously disturbed by the tumour.

Overall the results of interstitial radiosurgery in temporal low grade gliomas in the control of epilepsy compare favourably with the results of classical surgical resection of these epileptogenic tumours [6, 8, 9]. With the use of advanced imaging techniques, more and more temporal epilepsy syndromes which are subjected to surgery turn out to be truly lesional epilepsies and, with the demonstrated efficacy of interstitial radiosurgery in epileptogenic low grade gliomas, radiosurgery alone may be an attractive alternative treatment for lesional epilepsy in an even more refined and less invasive way than classical resection.

References

1. Abadie P, Baron JC, Bisserbe JC, Boulenger JP, Rioux P, Travère JM, Barré L, Petit-Taboué MC, Zarifian E (1992) Central benzodiazepine receptors in human brain: estimation of regional B_{max} and K_D values with positron emission tomography. Eur J Pharmacol 213: 107–115
2. Barcia Salorio JL, Vanaclocha V, Cerda M, Roldan P (1985) Focus irradiation in epilepsy. Experimental study in the cat. Appl Neurophysiol 48: 152
3. Barcia Salorio JL, Roldan P, Hernandez G, Lopez Gomez L (1985) Radiosurgical treatment of epilepsy. Appl Neurophysiol 48: 400–403
4. Cahan LD, Engel J (1986) Surgery for epilepsy: a review. Acta Neurol Scand 73: 551–560
5. Heikkinen ER, Konnov B, Melnikov L, Yalynych N, Zubkov YN, Garmashov YA, Pak VA (1989) Relief of epilepsy by radiosurgery of cerebral arteriovenous malformations. Stereotact Funct Neurosurg 53: 157–166
6. Kirkpatrick PJ, Honavar M, Janota I, Polkey CE (1993) Control of temporal lobe epilepsy following en bloc resection of low-grade tumors. J Neurosurg 78: 19–25
7. Kreth FW, Faist M, Warnke PC, Roßner R, Volk B, Ostertag CB (1995) Interstitial radiosurgery of low-grade gliomas. J Neurosurg 82: 418–429
8. Packer RJ, Sutton LN, Patel KM, Duhaime AC, Schiff S, Weinstein SR, Gaillard WD, Conry JA, Schut L (1994) Seizure control following tumor surgery for childhood cortical low-grade gliomas. J Neurosurg 80: 998–1003
9. Patrick S, Berg A, Spencer SS (1995) EEG and seizure outcome after epilepsy surgery. Epilepsia 36: 236–240
10. Rossi GF, Scerrati M, Roselli R (1985) Epileptogenic cerebral low-grade tumors: Effect of interstitial stereotactic irradiation on seizures. Appl Neurophysiol 48: 127–132

Correspondence: Dr. P. Warnke, Abteilung Stereotaktische Neurochirurgie, Neurozentrum, Breisacher Str. 64, D-79106 Freiburg, Federal Republic of Germany.

Acta Neurochir (1997) [Suppl] 68: 93–99

Functional Neurosurgery Aided by Use of an Electronic Brain Atlas

T. T. Yeo[1] and **W. L. Nowinski**[2]

[1] Department of Neurosurgery, Tan Tock Seng Hospital, Singapore and [2]Institute of Systems Science, National University of Singapore, Singapore

Summary

The authors present their experience in the use of an atlas-based computer system for preoperative functional neurosurgery planning and postoperative analysis. It has also some potential for intraoperative support. The system is based on a deformable electronic version of "Atlas of Stereotaxy of the Human Brain" by Schaltenbrand and Wahren. This atlas is used for interactive segmentation and labelling of clinical data in two- and three dimensions, and for definition of stereotactic targets. The Schaltenbrand-Wahren atlas microseries are digitized, enhanced, segmented, labelled, aligned and organized into atlas volumes. They are mutually preregistered, and three-dimensional models of the structures are constructed. The atlas may be interactively registered with an actual patient's data. A computer system is developed which provides data interpolation, reformatting, registration, visualization, navigation, mensuration and path display and editing in two- and three dimensions. The system increases the accuracy of target definition, reduces the time of planning and the time of the procedure itself. It also constitutes a research platform for the construction of more advanced neurosurgery supporting tools and brain atlases.

Keywords: Brain atlas; functional neurosurgery; microelectrodes; registration.

Introduction

Microelectrode studies have been carried out in the human brain to help the neurosurgeon localize brain sites to be manipulated for the control of movement disorders, epilepsy, chronic pain and psychiatric illness. In the traditional approach, indirect measurements based on the AC-PC line are used to define the target. Deformable brain atlases can also be useful for interactive segmentation and labelling of clinical data [13]. The authors have constructed a multiple brain atlas database followed by the development of the atlas-based neuroimaging system [3–7]. This neuroimaging system provides: interactive 3D atlas-data registration; 3D display and real-time manipulation of cerebral structures; continuous navigation in the multiple atlas-data space; 2D, 2.5, and 3D presentation; anatomical indexing; image processing; volume interpolation and reformatting; 3D quantification of structures; file handling and conversion. The combined anatomical index contains about 1000 structures per hemisphere, and over 400 sulcal patterns. This neuroimaging system is extended here for preoperative functional neurosurgery planning, intraoperative support and postoperative analysis.

Methods and Materials

The atlas-based functional neurosurgery planning procedure is shown schematically in Fig. 1. The actual patient's data is first reformatted, if not acquired in the intercommissural plane, and then registered with a deformable electronic brain atlas based on the Talairach global registration (i.e. proportional grid system transformation) [11]. The accuracy of registration within a region of interest can later be enhanced by using any local landmarks. After completing the registration procedure, the neurosurgeon is able to navigate in the atlas-data space, as well as to plan the target and the entry point(s) in two- and three dimensions.

Electronic Brain Atlas

A number of print brain atlases are available, such as Schaltenbrand and Bailey [9], Schaltenbrand and Wahren [10], Talairach and Tournoux [11], Referentially Oriented Talairach and Tournoux [12], Afshar-Watkins-Yip [1], Van Buren and Borke [14], Andrew and Watkins [2], Ono-Kubik-Abernathey [8]. The print atlases have several limitations including static knowledge; print representation not suitable for electronic handling, processing and storing; static presentation and no means of atlas-to-data registration. On the other hand, electronic brain atlases are more convenient and flexible to use. They can also provide

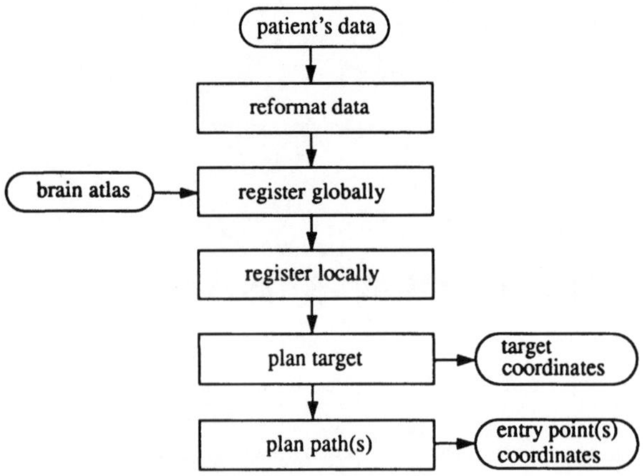

Fig. 1. Atlas-based neurosurgery planning: boxes denote operations and ovals represent data

additional and powerful features not available in the print atlases.

Ciemed* has developed electronic versions of the classic Thieme brain atlases: Talairach and Tournoux, Referentially Oriented Talairach and Tournoux, Schaltenbrand and Wahren, and Ono-Kubik-Abernathey [3, 5–7]. They feature high quality data, fully segmented and labelled structures, mutually preregistered atlases, registration with actual patient's data, three-dimensional extensions, among others. These atlases are also available on CD-ROM distributed by Thieme [4].

In order to define stereotactic targets, the authors use the "Atlas of Stereotaxy of the Human Brain" by Schaltenbrand and Wahren [10]. The Schaltenbrand-Wahren (SW) brain atlas is constructed based on 111 brains. It contains photographic plates of macroscopic and microscopic sections. The anatomical index has about 600 structures. The microscopic myelin-stained sections show in great detail cerebral deep structures.

The original microseries' photographic plates are digitized, aligned and organized into atlas volumes, i.e. stacks of atlas images corresponding to a given hemisphere [6]. The electronic images are extended in comparison to the print plates such that they cover both hemispheres (compare Fig. 2). The axial and coronal plates are mirrored along the AC-PC line, and the sagittal plates are replicated along the midsagittal plane. Three atlas volumes are built:

1. SW coronal: Brain LXVIII, right hemisphere (20 sections)
2. SW sagittal: Brain LXXVIII, left hemisphere (17 + 17 sections)
3. SW axial: Brain LXXVIII, right hemisphere (20 sections).

The SW overlays are also digitized, and then segmented (contoured), labelled, and preregistered with the SW atlas volumes. All structures on the microseries are contoured by manually tracing the digitized overlays. Each contour is assigned a label (or labels) consistent with the original overlays. The contours are suitably mirrored and replicated to cover both hemispheres. These contours are also utilized to reconstruct three-dimensional (3D) models of the SW structures which are useful for analysis and visualization of shapes as well as for neurosurgery planning [3]. All three SW atlas volumes are mutually preregistered such that any point in the SW stereotactic space can simultaneously be displayed on the axial, coronal and sagittal planes. The preregistered SW orthogonal images can be visualized together as the triplanar. The triplanar and 3D SW models are also preregistered and can be displayed jointly (see Fig. 2).

All the atlases are fully segmented and labelled in two- and three dimensions. The segmented atlas structures can be displayed as images with superimposed contours, contours alone or 3D models. The contours are useful for atlas-to-data registration since they do not obscure the actual patient's data (compare Fig. 3). The contours, atlas labels and 3D models are deformation independent. By conforming the atlases to the actual patient's data, this data can be segmented and labelled in two- and three dimensions in real-time.

Functional Neurosurgery Supporting System

The atlas-based computer system for functional neurosurgery supports preoperative planning, intraoperative procedures and postoperative analysis. Preoperative planning includes registration in multiple directions, target definition and target mensuration. The stereotactic path can be displayed and edited in two- and three dimensions.

The system facilitates postoperative evaluation of the patient. It displays the actual patient's data as the axial, coronal, sagittal views and the triplanar supported by continuous navigation in the atlas-data space and high accuracy mensuration. It can also be used off-line to collect and analyze the functional data

* Ciemed: Center for Information-enhanced Medicine, a joint center between the Institute of Systems Science in Singapore and Johns Hopkins University, Baltimore.

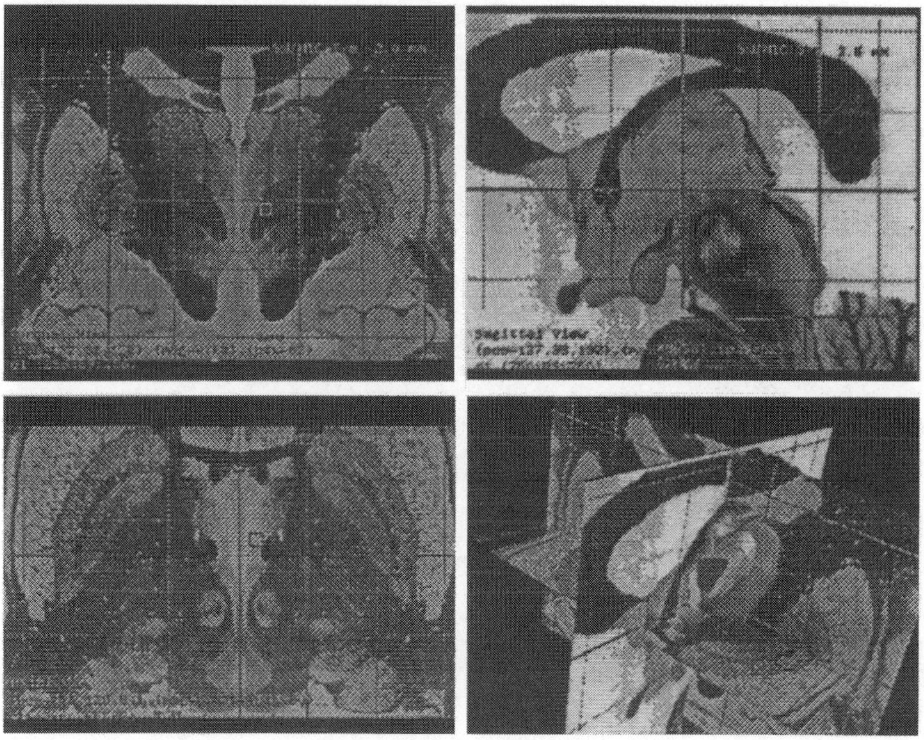

Fig. 2. Electronic Schaltenbrand-Wahren brain atlas: the axial (bottom-left), coronal (top-left) and sagittal (top-right) sections covering both hemispheres. Bottom-right: the SW triplanar the original of which corresponds to the location of the box cursor on the orthogonal sections; 3D thalamic structures preregistered with the SW triplanar

in order to construct more advanced tools and new brain atlases.

Load data and atlas. The atlas-based system inputs the actual patient's data, interpolates it and provides the neurosurgeon with its axial, coronal and sagittal views. Moreover, the triplanar view shows a 3D image of all three planes, along with 3D SW structures. These views are smoothly and continuously resizeable to allow the neurosurgeon to direct attention to a particular view.

The SW atlas volumes can be displayed individually or superimposed on the actual patient's data. The atlas images are overlayed onto the patient's data with a user controlled degree of blending. The 3D SW structures can also be presented individually or jointly with the data. The neurosurgeon may select any subset of these structures for displaying and real-time manipulation.

Register. The brain atlas constitutes a model suitable for data quantification. The atlas is conformed to an individual patient's brain scan by means of 3D landmark-based registrations [3]. The placement of landmarks is interactive, and the atlas deformation is a real-time operation. The SW brain atlas volumes, contours, triplanar and 3D models are mutually preregistered, and the registration of a single atlas volume with the actual patient's data automatically registers all other atlas volumes, contours and 3D models with this data. The atlas plates are piecewise-linearly warped and overlayed onto the data images. The contours are warped in a similar way and the 3D atlas structures are piecewise-linearly transformed to be visualized in relation to the triplanar (compare Figs. 3 and 4).

Measure and reformat. The position of a point target can be measured in the SW stereotactic space [10]. The locations of the reference axes in this space are defined by the registration grid displayed and editable on all three orthogonal views and in 3D (compare Fig. 4). High accuracy mensuration allows the neurosurgeon to set the coordinate system, get target coordinates and measure distances (compare Fig. 5).

Mensuration of angles is provided on all 2D views and is associated with data reformatting. The user can interactively measure the angle between the horizontal line and AC-PC line on the sagittal view, as well as the angles between the vertical line and longitudinal cerebral fissure on the coronal and sagittal views, and suitably reformat the data.

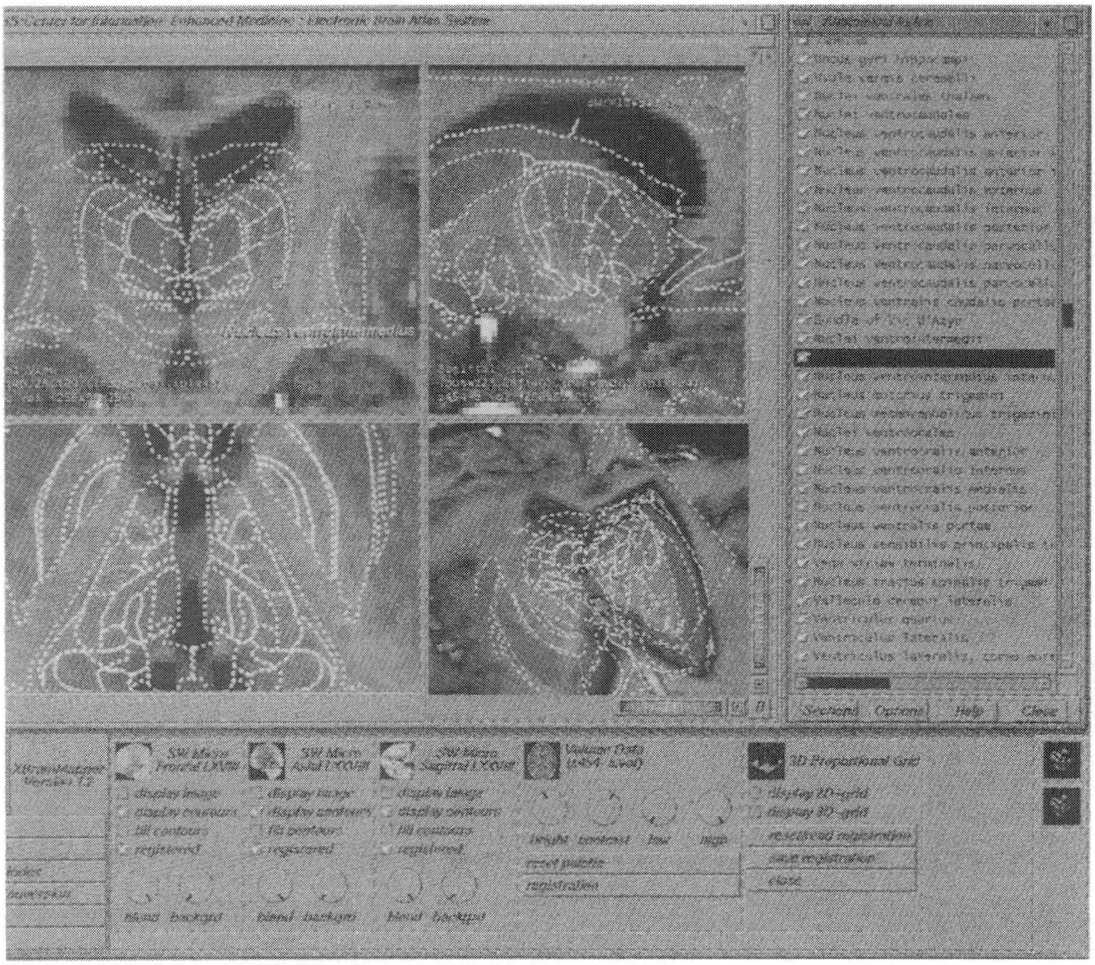

Fig. 3. System user interface. Top-left: main work window with four smoothly and continuously resizeable views containing orthogonal data sections registered with the SW contours, and the atlas/data triplanar (note the SW contours are also displayed on the data triplanar). Right: scrollable anatomical index with the selected Vim nucleus highlighted. Bottom: scrollable control panel providing multiple atlas and data operations

Path display and edit. The location of the stereotactic path is shown in relation to the atlas-segmented actual patient anatomy. The path is displayed and manipulated in 3D, and as its projections on the orthogonal views are drawn. The lists of structures encountered along the path are given for all three orientations. The 3D mono or stereo display of the path along with the actual data triplanar (with superimposed contours) and 3D SW structures assist the neurosurgeon in editing the entry point and enhancing the path.

Results

The atlas-based computer system providing operations as discussed in the previous section is developed, and its clinical validation is underway. Figure 3 shows the complete user interface with its main components: work window with four views, anatomical index, and control panel. The atlas-defined target structure (in this case the nucleus ventrointermedius externa) is contoured on the axial, coronal and sagittal planes, as well as on the triplanar.

By clicking on a 2D structure, its name is highlighted in the anatomical index, and the structure is contoured on all three orthogonal planes and on the triplanar (see the Vim nucleus in Fig. 3). By pointing to any 2D or 3D structure, its anatomical name is displayed.

The data and atlases are explored by means of continuous navigation [5]. The neurosurgeon is able to continuously navigate in the atlas-data space such that

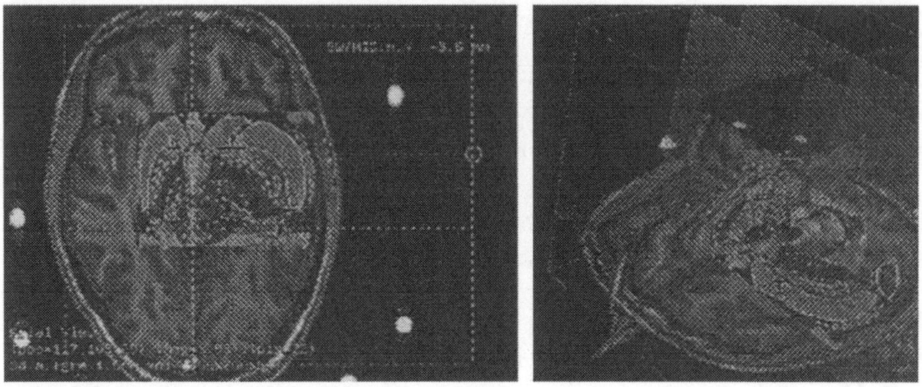

Fig. 4. Superimposition of the SW atlas onto an MRI data. Left: the axial view with the Talairach proportional grid. The SW atlas images, contours and 3D models (see on the right) are elongated laterally (compare e.g. the putamen) and dorsally to illustrate deformation capabilities. Any corner of the proportional grid is a movable landmark. When a corner is pointed to, the cursor turns into a circle. The neurosurgeon can then drag these circles to fit the grid to the data. Right: the reference planes along with the 3D bounding box in the 3D view containing the data/atlas triplanar and 3D SW models

any structure(s) from the anatomical index can be traced continuously in this space. The continuous navigation, fully controlled by the mouse buttons, includes continuous resizing of the views in the work window, continuous scaling of images in each view while maintaining the aspect ratio, continuous resizing of 3D structures and the triplanar, and continuous atlas – actual patient's data blending. Interactive operations are provided to rotate and move the triplanar or 3D structures in real-time.

The superimposition of the SW atlas onto an actual patient's data is shown in Fig. 4. The system displays the Talairach proportional grid in the orthogonal views and the reference planes along with the 3D bounding box in the 3D view. Any corner of the proportional grid is a movable landmark. By dragging these landmarks, the neurosurgeon conforms the atlas to the data.

High accuracy mensuration supported by continuous navigation allows the neurosurgeon to continuously resize the images. This way the neurosurgeon can magnify the image and measure it with high, subpixel accuracy.

Mensuration works in two modes: distance or readout. The readout measures the distance from the set origin, as well as giving the lateral, anterior and ventral coordinates of the target, see Fig. 5. The origin is set by the user, and it can be the intercommissural midpoint, anterior commissure, or user defined. In the latter case, for instance, by setting the microelectrode tip as a user defined origin, the neurosurgeon can easily measure the distances between the tip and its surrounding structures.

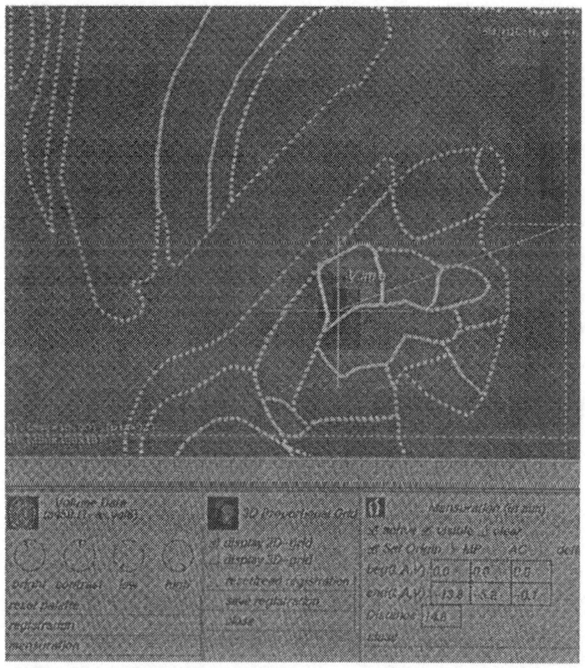

Fig. 5. Postoperative mensuration of the location of an electrode implanted in the right thalamus. Top: MRI image with the superimposed contours (the Vim.e nucleus is highlighted and labelled) and Talairach grids are highly magnified, and the target (marked by the cross) is measured with subpixel accuracy. Bottom-right: mensuration control panel segment. The intercommissural midpoint (MP) is set as the origin. The distance to the target, and the target lateral, anterior and ventral (L, A, V) coordinates are displayed

Discussion

The system provides the neurosurgeon with a very flexible and powerful display, and continuous yet simple navigation in the atlas-data space. The atlas and data are presented in the 2D and 3D views which are smoothly and continuously resizeable to allow the neurosurgeon directing attention to a particular detail in a chosen view.

The authors' registration procedure has numerous advantages, and is superior to MRI guided definition as well as traditional indirect measurements based on the AC-PC line. The scaling is done not only along the AC-PC distance but also dorso-ventrally and laterally. The registration landmarks can be determined on any of the axial, coronal and sagittal planes. This gives the neurosurgeon more flexibility in selecting clearly visible landmarks, increasing in this way the accuracy of registration. Three different, mutually preregistered SW atlas volumes are conformed to the actual patient's data enhancing the accuracy of target definition. The atlases are extended to cover both hemispheres and can also be used for planning bilateral cases. The deformation of images, contours and 3D objects is real-time, so the neurosurgeon can smoothly drag any landmarks and observe immediately the results. In addition, the registration can be supported by some other atlases preregistered with the SW atlas [6, 7]. The current user interface supports the placement of landmarks for the Talairach proportional grid system transformation. However any set of landmarks can be used with this approach, e.g. to compensate for the width of the third ventricle or internal capsule. The presentation of the contours on the orthogonal planes and on the triplanar and 3D shaded mono or stereo display of structures along with the stereotactic path facilitates neurosurgery planning.

Several factors limit the overall accuracy of atlas-to-data registration and target definition. They can be divided into two groups: inaccuracies of the print atlases, and inaccuracies of the electronic data and operations. The print atlas plates are sparse in some regions, the slice distance ranging from 0.5 mm to 4 mm. The SW axial plates are not exactly in the AC-PC plane. The shapes of the 3D models reconstructed from the original SW contours are convoluted and sometimes unrealistic. The sources of inaccuracy of the electronic version include digitization, image mirroring, construction of atlas volumes, contouring, preregistration of contours and preregistration of the atlas volumes with the overlays.

The system can be used intraoperatively to facilitate anatomico-physiological correlation. The intraoperative support displays the actual position of the microelectrode, constructs and draws a functional map, and assists the neurosurgeon to plan the insertion of the next microelectrode tracks.

The position of the microelectrode tip is displayed in 3D as well as on the orthogonal views. This gives the neurosurgeon a better correlation between the tip and its surrounding anatomy, and especially the location of some critical structures e.g. the optic tract during pallidotomy, the damage of which has to be avoided. By setting the tip as a user defined origin, the distances between the tip and its surrounding structures can be easily measures. The procedure usually requires insertion of multiple microelectrode tracks to fully map the area neurophysiologically. The functional map correlated with atlas-segmented actual patient anatomy guides the insertion of the next microelectrode track(s).

The system can also be used off-line to study postoperative cases (compare e.g. Fig. 5), as well as to collect and analyze the functional data in order to construct new brain atlases. The postoperative MRI scan contains the actual (functional) target which can be compared with the planned (atlas-derived) target. This information can be used for the enhancement of the registration procedure.

In summary, the atlas-based functional neurosurgery supporting system increases the accuracy of target definition, reduces the time of planning and the time of the procedure itself, and constitutes a research platform for the construction of more advanced neurosurgery supporting tools and brain atlases.

References

1. Afshar E, Watkins ES, Yap JC (1978) Stereotactic atlas of the human brainstem and cerebellar nuclei. Raven, New York
2. Andrew J, Watkins ES (1969) A stereotaxic atlas of the human thalamus and adjacent structures. A variability study. Williams and Wilkins, Baltimore
3. Nowinski WL, Fang A, Nguyen BT, Raphel JK, Jagannathan L, Raghavan R, Bryan RN, Miller G: Multiple brain atlas database and atlas-based neuroimaging system. J Image Guided Surg to appear
4. Nowinski WL, Bryan RN, Raghavan R (eds) (1996) The electronic clinical brain atlas: three dimensional navigation of the human brain. Thieme, Stuttgart
5. Nowinski WL, Fang A, Nguyen BT, Raghavan R, Bryan RN, Miller J (1995) Talairach-Tournoux/Schaltenbrand-Wahren based electronic brain atlas system. Lecture Notes in Computer Science, Vol 905. Springer, Proc. CVRMed'95, pp 257–261
6. Nowinski WL, Fang A, Nguyen BT (1995) Schaltenbrand-Wahren/Talairach-Tournoux brain atlas registration. Proc. SPIE Medical Imaging 1995: Image Display, San Diego, USA, Feb 1995, SPIE Vol 2431, pp 126–136

7. Nowinski WL, Raphel JK, Nguyen BT (1996) Atlas-based identification of cortical sulci. Proc. SPIE Medical Imaging 1996: Image Display, Newport Beach, USA, Feb. 1996, SPIE Vol 2707, pp 64–74
8. Ono M, Kubik S, Abernathey CD (1990) Atlas of the cerebral sulci. Thieme, Stuttgart
9. Schaltenbrand G, Bailey W (1959) Atlas of stereotaxy of the human brain. Thieme, Stuttgart
10. Schaltenbrand G, Wahren W (1977) Atlas of stereotaxy of the human brain. Thieme, Stuttgart
11. Talairach J, Tournoux P (1988) Co-planar stereotactic atlas of the human brain. Thieme, Stuttgart
12. Talairach J, Tournoux P (1993) Referentially oriented cerebral MRI anatomy. Atlas of stereotaxic anatomical correlations for grey and white matter. Thieme, Stuttgart
13. Toga AW, Mazziotta JC (1996) Brain mapping. The methods. Academic Press, San Diego
14. Van Buren JM, Borke RC (1972) Variations and connections of the human thalamus. Springer, Berlin Heidelberg New York

Correspondence: Dr. Wieslaw L. Nowinski, Center for Information Enhanced Medicine, Ciemed, Institute of Systems Science, National University of Singapore, Kent Ridge, 119597 Singapore.

Acta Neurochir (1997) [Suppl] 68: 100–104

Gene Transfer of Suicide Genes for the Treatment of Malignant Gliomas: Efficacy, Limitations, and Perspectives for a Combined Immunotherapy

S. Benedetti[1], **F. Di Meco**[2], **B. Pollo**[3], **M. G. Bruzzone**[4], **N. Cirenei**[1], **R. Spreafico**[5], **C. L. Solero**[2], **G. Broggi**[2], **St. Di Donato**[1], and **G. Finocchiaro**[1]

[1] Department of Biochemistry and Genetics, [2]Department of Neurosurgery, [3]Department of Neuropathology, [4]Department of Neuroradiology, and [5]Department of Experimental Neurophysiology, Istituto Nazionale Neurologico "Carlo Besta", Milano, Italy

Summary

The potential of gene therapy strategies for malignant gliomas that are based on retroviral-mediated transfer of a "suicide gene" such as Herpes Simplex Virus-thymidine kinase HSV-tk and subsequent treatment by a prodrug (ganciclovir, for example), has been emphasized by the promising results obtained by several groups. However, further experimental data as well as preliminary clinical results indicate that the low efficiency of retroviral-mediated gene transfer *in vivo* as well as difficulties for the diffusion of the prodrug inside the tumour mass can limit the efficacy of this form of gene therapy.

To achieve a more effective limitation of tumour growth other approaches may be combined with the "suicide gene" strategy and the enhancement of the immunological response to the tumour by cytokine gene transfer is prominent among these approaches. The authors' experiments in nude mice confirm the antineoplastic role of IL-4 and encourage testing the effects of the simultaneous transfer of IL-4 and HSV-tk genes in immunocompetent animals.

Keywords: Malignant gliomas; gene therapy; suicide gene; ganciclovir; retrovirus; interleukin-4.

Retroviral-Mediated Transfer of a Suicide Gene

The expression of the Herpes Simplex Virus thymidine kinase (HSV-tk) gene can make tumour cells sensitive to the nucleoside analogue ganciclovir (GCV). GCV phosphorylation by HSV-tk and by endogenous kinases causes the formation of GCV triphosphate which will compete with GTP during DNA synthesis. The incorporation of GCV triphosphate will stop the further elongation of DNA, and kill cells that are actively cycling, such as neoplastic cells. HSV-tk gene transfer and GCV treatment should therefore be able to selectively kill neoplastic cells in the brain, since these cells are actively growing in an environment of post-mitotic cells. A further contribution to the selectivity of this therapeutic system is by the use of retroviruses as vectors for gene delivery, since the DNA deriving from reverse transcriptase-mediated transcription of viral RNA will only integrate into actively dividing cells. Thus, the toxic effects of HSV-tk-metabolized GCV should only affect tumour cells and not the surrounding tissue.

Several groups have reported eradication of established gliomas by retroviral transduction *in vivo* of the HSV-tk gene and by subsequent GCV treatment [1, 8, 10]. On this basis, a phase I clinical trial in patients with glioblastoma multiforme has been performed in the US. The preliminary results of this trial as well as other pre-clinical experiments, have suggested that this novel therapy might be limited by the low-efficiency of *in vivo* gene transfer [7, 15].

The authors evaluated the therapeutic potential of the treatment with the Herpes Simplex Virus thymidine kinase (HSV-tk) gene and GCV in killing experimental rat gliomas grafted in the brain of Sprague-Dawley rats. Rats were anaesthetised, and 4×10^4 C6 cells (C6 is a highly malignant cell line derived from a rat glioblastoma) alone or mixed with the same number of viral producer cells were injected into the left striatum.

Two sets of experiments were performed to compare the efficacy of in vitro and in vivo transfer of the HSV-tk gene in tumour cells, inoculating either C6 cells selected in vitro for HSV-tk expression (C6.SBA cells) or mixtures of C6 and HSV-tk retroviral producer cells (SBA cells) in rat brain [6]. Even if rats injected with C6/SBA mixtures and treated by GCV survived longer than controls, the difference was not statistically significant.

This result may, at least partially, be caused by the low *in vivo* efficiency of retroviral-mediated transduction of the therapeutic gene. Recent *in vitro* experiments, based on the identification of antibiotic-resistant cells after replating cells from a tumour transduced *in vivo*, indicated that not more than 10% of neoplastic cells had been reached by the retroviral particles [16]. Data from other laboratories were in the same range [7]. To increase transduction efficiency adenoviruses are presently the most attractive candidates, since they are more stable than retroviruses and can be obtained in very high concentrations: titres of 10^{10}–10^{11} pfu/ml can be reached while for retroviruses titres do not go beyond 10^7.

The poor diffusion of GCV into the tumour mass might also be a limiting factor for this form of gene therapy. This is well explained by the observation that although GCV treatment of tumours obtained from C6 cells previously engineered to express HSV-tk (C6.SBA cells) caused a significant prolongation of rat survival [3], these tk+ tumours could not be completely eradicated. Interestingly, C6.SBA cells, replated after *in vivo* growth and GCV treatment, retained GCV sensitivity *in vitro*. This experiment suggests that an impaired diffusion of the drug into the tumour, rather than mutations or inactivations of HSV-tk, are responsible for the lack of a cure of HSV-tk tumours. One way to deal with such a limited diffusion is suggested by the possibility of administering GCV more directly either through reservoirs that are communicating directly with tumour cavities or through drug releasing devices, named "wafers" [17].

Bystander Effect and Immunological Responses Against the Tumour

To have a more complete picture of the features related with the HSV-tk/GCV system for the treatment of malignant gliomas one should also consider other factors that might enhance the efficacy of this system. These factors are part of the so-called bystander effect, the phenomenon by which HSV-tk negative tumour cells nearby HSV-tk-positive cells are also killed by GCV administration [8]. Gap junctional intercellular communication (GJIC) seems to be one component of this effect. Gap-junctions are inter-cellular channels constituted by juxta-position of connexons. Each connexon is constituted by six units of connexins, membrane proteins with different tissue-specificity that are characterized by the presence of four membrane-spanning domains, highly conserved among different species and in different tissues, and by a cytoplasmic tail [4]. GJIC allows the passage of GCV-triphosphate from tk-positive to tk-negative contiguous cells [11].

The authors previously confirmed that *in vivo* delivery of the HSV-tk gene and GCV treatment can restrain the growth of U-87 gliomas in nude mice and investigated some of the molecular features of the bystander effect in this model [6]. This data suggested that the release of apoptotic vesicles caused by GCV-mediated death of glioma cells can co-operate with the presence of gap-junctions to spread GCV-triphosphate to surrounding cells and the present investigation continues into whether the combined transfer of connexins and HSV-tk genes is a way to increase the efficacy of GCV administration.

Immunological reactions linked to GCV-induced tumour death might also have a role in the generation of the bystander effect and "combination" therapies, attempting to enhance such a role, have recently been proposed [2]. These approaches are based on the contemporaneous delivery of HSV-tk and cytokine genes to the tumour. The combined transfer of HSV-tk and interleukin-2 genes, for instance, allowed the development of a systemic anti-tumoural immunity, associated with the presence of tumour-specific $CD8^+$ T lymphocytes [21], against challenges of parental tumour cells inoculated at distant sites. On the contrary, no enhancement of tumour eradication was observed by adding the IL-2 gene in the HSV-tk vector used for the transduction of 9L gliomas [15], a finding that could be related partly to the low expression of the p55 subunit of the IL-2 receptor in gliomas.

Interleukin 4 (IL-4) is a cytokine whose anti-tumour effects have been described in different tumours [18, 19]. In particular, Yu *et al.* [23] observed a significant growth inhibition of U-87 human gliomas inoculated subcutaneously and intracerebrally in athymic nude mice in association with an IL-4 secreting cell line. More recently, Wei *et al.* [22] demonstrated the higher therapeutic efficacy of the intratumoural grafting of retroviral producer cells that transduce the IL-4 gene compared to the implantation of fibroblasts engineered to express and release IL-4. These data, obtained in athymic mice, confirm that the activation of the IL-4-mediated immune reaction is not strictly dependent on T lymphocytes and can be suitable for the treatment of glioblastoma patients, who suffer

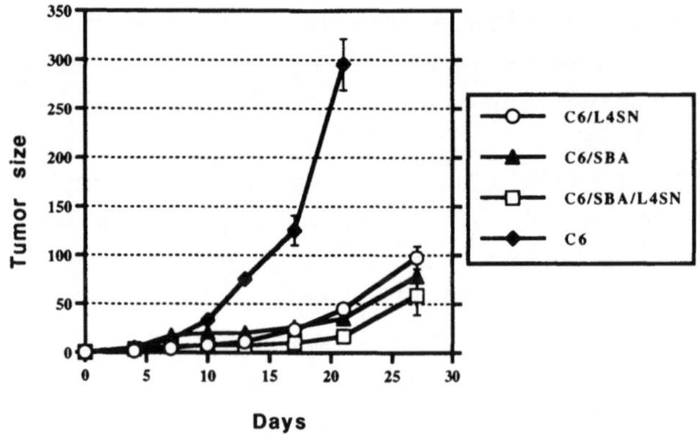

T- test (2 tails, unpaired)

Day	L4SN/SBA vs SBA	L4SN/SBA vs L4SN	SBA vs L4SN
0	-	-	-
4	n.s.	n.s.	n.s.
7	p<0.001	n.s.	p<0.001
10	p<0.005	n.s.	p<0.005
13	p<0.005	p<0.02	p<0.05
17	p<0.005	p<0.0001	n.s.
21	p<0.05	p<0.0001	n.s.
27	n.s.	n.s.	n.s.

Fig. 1. In vivo growth of C6 gliomas injected sub-cutaneously in nude mice. The graph is showing the growth rate of C6 cells (American Type Culture Collection) alone or injected in combination with retroviral producer cells expressing the HSV-tk gene (SBA cells; [6]), the IL-4 gene (L4SN cells; [14]) or both. Nude mice (Charles-River Italia) were inoculated subcutaneously in one flank with 3×10^5 C6 cells, alone or mixed in a 1:1 ratio with SBA or L4SN cells. Osmotic pumps (Alzet, Charles River Italia) were used to deliver GCV at 30 mg/kg/die for about two weeks. The size of subcutaneous tumours was evaluated by multiplying the two major diameters (cross-sectional area). The statistical analysis of the results is presented below the graph

from a well-documented depression of the T cell arm of the immune response [5, 12, 20].

The authors evaluated whether the transfer of the IL-4 gene can strengthen the anti-tumour immune response elicited by the treatment with HSV-tk and GCV [2, 21] and mediate a long-term tumour rejection. Preliminary experiments were performed in athymic nude mice to evaluate the role of the initial, T lymphocyte-independent, response induced by in vivo transduction of IL-4 gene and to test the effects of the combined transduction with the HSV-tk gene. Three groups of mice were inoculated subcutaneously with C6+IL-4 retroviral producer cells (L4SN cells, derived from the psi-two packaging cell line [14], C6+SBA or C6+L4SN+SBA cells and the last two groups were treated with GCV. It was found that transduction of the IL-4 gene could restrain tumour growth similarly to HSV-tk/GCV. The combined transduction of IL-4 and HSV-tk provided a higher anti-tumour effect compared to the transfer of a single therapeutic gene, but the differences were only significant for the first three weeks (Fig. 1). This could be explained by the two-step response induced by IL-4: the initial tumour destruction is, in fact, mediated by the cytotoxic and phagocytic activity of eosinophils and macrophages and is therefore aspecific, while the delayed and specific response, which requires the activation of T and B lymphocytes, can lead to a definitive tumour rejection and to the establishment of a long term immunological memory [9, 14]. In nude mice, only the early and aspecific response can take place and the antitumour effect observed is therefore limited in time. On the other hand, HSV-tk expression also restrains tumour growth for a limited period after GCV administration. These two observations can explain why the neoplastic proliferation re-occurs after the combined transfer of HSV-tk and IL-4 genes.

Preliminary Observations on IL-4 Gene Transfer in Immunocompetent Rats

The authors expected that in immunocompetent animals the immune response elicited by IL-4 transduction could induce a stronger anti-tumour reaction and ensure a long term survival of the treated animals. To test this, stereotactic injections were performed in the brain of 13 rats with equal amounts of C6 and L4SN cells and their survival compared to that of a control group inoculated with C6 cells alone (n = 17).

Tumour growth was demonstrated by histological analysis and/or MRI. Initially, a good correlation was found between MRI and the normal anatomy of the rat brain, as defined by a stereotactic atlas. MRI could demonstrate the presence of tumour growth as early as 10 days after the injection of 4×10^4 C6 cells in rat brain. Thus, MRI follow-up was instrumental in establishing the presence and the growth of the tumour (Fig. 2), since in 15–20% of the animals such growth

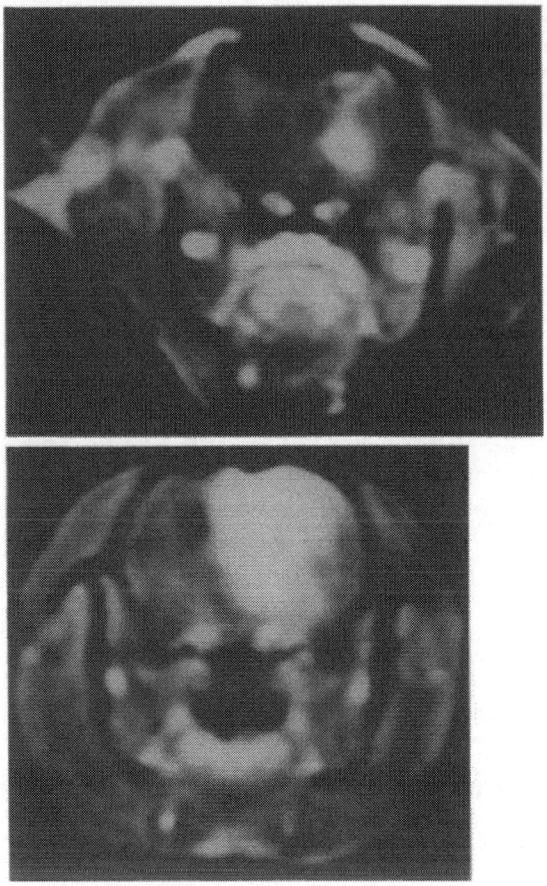

Fig. 2. Magnetic resonance imaging (MRI) of a control rat brain injected in the left hemisphere with 4×10^4 C6 cells 12 (part A) and 21 (part B) days, respectively, after the injection. MRI was performed using a 1.5 T equipment with a 10 cm surface coil. Coronal and sagittal Vol 2 mm-T1-FFE, Vol 2 mm T2-TSE and intermediate and T2-WSE sequences were obtained. The FOV was 160 and the acquisition matrix 256×256. Part A: vol T1 FFE 2 mm image showing a tumoral enhancement in the left hemisphere. Lateral ventricles are also recognizable. The few artifacts are due to the previous injection. Part B: post-contrast T1 FFE 2 mm image demonstrating the dramatic growth of the tumour with intense dishomogeneous enhancement. The arrow points to a displaced and enlarged ventricle

Fig. 3. Haematoxylin Eosin staining of a C6 brain glioma in one animal injected with C6 and L4SN cells. Rat brains were fixed by Carnoy, embedded in paraffin and examined by light microscopy. In addition, immunohistochemical analysis was performed using antibodies against GFAP (gliofibrillary acidic protein) and vimentin (not shown here). The rat died 66 days after injection: lymphocytes infiltrating the neoplastic cells are clearly visible

does not take place. The feasibility of further evaluations to size the tumours in the presence of different therapeutic modalities is presently under scrutiny. The analysis of this group of animals demonstrated that C6+IL-4-treated rats, overall, lived significantly longer than controls (52.6+/−9.6 days vs 25.3+/−1.8, $p = 0.0038$). Histological analysis of some of the long term survivors by hematoxylin-eosin staining, revealed the presence of a lymphocytic infiltrate at the borders of the neoplastic lesion (Fig. 3), demonstrating the occurrence of an inflammatory reaction which, at least for several weeks, counteracted tumour growth.

Perspectives

The therapeutic potential of the "suicide gene" strategy, based on the treatment with HSV-tk and GCV for the cure of malignant gliomas, has been emphasized by the promising results described by some authors [1, 2, 8, 10], but the outcome of clinical studies [15] as well as the results obtained by Cool *et al.* [7] and by the authors' concur to define the limits of this system.

To achieve a complete tumour eradication other approaches may be combined with the "suicide gene" strategy and the enhancement of the immunological response to the tumour by cytokine gene transfer seems to offer an interesting perspective. The authors' experiments in nude mice seem to confirm the antineoplastic role of IL-4 [3] and encourage the testing of co-transduction of IL-4 and HSV-tk genes in immunocompetent animals. However, since the retroviral producer cell line L4SN is derived from first generation "psi-two" packaging cells, recombination events can take place and lead to the formation of a replication competent virus (helper virus), facilitating the spreading of IL-4 and HSV-tk genes, but considerably increasing the risk of insertional mutagenesis. The preparation of retroviral producer cell lines derived from third generation packaging cells [13], currently underway in this laboratory, should efficiently counteract the occurrence of replication competent retroviruses.

The authors hypothesised that in immunocompetent rats a lymphocyte-mediated response against the tumour could be activated by IL-4 transduction and ensure a longer survival of treated animals. Preliminary results seem to confirm this hypothesis, but the anti-neoplastic effect of IL-4 was only observed in a fraction of the treated rats. It is not known whether this different response is due to a diverse individual reaction of the animals to the treatment or to the low amount of IL-4 secreted in the tumour microenviroment. This second hypothesis will be tested by using another IL-4 viral producer cell line, able to release higher levels of the cytokine. In addition there will be an evaluation as to whether the combined in vivo transduction of HSV-tk and IL-4 genes can strengthen the anti-tumour effect of the IL-4 transfer alone. Preliminary results seem to be promising and encourage the use of similar combination therapies for the treatment of gliomas.

Acknowledgements

We thank Dr. M. Colombo of the Istituto Nazionale dei Tumori for making available L4SN cells, Mrs. C. Regondi for helping in the follow-up of nude mice, Mrs. L. Caposio and Dr. N. Florio for collaborating with the MRI analysis of rat brains.

Dr. S. Benedetti has been supported by a fellowship of the Associazione Italiana per la Ricerca sul Cancro (AIRC).

References

1. Barba D, Hardin J, Jasodhara R, Gage FH (1993) Thymidine kinase-mediated killing of rat brain tumors. J Neurosurg 79: 729–735
2. Barba D, Hardin J, Sadelain M, Gage FH (1994) Development of anti-tumor immunity following thymidine kinase-mediated killing of experimental brain tumors. Proc Natl Acad Sci USA 91: 4348–4352
3. Benedetti S, DiMeco F, Colombo BM, Cirenei N, Pollo B, Bruzzone MG, Vescovi A, Colombo MP, DiDonato S, Finocchiaro G: Limits of the HSV-TK/GCV system for gene therapy of malignant gliomas: perspectives for the combined transduction of the IL-4 gene. Submitted
4. Beyer EC, Paul DL, Goodenough DA (1990) J Membr Biol 116: 187–194
5. Brooks WH, Markersbery WR, Gupta D, Roszman TL (1978) Relationship of lymphocyte invasion and survival of brain tumor patients. Ann Neurol 2: 219–224
6. Colombo BM, Benedetti S, Ottolenghi S, Poli G, Pollo B, Mora M, Finocchiaro G (1995) The "bystander effect": association of U-87 cell death with ganciclovir-mediated apoptosis of nearby cells and lack of effect in athymic mice. Hum Gene Ther 6: 763–772
7. Cool V, Pirotte B, Gérard C, Dargent J-L, Baudson N, Levivier M, Goldman S, Hildebrand J, Brotchi J, Velu T (1996) Curative potential of Herpes Simplex virus thymidine kinase gene transfer in rats with 9L gliosarcoma. Hum Gene Ther 7: 627–635
8. Culver KW, Ram Z, Wallbridge S, Ishii H, Oldfield EH, Blaese RM (1992) In vivo gene transfer with retroviral vector-producer cells for treatment of experimental brain tumors. Science 256: 1550–1552
9. Golumbek PT, Lazenby AJ, Levitsky HI, Jaffee LM, Karasuyama H, Baker M, Pardoll DM (1991) Treatment of established renal cancer by tumor cells engineered to secrete interleukin-4. Science 254: 713–716
10. Izquierdo M, Cortes M, de Felipe P, Martin V, Diez-Guerra J, Talavera A, Perez-Higuera A (1995) Long-term rat survival after malignant brain tumor regression by retroviral gene therapy. Gene Therapy 2: 66–69
11. Li Bi W, Parysek LM, Warnick R, Stambrook PJ (1993) Hum Gene Ther 4: 725–731
12. Mahaley MS jr, Brooks WH, Roszman TL (1977) Immunobiology of primary intracranial tumors. I. Studies of the cellular and humoral general immune competence of brain tumor patients. J Neurosurg 46: 467–476
13. Markowitz D, Goff S, Bank A (1988) Construction and use of a safe and efficient amphotropic packaging cell line. Virology 167: 400–406
14. Pericle F, Giovarelli M, Colombo MP, Ferrari G, Musiani P, Modesti A, Cavallo F, DiPierro F, Novelli F, Forni G (1994) An efficient Th2-type memory follows $CD8^+$ lymphocyte-driven and eosinophil-mediated rejection of a spontaneous mouse mammary adenocarcinoma engineered to release IL-4. J Immunol 153: 5659–5673
15. Ram Z, Culver K, Oshiro E, Viola J, de Vroom H, Otto E, Long Z, McGarrity G, Muul G, Katz D, Blaese RM (1995) Summary of results and conclusion of the gene therapy of malignant brain tumors: clinical study. J Neurosurg 82: 343A
16. Sacco MG, Benedetti S, Duflot-Dancer A, Mesnil M, Bagnasco L, Strina D, Fasolo V, Villa A, Macchi P, Faranda S, Vezzoni P, Finocchiaro G (1996) Partial regression, yet incomplete eradication of mammary tumors in transgenic mice by retroviral mediated HSV-TK transfer in vivo. Gene Ther in press
17. Schold SC (1995) Placebo controlled trial of safety and efficacy of intraoperative controlled delivery by biodegradable polymers of chemotherapy for recurrent gliomas. Lancet 345: 1008–1012
18. Tepper RI, Pattengale PK, Leder P (1989) Murine Interleukin-4 displays potent anti-tumor activity in vivo. Cell 57: 503–512
19. Tepper RI, Coffman RL, Leder P (1992) An eosinophil-dependent mechanism for the antitumor effect of interleukin-4. Science 257: 548–551
20. Thomas DG, Lannigan CB, Behan PO (1975) Impaired cell mediated immunity in human brain tumors. Lancet 1: 1389–1390
21. Vile RG, Nelson JA, Castleden S, Chong H, Hart IR (1994) Systemic gene therapy of murine melanoma using tissue specific expression of the HSVtk gene involves an immune component. Cancer Res 54: 6228–6234
22. Wei MX, Tamiya T, Hurford RK, Boviatsis EJ, Tepper RI, Chiocca EA (1995) Enhancement of interleukin 4-mediated tumor regression in athymic mice by in situ retroviral gene transfer. Hum Gene Ther 6: 437–443
23. Yu JS, Wei MX, Chiocca EA, Martuza L, Tepper RI (1993) Treatment of glioma by engineered interleukin 4-secreting cells. Cancer Res 53: 3125–3128

Correspondence: Gaetano Finocchiaro, M.D., Istituto Nazionale Neurologico "C. Besta", Divisione di Biochimica e Genetica, via Celoria 11, 1-20133 Milano, Italy.

Acta Neurochir (1997) [Suppl] 68: 105–110

Anti-Angiogenic Gene Therapy of Malignant Glioma

A. Stratmann, M. R. Machein, and **K. H. Plate**

Department of Neuropathology, Neurozentrum, University of Freiburg Medical School, Freiburg, Federal Republic of Germany

Summary

Glioblastoma, one of the best vascularized tumours in humans, appears well suited for an antiangiogenic therapy. VEGF (vascular endothelial growth factor), the most important angiogenesis factor identified to date, is highly expressed in glioblastoma. VEGF is particulary upregulated in palisading cells adjacent to necroses and has subsequently been shown to be hypoxia-inducible in glioma cells in vitro. VEGF-receptor tyrosine kinases, VEGF-R1 (flt-1) and VEGF-R2 (flk-1), are induced in a tumour stage dependent manner during glioma progression and are exclusively expressed in tumour vascular endothelial cells.

These observations suggest that VEGF-receptors are promising targets for tumour endothelial cell specific therapy. The ability to block VEGF signalling by the VEGF R2 dominant negative mutant identifies the VEGF/VEGF-R2 system as a major regulator of glioma angiogenesis. Several experimental approaches demonstrate that in rat gliomas tumour growth can be prevented by the inhibition of angiogenesis. These findings are of pivotal importance for the development of anti-angiogenic therapies in glioblastoma patients.

Keywords: Glioblastoma; tumour angiogenesis; angiogenic growth factors; VEGF-R2 (flk).

Introduction

The molecular tumour genetics of gliomas pose many unanswered questions.

Are Malignant Gliomas Suitable for Anti-Angiogenic Therapy?

Malignant gliomas are neuroectodermal tumours which most commonly arise in the white matter of the cerebral hemispheres [1]. They are rapidly dividing and highly invasive tumours. Glioblastoma is the most common and most malignant brain tumour in humans and up to date is incurable because of its resistance to all available therapies. Histologically, glioblastomas are highly vascularised tumours and display large areas of necrosis. An event that accompanies glioma progression is the onset of angiogenesis [21, 23]. During development from a low-grade to a high grade glioma an increase in vessel density can be observed. Low-grade gliomas are moderately vascularised whereas high-grade gliomas display areas of high vascular density. Therefore, glioblastoma growth seems to be angiogenesis-dependent. The authors are interested in the molecular mechanisms underlying tumour angiogenesis and in the development of therapeutic strategies based on angiogenesis inhibition.

How is Angiogenesis Regulated in the Developing Brain and in Brain Tumours?

Angiogenesis is defined as the sprouting of capillaries from pre-existing vessels. Angiogenesis is observed during embryonic brain development but is downregulated in the adult brain. Angiogenesis may be reinduced under pathological conditions such as brain tumour growth [19], reviewed in [9, 24]. Folkman et al. have proposed that tumours require the formation of new blood vessels to grow beyond a minimum volume [8]. The most common model of tumour angiogenesis is that tumour cells secrete angiogenic factors that act on endothelial cells [21]. In addition, the expression of growth factor receptors must be induced on the endothelial cell surface. The angiogenesis factor secreted by the tumour cell binds to endothelial cells which express the respective receptor(s) and via receptor-signalling the endothelial cell becomes activated. Endothelial cell activation is characterised by the synthesis of proteolytic enzymes which serve for the degradation of the extracellular matrix, and by subsequent migration and proliferation of the endothelial cell. This process results in the formation of new capillaries which supply the tumour with oxygen and nutrients.

Which Molecules are Involved in Endothelial Cell Growth and Differentiation?

At present, four receptors have been identified which are known to be exclusively expressed on the endothelial cell surface. Two of them, flt-1 and flk-1 (KDR) belong to the PDGF-receptor family of receptor tyrosine-kinases. Both consist of an extracellular part characterised by seven immunoglobulin-domains, a transmembrane domain and an intracellular split kinase domain. The ligand of both receptors is VEGF (vascular endothelial growth factor) [6, 30]. Therefore flt-1 and flk-1/KDR are also denominated VEGF-receptor 1 (VEGF-R1) and -2 (VEGF-R2), respectively.

The two other endothelial cell specific receptors, tie-1 and tie-2 (tek) belong to a new class of receptor tyrosine kinases with an unusual structure of the extracellular part containing three fibronectin type III domains and three domains with epidermal growth factor homology [18, 27]. The ligand(s) for these two receptors are still unknown.

Results

VEGF and its Receptors flt-1/flk-1 (KDR) are the Prime Candidates for the Molecules which Regulate Glioma Angiogenesis

In contrast to other angiogenesis factors, VEGF is a secreted endothelial cell specific mitogen and potently stimulates angiogenesis in vivo [5, 14].

The important role of VEGF and its receptors in developmental angiogenesis was demonstrated by several groups. A transient expression of VEGF during mouse brain development was observed. VEGF-transcripts were abundant in the ventricular neuroectoderm of embryonic and postnatal brain but were reduced in the adult brain [2]. Correspondingly, VEGF-receptors were highly expressed in proliferating endothelial cells of vascular sprouts and branching vessels of embryonic and early postnatal brain but were drastically downregulated in adult brain [15].

The authors addressed the question of whether VEGF and its receptors are involved in the regulation on angiogenesis in human gliomas [19, 22]. In situ-hybridisation analysis of VEGF-R1 expression revealed that VEGF-R1 was upregulated in a tumour stage dependent manner in glioma endothelial cells, since VEGF-R1-mRNA was not detectable in normal adult brain but was present in low grade glioma and was highly expressed in the vasculature of glioblastoma. VEGF-R2 analysis showed a similar expression pattern as VEGFR-1. VEGF-R2-mRNA could not be detected in the vasculature of normal brain and of low-grade gliomas but was highly expressed in the endothelial cells of glioblastomas.

The expression of the ligand of both receptors was also analysed. VEGF, like its corresponding receptors, is highly expressed in glioblastoma but to a lower extent in glioma WHO-grade II and even lower in normal brain.

Interestingly, only a subset of glioblastoma cells expressed VEGF. VEGF was upregulated in a specific subset of tumour cells which were located immediately adjacent to necrosis. Due to their characteristic morphology, these cells have been denominated palisading cells.

The above findings suggested that VEGF-expression in glioblastoma is regulated by oxygen-tension. Hypoxia-inducibility of VEGF was demonstrated in C6 glioma cells in vitro [12, 20]. Northern blot analysis of RNA isolated from C6 cells which were incubated either under normoxic conditions or under hypoxic conditions showed that VEGF-mRNA expression is drastically upregulated in response to hypoxia. Western blot analysis confirmed that VEGF-protein is hypoxia-inducible in C6 glioma cells in vitro. The question was then addressed whether palisading cells represent hypoxic glioma cells in vivo. Rat glioma cells, stably transfected with a lacZ-expression vector under control of hypoxia-responsive elements of the VEGF gene, showed a strong reporter gene expression in pernecrotic palisading cells, but not in cells distant from necrosis (A. Damert, M. R. Machein, W. Risau, K. H. Plate, personal communication). These findings support the hypothesis that palisading cells are hypoxic glioma cells and suggest that hypoxia is a major regulator of VEGF-expression in glioma cells in vivo.

The authors suggest that glioma cells try to overcome tissue hypoxia by upregulating VEGF in order to induce angiogenesis and increase their blood supply. VEGF secreted by the glioma cells acts as a paracrine growth factor that binds to endothelial cells which express VEGF-receptors. Therefore VEGF receptors represent a promising target for endothelial cell specific anti-angiogenic therapy.

Development of an Animal Model for Glioblastoma Angiogenesis

To study the possibility of anti-angiogenic glioma therapy an animal model of tumour angiogenesis was developed by the authors [20]. Rat C6 glioma cells were transplanted intracerebrally into syngeneic rats. The resulting C6 gliomas exhibited morphological characteristics of human glioblastoma such as necrosis and high vascularisation. Analysis of VEGF-receptor expression by in situ-hybridisation revealed that both receptors VEGF-R1 and VEGF-R2 were upregulated in C6-tumour endothelial cells as they were in human glioblastoma. Tumour cells did not express VEGF-receptors. VEGF-receptors were specifically expressed in the endothelial cells of C6 tumour but not in those of the surrounding normal brain. Blood vessels in normal brain outside the tumour did not express VEGF receptors whereas vessels immediately at the tumour-brain-interface and vessels in the tumour did express VEGF-receptors. The expression of the ligand VEGF was also analysed in C6 glioma. VEGF-expression was low in normal brain and in tumour cells at the periphery of the tumour. However VEGF was highly upregulated in glioma cells lying close to necrotic areas in the centre of the tumour. Similar to human glioblastoma, only tumour cells located at the border of necrotic tumour areas expressed high levels of VEGF.

Since the expression pattern of VEGF and its corresponding receptors in rat glioma was indistinguishable from human glioblastoma this animal model provided an excellent tool to study the putative effects of an anti-angiogenic therapy.

Anti-Angiogenic Gene-Therapy by Dominant-Negative Inhibition of flk-1

This anti-angiogenic gene therapy approach [15–17] is aimed to inhibit tumour-angiogenesis by specifically inhibiting signal transduction in tumour endothelial cells which express VEGF-R2 (flk-1). The strategy used is called trans-dominant-negative inhibition of receptor signalling. This was achieved by the construction of a mutant VEGF-R2 (called flk-1 TM) which in contrast to the wild-type-receptor lacks the intracellular kinase domain and therefore is signalling-defective [16].

A recombinant retrovirus was used for in vivo gene-transfer of the dominant-negative VEGF-R2 deletion mutant flk-1 TM. Retrovirus producing cells deliver the virus particles which infect proliferating endothelial cells. For mediating signal transduction the wild-type receptor must form dimers on the endothelial cell surface upon ligand-binding. The truncated receptor is able to bind VEGF and to dimerise with the wt-receptor but the resulting heterodimers are inactive and signal transduction is not possible. It was expected that disruption of receptor-signalling achieved by overexpression of mutant VEGF-R2 in tumour-invading endothelial cells should prevent vascularisation of the tumour and consequently suppress tumour growth. For the analysis of the efficacy of flk-1 TM retrovirus therapy two different glioma cell lines, C6 and GS-9L, were tested. Tumours were either transplanted subcutaneously into nude mice or stereotactically implanted into the brains of syngeneic rats. The effect of retrovirus treatment on tumour growth, tumour angiogenesis and survival time of the animals was examined. Co-transplantation of virus producer cells together with rat C6 glioma cells into nude mice led to a dramatic inhibition of tumour growth as compared to the control groups. In control groups animals were either not treated with virus producing cells or a virus producing a mutated form of c-fms (c-fms TM) was used which has no function in angiogenesis. In both control groups tumours showed the same growth behaviour [16].

In a second experiment GS-9L glioma cells were transplanted either alone (untreated control) or together with the retrovirus producing cells subcutaneously into syngeneic host rats. The reduction in tumour size in the flk-1 TM retrovirus treated animals was directly correlated with the inhibition of tumour angiogenesis. In untreated mice the border zone between infiltrating tumour and normal skin was well vascularised displaying capillaries and larger vessels whereas in the growth inhibited tumours this zone was completely devoid of blood vessels [17].

In a third set of experiments, C6 or GS-9L glioma cells were implanted stereotactically into the brains of syngeneic rats. Animals with C6 gliomas which were co-implanted with the virus producer cells developed smaller tumours than rats implanted with C6 cells alone. Moreover the survival time of rats with intracranial 9L-gliomas was prolonged by dominant-negative inhibition of the flk-receptor signalling. Twenty days after tumour implantation, survival was 50% in the untreated group, compared to 100% in the retrovirus-treated group. After 29 days all animals succumbed in the control group, while in the treated group 80% were still alive and stayed alive until the end of the study on day 39.

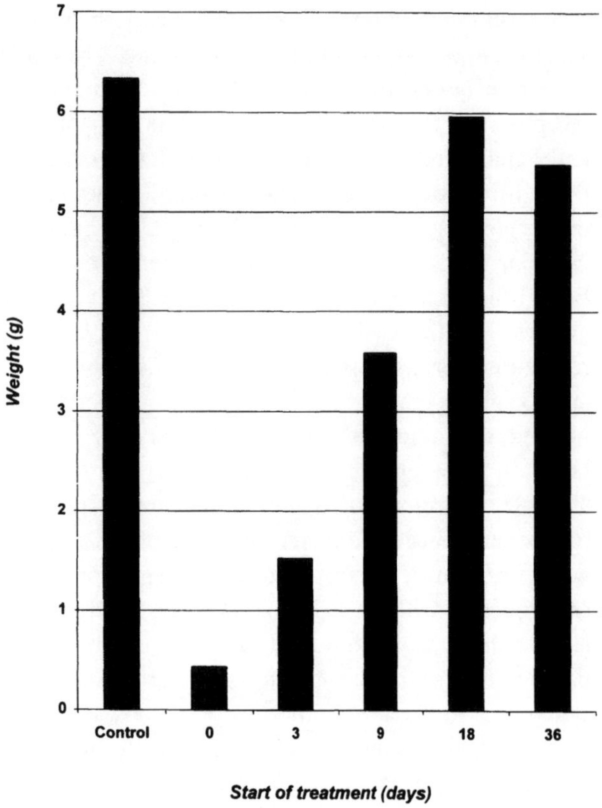

Fig. 1. Effect of different starting points of flk 1-TM retrovirus treatment on tumour weight increase

In addition, the authors examined the influence of tumour size on the therapeutic efficacy of the flk-1 dominant-negative retroviral treatment (Fig. 1). When 10^6 tumour cells and 10^6 virus producing cells were cotransplanted at the beginning of the study, they observed a 92% decrease in tumour weight compared to untreated control animals during a period of 39 days. When the treatment with 10^6 virus-producing cells started 9 days after transplantation of 10^6tumour cells, a 43% decrease in tumour weight was observed as compared to controls. However, tumour growth could not be significantly inhibited when treatment with 10^6 virus-producing cells started on day 18 or later after tumour cell transplantation. In these animals (which were designated "late treatment group"), no growth-inhibitory effect could be observed as compared to untreated control tumours (Fig. 1).

Discussion

The above experiments demonstrate that the inhibition of VEGF-mediated signal transduction by the dominant negative VEGF-R2 inhibits tumour growth and prolongs survival in rats with intracranial gliomas. These results are consistent with observation by Kim *et al.* [13] who used neutralizing anti-VEGF-antibodies to treat nude mice with subcutaneous gliomas. The authors observed inhibition of tumour growth and decreased vascular density.

Similar results were obtained from a recent experimental approach used by Cheng *et al.* [3] and Saleh *et al.* [25] who introduced an antisense-VEGF expression construct into glioblastoma cells. These cells were not able to sustain tumour growth in immunodeficient mice and the density of in vivo blood vessel formation was reduced. Claffey *et al.* [4] used the same approach to demonstrate reduced melanoma growth in nude mice after introduction of an antisense VEGF-construct into human melanoma cells. Flk-1 as a target for tumour growth inhibition was also proposed by Strawn *et al.* [29] who recently identified anti-angiogenic compounds that specifically inhibited flk-1 tyrosine kinase activity and subsequently blood vessel formation in the chorio-allantoic membrane assay. In summary, there is accumulating evidence that specific inhibition of tumour angiogenesis is possible by targetting VEGF or its receptors and that this inhibition will significantly reduce tumour growth.

At present, there are four major questions which need to be considered in more detail before the above described dominant-negative anti-angiogenic gene therapy approach can be transferred to the clinics. Firstly, is flt-1, the other VEGF-receptor, involved in glioma angiogenesis? Secondly, what is the function of the two other endothelial cell specific receptors, tie-1 and tie-2 (tek), whose ligands are still unknown? Thirdly, can stereotactically transplanted retrovirus-particles leave the brain and infect other organs or other organisms? Finally, the low infection rate of retroviruses in vivo represents a major problem.

The function of flt-1, the other VEGF-receptor, in tumour angiogenesis is unknown. However since flt-1 is highly upregulated in glioma vessels, a role in tumour angiogenesis seems likely. One possibility is, that in the dominant-negative experiments, flt-1 function was inhibited via heterodimerisation of the wild-type flt-1 with the mutant flk-1 receptor.

There is also limited information about the other two endothelial tyrosine kinase-receptors tie-1 and tie-2 (tek) the ligands of which have not yet been identified. Upregulation of tie-1 was described in glioma endothelial cells [11] but in vivo inhibition data in a tumour model are not yet available. It is important to

Table 1. *Endothelial Cell Specific Receptor Tyrosine Kinases (EC endothelial Cells)*

RTK	flt-1 (VEGF-R1)	flk-1 (VEGF-R2)	tie-1	tie-2 (tek)
Ligand	VEGF PlGF	VEGF VEGF-C	?	?
Expression during mouse embryonic development	in EC from E 8.0	in EC and hemangioblasts from E 7.0	in EC from E 8.5	in EC from E 8.0
K. O. mice	die at E 8.5	die at E 8.5–9.5	die at P 0	die at E 10.5
Phenotype of k. o. mice	disorganized blood vessels, EC migrate and proliferate, EC phenotypically abnormal	no vasculogenesis, no angiogenesis, no hematopoiesis	normal vascular network, "leaky vessels" oedema, hemorrhage	dilated vessels, no capillary sprouts, malformations of vascular network
Expression in tumour vascular EC	yes	yes	yes	?
Tumour reduction by receptor-inhibition	?	yes	?	?

identify putative functions of these receptors in tumour angiogenesis, since tie-1 and tie-2, as well as flt-1 and flk-1, are necessary for normal blood vessel formation during embryonic development and distinct roles for each receptor were shown recently in transgenic knock-out mice (Table 1) [7, 10, 26, 28].

Dominant-negative inhibition of flk-1 may interfere with physiological flk-1 function in the kidney or with wound healing. Although there is no evidence so far that intracerebral injection of virus producing cells into the brain leads to infection of other organs, this point needs to be carefully considered. The authors have however so far been unable to observe any undesired effects which could be attributed to flk-1 inhibition.

In the dominant-negative flk-1 experiments described, gene transfer efficacy was a limiting factor of the retrovirus-mediated therapy, since a 20-fold excess of virus producing cells to tumour cells was necessary to reach a maximal effect in the nude mouse model [16]. The authors observed a significant (e.g. more than 90%) growth inhibition with an equal ratio of tumour cells and virus producing cells. In these experiments, failure of tumour growth inhibition in the late treatment groups (e.g. treatment of 10^6 transplanted tumour cells grown in vivo for 18 days or more) most likely represents inadequate gene transfer rates, since the number of tumour cells was in large excess compared to the number of virus producer cells. It needs to be seen whether improved vector systems or the use of specific low molecular weight inhibitors will help to overcome these problems in the future.

Acknowledgements

Our studies are carried out in collaboration with Dr. Werner Risau, Bad Nauheim and Dr. Axel Ullrich, Martinsried. We gratefully acknowledge Richard Haas for technical assistance. Our work is supported by grants from the Deutsche Krebshilfe and the Bundesministerium für Bildung und Forschung.

References

1. Barnard RO (1986) The pathology of brain tumours. In: Beehen NM (ed) Tumours of the brain. Springer, Berlin Heidelberg New York Tokyo, pp 60–70
2. Breier G, Albrecht U, Sterrer S, Risau W (1992) Expression of vascular endothelial growth factor during embryonic angiogenesis and endothelial cell differentiation. Development 114: 521–532
3. Cheng SY, Huang HJS, Nagane M, Ji XD, Wang DG, Shih CCY, Arap W, Huang CM, Cavenee WK (1996) Suppression of glioblastoma angiogenicity and tumourigenicity by inhibition of endogenous expression of vascular endothelial growth factor. Proc Natl Acad Sci USA 93: 8502–8507
4. Claffey KP, Brown LF, Delaguila LF, Tognazzi K, Yeo KT, Manseau EJ, Dvorak HF (1996) Expression of vascular permeability factor/vascular endothelial growth factor by melanoma cells increases tumour growth, angiogenesis, and experimental metastasis. Cancer Res 56: 172–181
5. Conolly DT, Heuvelman DM, Nelson R, Olander JV, Eppley BL, Delfino JJ, Siegel NR, Leimgruber RM, Feder J (1989) Tumour vascular permeability factor stimulates endothelial cell growth and angiogenesis. J Clin Invest 84: 1470–1478
6. De Vries C, Escobedo JA, Ueno H, Houck K, Ferrara N, Williams LT (1992) The fms-like tyrosine kinase, a receptor for vascular endothelial growth factor. Science 255: 989–991
7. Dumont DJ, Gradwohl G, Fong GH, Puri MC, Gertsenstein M, Auerbach A, Breitman ML (1994) Dominant-negative and targeted null mutations in the endothelial receptor tyrosine kinase, tek, reveal a critical role in vasculogenesis of the embryo. Genes Dev 8: 1897–1909
8. Folkman J (1990) What is the evidence that tumours are angiogenesis dependent? J Natl Cancer Inst 82: 4–6
9. Folkman J (1995) Angiogenesis in cancer, vascular, rheumatoid and other disease. Nat Med 1: 27–31
10. Fong GH, Rossant J, Gertsenstein M, Breitman M (1995) Role of the flt-1 receptor tyrosine kinase in regulating the assembly of vascular endothelium. Nature 376: 66–70
11. Hatva E, Kaipainen A, Mentula P, Jääskeläinen J, Paetau A, Haltia M, Alitalo K (1995) Expression of endothelial cell-

specific receptor tyrosine kinases and growth factors in human brain tumours. Am J Pathol 146: 368–378
12. Ikeda E, Achen MG, Breier G, Risau W (1995) Hypoxia-induced transcriptional activation and increased mRNA stability of vascular endothelial growth factor in C6 glioma cells. J Biol Chem 270: 19761–19766
13. Kim JB, Li B, Winer J, Armanini M, Gillet N, Philipps HS, Ferrara N (1993) Inhibition of vascular endothelial growth factor-induced angiogenesis suppresses tumour growth in vivo. Nature 362: 841–844
14. Leung DW, Cachianes G, Kuang WJ, Goeddel DV, Ferrara N (1989) Vascular endothelial growth factor is a secreted angiogenic mitogen. Science 246: 1306–1309
15. Millauer B, Wizigmann-Voos S, Schnürch H, Martinez R, Moller N, Risau W, Ullrich A (1993) High affinity VEGF binding and developmental expression suggest flk-1 as a major regulator of vasculogenesis and angiogenesis. Cell 72: 835–846
16. Millauer B, Shawver LK, Plate KH, Risau W, Ullrich A (1994) Glioblastoma growth inhibited in vivo by a dominant-negative flk-1 mutant. Nature 367: 576–579
17. Millauer B, Longhi MP, Plate KH, Shawver LK, Risau W, Ullrich A, Strawn LM (1996) Dominant-negative inhibition of flk-1 suppresses the growth of many tumour types in vivo. Cancer Res 56: 1615–1620
18. Partanen J, Armstrong E, Mäkelä TP, Korhonen J, Sandberg M, Renkonen R, Knuutila S, Huebner K, Alitalo K (1992) A novel endothelial cell surface receptor tyrosine kinase with extracellular epidermal growth factor homology domains. Mol Cell Biol 12: 1698–1707
19. Plate KH, Breier G, Weich HA, Risau W (1992) Vascular endothelial growth factor is a potential tumour angiogenesis factor in human gliomas in vivo. Nature 359: 845–847
20. Plate KH, Breier G, Millauer B, Ullrich A, Risau W (1993) Up-regulation of vascular endothelial growth factor and its cognate receptors in a rat glioma model of tumour angiogenesis. Cancer Res 53: 5822–5827
21. Plate KH, Breier G, Risau W (1994) Molecular mechanisms of developmental and tumour angiogenesis. Brain Pathol 4: 207–218
22. Plate KH, Breier G, Weich HA, Mennel HD, Risau W (1994) Vascular endothelial growth factor and glioma angiogenesis: coordinate induction of VEGF receptors, distribution of VEGF protein and possible in vivo regulatory mechanisms. Int J Cancer 59: 520–529
23. Plate KH, Risau W (1995) Angiogenesis in malignant gliomas. Glia 15: 339–347
24. Rak JW, St Croix BD, Kerbel RS (1995) Consequences of angiogenesis for tumour progression, metastasis and cancer therapy. Anticancer Drugs 6: 3–18
25. Saleh M, Stacker SA, Wilks AF (1996) Inhibition of growth of C6 glioma cells in vivo by expression of antisense vascular endothelial growth factor sequence. Cancer Res 56: 393–401
26. Sato TN, Tozawa Y, Deutsch U, Wolburg-Buchholz K, Fujiwara Y, Gendron-Maguire M, Gridley T, Wolburg H, Risau W, Quin Y (1995) Distinct roles of the receptor tyrosine kinases tie-1 and tie-2 in blood vessel formation. Nature 376: 70–74
27. Schnürch H, Risau W (1993) Expression of tie-2, a member of novel family of receptor tyrosine kinases, in the endothelial cell lineage. Development 119: 957–968
28. Shalaby F, Rossant J, Yamaguchi TP, Gertsenstein M, Wu XF, Breitman ML, Schuh AC (1995) Failure of blood-island formation and vasculogenesis in flk-1-deficient mice. Nature 376: 62–66
29. Strawn LM, McMahon G, App H, Schreck R, Kuchler WR, Longhi MP, Hui TH, Tang C, Levitzki A, Gazit A, Chen I, Keri G, Orfi L, Risau W, Flamme I, Ullrich A, Hirth KP, Shawver LK (1996) Flk-1 as a target for tumour growth inhibition. Cancer Res 56: 3540–3545
30. Terman BI, Dougher-Vermazen M, Carrion ME, Dimitrov D, Armellino DC, Gospodarowicz C, Böhlen P (1992) Identification of the KDR tyrosine kinase as a receptor for vascular endothelial growth factor. Biochem Biophys Res Commun 187: 1579–1586

Correspondence: Karl H. Plate, M.D., Department of Neuropathology, Neurozentrum, University of Freiburg, Breisacherstr. 64, D-79106 Freiburg, Federal Republic of Germany.

Acta Neurochir (1997) [Suppl] 68: 111–117

Gene Therapy in Brain Tumours: Implications of the Size of Glioblastoma on its Curability

M. Izquierdo[1], M. L. Cortés[1], V. Martín[1], P. de Felipe[1], J. M. Izquierdo[2], A. Pérez-Higueras[3], J. F. Paz[4], A. Isla[4], and M. G. Blázquez[4]

[1] Departamento de Biología Molecular/Centro de Biología Molecular Severo Ochoa, Facultad de Ciencias, Universidad Autónoma de Madrid, Cantoblanco, Madrid, [2]Servicio de Neurocirugía, Hospital Universitario Marqués de Valdecilla, Santander, [3]Servicio de Neuroradiología, Clínica de la Concepción, Fundación Jiménez Díaz, Madrid, and [4]Servicio de Neurocirugía, Hospital "La Paz", Instituto Nacional de la Salud, Madrid, Spain

Summary

The authors have used the thymidine kinase/ganciclovir system to block glioblastoma multiforme neoplastic cells in vivo, both in experimental animals and in two patients in which the more conventional therapies had been unsuccessful. In the Wistar rat it was found that the curability potential of the system is correlated with tumoral volume. Tumours smaller than 20 mm^3 can be cured with defective retrovirus that do not carry the Herpes simplex thymidine kinase (Hsvtk) gene. While tumours smaller than 150 mm^3 can regress totally by the kinase/ganciclovir system, those above that size cannot be cured by this treatment. In humans the situation seems very similar in that the authors have been unable either to reduce the tumour size of recurrent patients with tumour volumes larger than 100 cm^3 applying the standard thymidine kinase/ganciclovir gene therapy or to prolong their survival time more than 8 months [7]. When a combination of size reduction by neurosurgery and gene therapy was used the survival time increased considerably. Two patients have been treated by partial surgery and repeated treatment with thymidine kinase/ganciclovir through an Ommaya reservoir connected to a catheter leading into the tumour cavity. The magnetic resonance imaging (MRI) of these patients show only a residual tumoral growth along side the tumoral bed. The procedure may be partially controlling the proliferation of cancerous cells, because, these two patients having recurrent glioblastoma, are alive 11 and 17 months after the beginning of the treatment.

Keywords: Gene therapy; glioblastoma; Hstk/ganciclovir system; tumour size-curability.

Introduction

Glioblastoma patients have an average survival time of 12 to 18 months despite surgery, radiation therapy and/or chemotherapy. Within that time, recurrence is associated with a 100% mortality and a life expectancy of about 3–6 months. The tumour appears with a frequency of 1/50.000 inhabitants/year. Most of the brain cells in an adult do not divide. Since retrovirus only integrate into the genome of dividing cells, they provide a potential means of infecting selectively neoplastic cells in an adult brain which harbour a tumour. The conversion of an ordinary retrovirus to a therapeutic vector involves the substitution of the viral genes by the therapeutic one. The authors have constructed vectors carrying the thymidine kinase (tk 1) gene from Herpes simplex (Hsvtk). These vectors produced therapeutic viruses upon their introduction into retrovirus packaging cells [6]. The thymidine kinase gene from Herpes simplex virus encodes an enzyme, not as strict as the mammalian counterpart, which can phosphorylate nucleoside analogues, such as ganciclovir, that would not be a substrate for the cell host thymidine kinase. Phosphorylated ganciclovir can be incorporated into the growing DNA chain and block replication, killing, as a consequence, the dividing cell.

The authors had previously observed total regression of malignant brain tumours up to a size of 150 mm^3 in Wistar rats after retroviral-mediated gene therapy [6], and present here an extension of that study in which they analyze the possibility of curing glioblastoma tumours smaller than 20 mm^3 by intratumoral injection of murine defective retrovirus producer cells of high titre (10^5–2×10^6 colony forming units). The retrovirus produced by these cells lack Hstk, all retroviral genes (gag, pol, env) and only carry the selection gene puro that confers resistance to puromycin.

The Herpes simplex thymidine kinase (Hsvtk)/

ganciclovir system has been also used in five patients with large glioblastoma, in two of whom, a reduction of the tumoral mass followed the gene therapy treatment [7]. An up date on those experiments in which two recurrent patients are alive 17 and 11 months after initiation of a combination of neurosurgery (to reduce the tumoral mass) and gene therapy treatment (to kill the remaining cancerous cells) is presented below.

Methods and Material

Retroviral Vector

The plasmid pBabepuro was used [12] and a derivative new construct in which the Hsvtk. gene was inserted via Eco Rl-Sal 1. The synthesis of the protein is directed by the viral LTR (long terminal repeat) having been removed from its own promoter. The new retroviral plasmid has been called pBabetk puro.

Wistar Rat C6 Brain Inoculation, Producer Cell Injection and Ganciclovir Administration

The authors have essentially followed procedures described previously [6]. Wistar male rats weighing 250–300 grams were anaesthetized with a mixture of ketamine (50 mg/ml), valium (5 mg/ml) and atropine (1mg/ml) in a 5:4:1 ratio, by volume at a dose of 0.3 ml/100g of body weight before placing them in a stereotaxic apparatus. C6 or L9 glioma cells were injected at a concentration of 10^5 cells/μl in complete PBS (with calcium and magnesium) supplemented with 0.1% glucose. With the aid of the manipulating arm of the stereotaxic apparatus a total of 5 μl were introduced, over a 5 minute interval, into the fronto-parietal lobe of the right cerebral hemisphere (4 mm to the right from Bregma and 4.5 mm deep from the skull) using a 10 μl Hamilton syringe connected to a 25 gauge needle; the needle was kept in place 3 minutes before and after injection. Control rats received saline solution and did not develop any tumour. All rats received tetracycline in the drinking water (approximately 75 mg/kg) and dexamethasone (0.5 mg/kg/20ml) for one week after surgery.

The producer cells were injected over a 10 min. period and slow 5 min. needle insertion and retraction before and after injection, at a concentration of 10^5 cells/μl in complete PBS, 0.1% glucose; a total of 5×10^6 cells of titres between 5×10^5–2×10^6 colony forming units (c.f.u.) were injected. Ganciclovir treatment was started 7 days later and was administered intraperitoneally at 15 mg/kg twice daily (1 ml/injection) for 14 days.

Producer Cells for Human Gene Therapy

Murine therapeutic retroviruses producing cells (MPC) were prepared as described previously [6, 8]. Essentially, DNA from plasmid pBabetk puro [6] was introduced to ecotropic Ψ CRE packaging cells using lipofectin®. Viral supernatants from transfected cells were used to infect amphotropic Ψ CRIP packaging cells. After selection with puromycin (2 μg/ml), colonies were isolated using cloning rings. These clonal lines were then assayed for vector titre and recombinant-competent retrovirus. Titres were estimated as follows: on day 1, NIH-3T3 cells were seeded at $5 \cdot 10^5$ cells/10-cm plate. On day 2, cells were infected with viral supernatants (filtered through a 0.45-μm filter) in the presence of 8 μg/ml polybrene. On day 4, cells were split 1:10 and 1:20 and selected with medium containing puromycin (2 μg/ml), medium changed 3 times/week until day 12 when colonies were stained with methylene blue. The titre expressed in c.f.u./ml was calculated multiplying by factors to correct dilutions, and dividing by 2.5 to correct cell proliferation before split. Marker rescue/mobilization assay for recombinant-competent retrovirus [3, 9] was as follows: viral supernatants from producer Ψ CRIP clones were used to infect 3T3-BAG and Mus dunni-BAG cells (MDTF-BAG). On day 1, $5 \cdot 10^5$ 3T3-BAG and MDTF-BAG were seeded in 10-cm plates. On day 2, plates were infected with 1 ml of pure viral supernatants (filtered through a 0.45-μm filter) from confluent 10-cm plates of Ψ CRIP producer cells in the presence of 8 μg/ml polybrene. Infected cells were cultured for a week (allowing amplification of possible RCR) in medium containing 1 mg/ml G418. The medium was then changed, harvested about 20 hours later, filtered and used to infect NIH-3T3 $5 \cdot 10^5$ cells/10-cm plates with 2 ml in the presence of 8 μg/ml polybrene. Detection of possible mobilized BAG virus was visualized by X-Gal stain directly and by selection with puromycin for one week before staining with X-Gal.

Large quantities of murine therapeutic retrovirus producer cells (MPC) were cultured in triple flasks (Nunc, 500 cm^2 growth area) with 100 ml per flask of DMEM supplemented with 10% calf serum. The cells were harvested just before use, washed and resuspended in a small volume of complete PBS (supplemented with calcium and magnesium) and glucose 0.1%.

Clinical and Surgical Procedures

Patients suffering from recurrent glioblastoma multiforme were reoperated on by re-opening their previous craniectomy to remove part of the tumoral mass and locally to inject the tumour bed with 8–10 ml of MPC at different points. During the surgical intervention an Ommaya reservoir was placed under the skin and connected to a catheter leading into the surgical cavity. Ganciclovir (Cymevene-Syntex) was administered intravenously at 5 mg/kg in 100 ml saline over one hour twice daily for 14 days. Blood and urine analysis performed at several points after treatment was normal. Patients received standard medication such as dexamethasone, antibiotics or anticonvulsants according to the usual neurosurgical guidelines. No increase of the brain oedema or intracranial pressure was observed. PCR on peripheral blood did not detect vector sequences in any of the patients. Magnetic resonance imaging (MRI) was performed at different times before and after surgery. Imaging was done in a 0.5 Tesla MR unit using Spin Echo T1 and T2 weighted images enhanced by treatment with 0.1 ml/Kg of Gadolinium in the three spatial planes.

MPC cells were administered through the Ommaya reservoir in a total volume of 6–8 ml. A 2 ml rinsing with sterile normal saline was added before and after injection of the cells (Table 1).

Results

Curability of Different Volume Size Tumors in the Wistar Rat

Tumour induction was achieved by direct injection of 5×10^5 cells into the right hemisphere of recipient

Table 1. *Treatment Scheme for the Two Patients*

No. patient	Treatment	No. producer cells	Titre (cfu/ml)[a]	Date
Patient 1	Partial resection with Ommaya reservoir placement	4.4×10^8	5×10^5	4.4.1995
Cycle 1	Intra-Ommaya injection	4×10^8	5×10^5	1 week later
	GCV intravenous	—	—	2 weeks
Cycle 2	idem	idem	idem	12.6.1995
Cycle 3	idem	idem	idem	3.11.1995
Patient 2	Partial resection with Ommaya	3×10^8	5×10^5	27.10.1995
Cycle 1	reservoir placement			
	Intra-Ommaya injection	4×10^8	5×10^5	1 week later
	GCV intravenous	—	—	2 weeks
Cycle 2	idem	idem	idem	2 months later

[a] c.f.u./ml: colony forming units per ml.

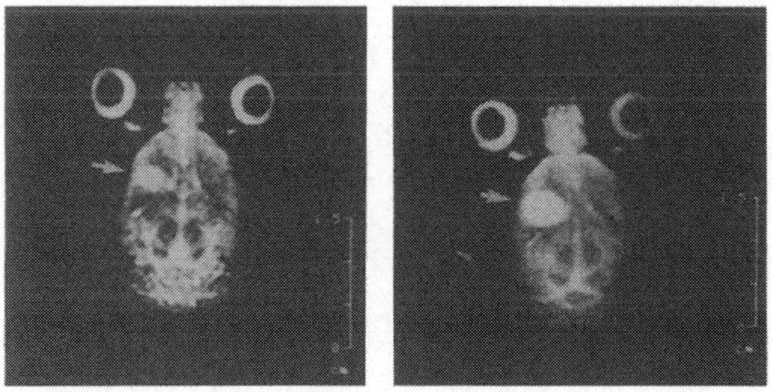

Fig. 1. Axial views of magnetic resonance images showing the progression of a rat brain tumour. Left picture: image obtained three weeks after C6 inoculum showing hyperintense signal at the site of injection (arrow, right hemisphere, left side of the picture). Right: the same rat two weeks later. The day after the first image was taken, 5×10^6 murine packaging cells were introduced into the tumour without apparent halt in tumour expansion (arrow)

rats in batches of 6 at a time, with the help of a stereotaxic apparatus. All the animals tolerated surgery very well and a few weeks after the injection about 70% of the animals inoculated with C6 and 90% of those receiving L9 harboured a tumour of variable size. Some of the rats were sacrificed for histopathology section study. The comparison of the two glioma cell lines indicates some differences mainly in two points: the mitotic index is slightly higher in L9 than C6 and lymphocytes and macrophages were found exclusively in some of the tumours induced by C6. The degree of infiltration is also higher for C6. Most of the experiments described below have been performed with C6.

The whole process can be followed by magnetic resonance performed at convenient time intervals. The majority of the C6 tumours can double their volume in about two weeks. As an example, a control animal is presented with a volume size tumour of 14 mm^3 treated with murine packaging cells and having two weeks later a volume of 32 mm^3 (Fig. 1). The result shows that murine packaging cells alone are not able to stop tumoral growth. A different result can be obtained if, instead of packaging cells which are unable to produce retroviral particles, high titre defective retrovirus producer cells are inoculated. A retrovirus carrying only the selection gene puro under the control of the LTR promoter (pBabepuro) was used for this purpose. In these conditions, about 60% of the tumours not larger than 20 mm^3 regressed when treated with pBabepuro producer cells with titres higher than 5×10^4 c.f.u. (colony forming units) (Fig. 2). When the brain tumour gets too large and extends beyond 150 mm^3, the conventional therapy of Hsvtk producer cells/ganciclovir system is not sufficient to stop the progression of the illness. The authors have been unable to cure a rat with a tumour size of 212 mm^3 using the same conditions and retroviral clones which can cure smaller size tumours (Fig. 3).

From the results obtained three volume dependent stages can be distinguished which would respond differently to conventional HSVtk/ganciclovir therapy (Table 2).

During the first stage, when the volume/size of the intracranial tumour is not greater than approximately 20 mm^3, an intracranial injection of retroviral producer cells with titres higher than 10^5 is sufficient to eradicate the tumour. The tumour infected cells are

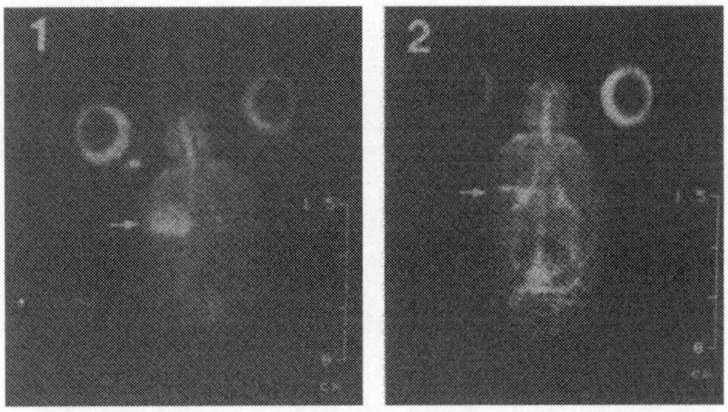

Fig. 2. Magnetic resonance images showing: *1* small and somewhat diffuse tumor *2* (arrow, right hemisphere, left side of the picture) obtained three weeks after a C6 inoculum, that can be cured by injection of 5×10^6 murine producer cells (MPC). The arrow indicates the regression of the original tumour two weeks after the MPC injection

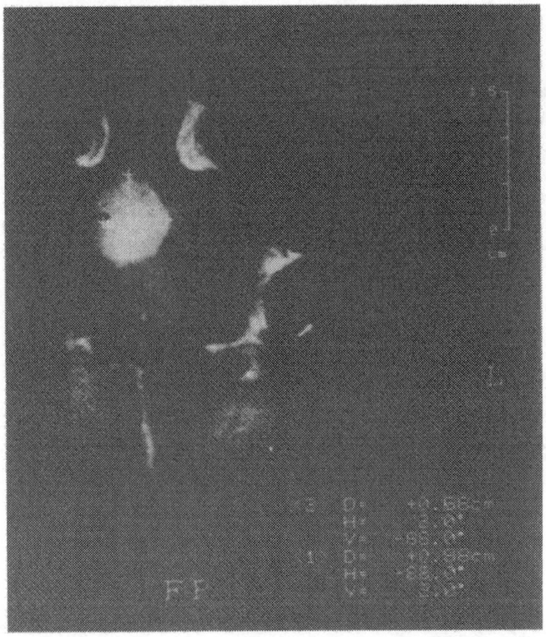

Fig. 3. Magnetic resonance image of a large tumour (V = 212 mm^3) on the right hemisphere of the animal (left side of the picture) unable to stop its growth and regression by ordinary Hstk/ganciclovir gene therapy

probably eliminated as a result of the immune system stimulation by retrovirus. This stage is particularly sensitive to retrovirus.

The second stage would include tumours of between 20 and 150 mm^3 volume. In this category retrovirus producer cells alone may be able to slow down the growing tumour, but never to eradicate it. Nevertheless retrovirus producing cells, carrying the thymidine kinase gene of the Herpes simplex virus, followed

Table 2. *Curability Potential at Different Volume Sizes in the Wistar Rat.* More than 10 tumours in each volume-size class have been analyzed

Stages	Rat	Humans
	Critical volume	(Diameter) = critical volume
1. Retroviral sensitivity	20 mm^3	1 cm = 0.5 cm^3
2. Gene therapy sensitivity	150 mm^3	(5–6 cm) = 100 cm^3
3. Irreversible insensitivity	more than 150 mm^3	>6 cm = more than 100 cm^3

$V = 4/3\pi r_1 \times r_2^2$; r_1 = length/2, r_2 = width/2.

by ganciclovir administration (Hsvtk/ganciclovir killer-suicide system), is very efficient in eradicating the tumours completely [6]. Within this stage (gene therapy sensitive) there is a correlation between the tumour size curability and the retroviral titre of producer cells. The volumes must be taken as approximate values. At the border line it would be difficult to predict the final outcome depending mainly upon the retroviral titre of producer cells.

Tumours with volumes higher than 150 mm^3 come into a final stage which is insensitive to gene therapy, perhaps due to the inability of obtaining producer cells with titres high enough to infect all the tumour cells as well as to the slow diffusion of particles across the solid tumour mass.

Human tumours are very likely to follow a similar pattern so that tumours larger than about 100 cm^3 would be unsuccessfully treated by the conventional thymidine kinase/ganciclovir system. Previous results of the authors in treating five patients, four of whom had tumours larger than 100 cm^3, confirm this interpretation. A correlation between the size of the tumour and the effectiveness of the treatment was established with the greatest effect in the smaller tumours, and vice versa [7]. The possibility of reducing the real tumour size by neurosurgery at the time of thymidine kinase/ganciclovir treatment was next explored.

Human Gene Therapy Response Using the Thymidine Kinase/Ganciclovir System

Three patients were originally selected to be treated by the combination of neurosurgery and thymidine kinase/ganciclovir. All three patients suffered from a relapsing glioblastoma and partial surgical removal of

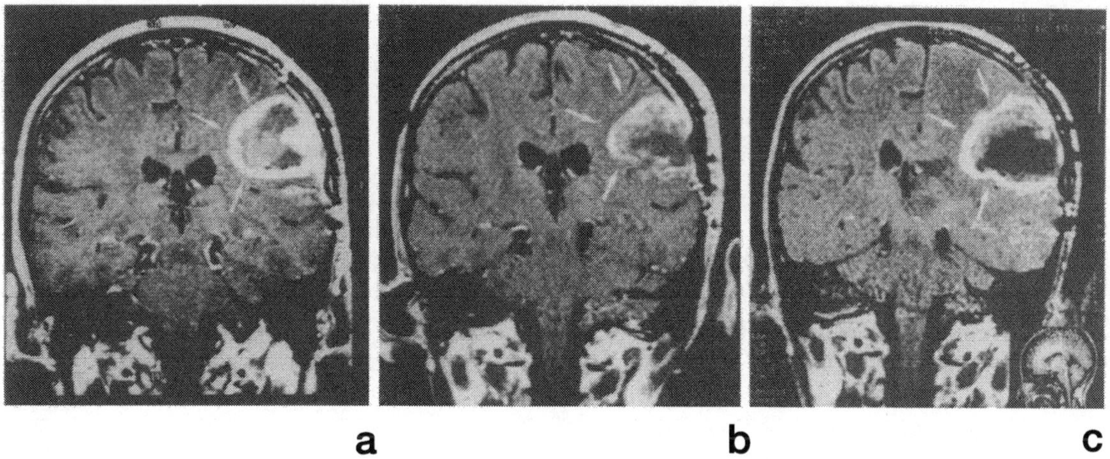

Fig. 4. Magnetic resonance imaging before and after gene therapy. Axial contrast enhanced T1W1 image of a large recurrent glioblastoma, (a) before partial resection and MPC injection, (b) after reoperation, (c) after one dose of gene therapy, showing a large necrotic area and persistent residual tumour (arrows)

the tumour mass was combined with the imbedding of the surgical cavity with murine Hsvtk producer cells (MPC) (5×10^8 cells), with a simultaneous insertion of an Ommaya reservoir for subsequent dose administration (Fig. 4) [2]. Seven days after surgery the first dose of MPCs was given via the reservoir and a week later ganciclovir treatment was initiated for two more weeks. Patients were followed by magnetic resonance imaging (MRI) before and after gene therapy. One of the patients developed a large haematoma after the intervention and the treatment was not completed; the patient died two months later. One of the other two patients developed fever which resolved 24 hours later. The two patients are still alive 11 (the first) and 17 months (the second) after the first gene therapy treatment during which 2 and 3 doses respectively of 5×10^8 MPCs were administered through their Ommaya reservoir at different times. The patients are followed up by magnetic resonance every three months and the new treatments have been performed in an attempt to eliminate any remaining neoplastic cells or new growths (Fig. 4). Total elimination of the residual tumour has not been achieved and the patients will probably not receive more intra-Ommaya injections of retroviral producer cells. The survival time of both patients has increased considerably suggesting a partial control of the tumoral growth by the treatment. The presence of residual tumour nevertheless indicates that the risk of a new outburst of growth persists despite several cycles of thymidine kinase/ganciclovir treatment.

Discussion

Gene therapy has been proved to be a valid and effective method to eradicate malignant brain tumours in experimental animal models mainly in the rat [1, 6, 11, 14–17]. Total disappearance of the tumour can be achieved by direct injection at the site of the growing mass of a large quantity of murine Hstk producer cells (5×10^6) and subsequent ganciclovir treatment. A period of 7 days is allowed between the producer cell injection and the ganciclovir treatment in order to allow the recombinant virus, which contains the Hsvtk gen, to infect the cancerous cells. Experimental data have shown that it is not strictly necessary to infect every single neoplastic cell with the retroviral killer-suicide vector to destroy the whole tumour, because there is a "bystander effect" that magnifies the response [5, 8, 18]. As little as 10% of the cancerous cells may need to be expressing the Hstk gen to cause the total destruction of the tumour. There is direct evidence to suggest that gap junctions play an important role in mediating the bystander response [4]. There may be also a role for a cell mediated immune response [5]. The cell line the authors have mainly used, C6, is known to express no detectable levels of connexins and form less compact and more infiltrating type of tumours than, for example, L9. Additionally, the L9 gliosarcoma cell line, but not the C6, has lost its ability to invade the parenchyma of the brain, perhaps due to the inability of the L9 cells to effect neovascularity [11]. In general, C6 is closer in properties to human glioblastomas than L9 and that is the reason why it was preferred for the present study. Nevertheless, if the bystander effect is mainly mediated by gap junctions, neither in the C6 animal model nor in human glioblastoma (closer in properties to C6) would such an effect be very strong.

The contribution of retroviral stimulation of the immune response in the regression of small tumours was studied despite the fact that the brain in general is a very poor immunogenic organ due to the blood-brain barrier. More than half of the induced tumors, if stimulated by the presence of defective retrovirus, disappear in two weeks from the time retroviral producer cells are injected at the site of the tumour. The authors have estimated that the titre of the producer cells has to be higher than 10^5 c.f.u. because in the 40% of the cases in which the tumours were not totally eliminated the titre of the producer cells was lower than that value. In these cases there is a delay in tumour growth but no appreciable regression.

This study has found in experimental animals, that tumours above a certain size (about 150 mm^3) cannot be cured by the ordinary thymidine kinase/ganciclovir system. It is not known whether in those conditions there is not enough retrovirus to infect a sufficient proportion of the tumour cells to provoke its regression, or, on reaching a certain tumour size, the progress of the illness is faster than gene therapy, which needs three weeks to complete. In humans it is very likely that also there are volume-size barriers as suggested in Table 2. In general, by the time a human tumour reaches the volumes considered, it has grown to form a mass of 5×10^{10} cells or more. The 5×10^8 producer cells delivered to the tumour will not be able to supply the amount of retroviral particles needed to infect every cancerous cell. The previous reduction of the tumoral mass by surgery, seems to be the best choice for the treatment of large human tumours. Two patients in which gene therapy was combined with neurosurgery are alive 11 and 17 months after the first cycle of thymidine kinase/ganciclovir respectively was given. Nevertheless total disappearance of the residual tumour has not been achieved despite several MPC injections. No side-effects have been observed and the survivors are followed up every three months as outpatients. The treatment so far has been safe and the results are encouraging. Achieving higher titres on producer cells, treating smaller tumours or changing the thymidine kinase gene to a more potent killer-suicide gene may be some of the improvements to be tried in the very near future.

Acknowledgments

We gratefully acknowledge Hartmut Land for the plasmid pBabepuro and Jean-Michael Heard for the packaging cell lines Ψ CRIP, Ψ CRE and for 3T3-BAG and Dunni-BAG. We are also very grateful to Drs. Felipe Sanz and Felipe Trigueros (Hospital Valdecilla) whose collaboration in this project has been extremely valuable. The work was supported by the Fondo de Investigaciones Sanitarias (FIS grant number 94/0417) Spain and by an institutional grant from the Fundación Ramón Areces to the Centro de Biología Molecular.

References

1. Culver KW, Wallbridge S, Ishii H, Oldfield EH, Blaese RM (1992) In vivo gene transfer with retroviral vector-producer cells for treatment of experimental brain tumors. Science 256: 1550–1552.
2. Culver K *et al* (1994) Gene therapy for the treatment of malignant brain tumors with in vivo tumor transduction with herpes simplex thymidine kinase gene/ganciclovir system (clinical protocol). Hum Gene Ther 5: 343–379
3. Danos O (1991) Construction of retroviral packaging cell lines. Methods Mol Biol 8: 17–27
4. Elshami AA *et al* (1996) Gap junctions play a role in the "bystander effect" of the herpes simplex virus thymidine kinase/ganciclovir system in vitro. Gene Ther 3: 85–92
5. Freeman SM *et al* (1993) The "bystander effect": tumor regression when a fraction of the tumor mass is genetically modified. Cancer Res 53: 5274–5283
6. Izquierdo M Cortés M, de Felipe P, Martín V Diéz-Guerra J, Talavera A, Perez-Higueras A (1995) Long term rat survival after malignant brain tumor regression by retroviral gene therapy. Gene Ther 2: 66–69
7. Izquierdo M, Martín V, de Felipe P, Izquierdo JM, Pérez-Higueras A, Cortés ML, Paz JF, Isla A, Blázquez MG (1996) Human malignant brain tumor response to Herpes Simplex thimidine kinase (HSVtk)/ganciclovir gene therapy. Gene Ther 3: 491–495
8. Li Bi W, Parysek LM, Warnick R, Stambrook PJ (1993) In vitro evidence that metabolic cooperation is responsible for the bystander effect observed whith HSVtk retroviral gene therapy. Hum Gene Ther 4: 725–731
9. Miller AD, Miller DG, García JV, Lynch CM (1993) Use of retroviral vectors for gene transfer and expression. Meth Enzymol 217: 581–599
10. Miller AD, Rosman GJ (1989) Improved retroviral vectors for gene transfer and expression. BioTechniques 7: 980–990
11. Moolten FL (1986) Tumor chemosensitivity conferred by inserted herpes thymidine kinase genes: Paradigm for a prospective cancer control strategy. Cancer Res 46: 5276–5281
12. Morgenstern J, Land H (1990) Advanced mammalian gene transfer: high titre retroviral vectors with multiple drug selection markers and a complementary helper-free packaging cell line. Nuc Acid Res 18: 3587–3596
13. Peterson DL, Sheridan PJ, Brown WE (1994) Animal models for brain tumors: historical perspectives and future directions. J Neurosurg 80: 865–876

14. Ram Z, Culver KW, Walbridge S, Blaese RM, Oldfield EH (1993) In situ retroviral-mediated gene transfer for the treatment of brain tumors in rats. Cancer Res 53: 83–88
15. Ram Z, Culver KW, Walbridge Frank JA, S, Blaese RM, Oldfield EH (1993) Toxicity studies of retroviral-mediated gene transfer for the treatment of brain tumors. J Neurosurg 79: 400–407
16. Short MP, Choi BC, Lee JK, Malick A, Breakefield XO, Martuza RL (1990) Gene delivery to glioma cells in rat brain by grafting of a retrovirus packaging cell line. J Neurosci Res 27: 427–433
17. Takamiya Y, Short MP, Ezzeddine ZD, Moolten FL, Breakefield XO, Martuza RL (1992) Gene therapy of malignant brain tumors: a rat glioma line bearing the herpes simplex virus type 1-thymidine kinase gene and wild type retrovirus kills other tumor cells. J Neurosci Res 33: 493–503
18. Wu JK *et al* (1994) Bystander tumoricidal effect in the treatment of experimental brain tumors. Neurosurgery 35: 1094–1102

Correspondence: Marta Izquierdo, M.D, Departamento de Biología Molecular/Centro de Biología Molecular Severo Ochoa, Facultad de Ciencias (modu 10-C-X), Universidad Autónoma de Madrid, Cantoblanco, E-28049 Madrid, Spain.

Acta Neurochir (1997) [Suppl] 68: 118–123

Risk Analysis of LINAC Radiosurgery in Patients with Arteriovenous Malformation (AVM)

J. Voges[1], H. Treuer[1], R. Lehrke[1], M. Kocher[2], S. Staar[2], R.-P. Müller[2], and V. Sturm[1]

[1] Departments of Stereotactic and Functional Neurosurgery and [2]Radiation Oncology, The University of Cologne, Federal Republic of Germany

Summary

The purposes of this analysis were the evaluation of the toxicity of stereotactic single dose irradiation in patients with an arteriovenous malformation (AVM) and the comparison of the authors' own results with already existing risk prediction models. Computed-tomography (CT) or magnetic-resonance (MR) images, and clinical data of patients treated with linear accelerator radiosurgery for an AVM were analysed retrospectively. Using the Cox proportional hazards model (1), the relevance of treatment parameters and dose-volume relationships to the occurrence of radiation-induced tissue changes (oedema and localised blood-brain-barrier breakdown) were assessed. The 81 patients selected for analysis had a mean follow-up of 28.9 months (range: 9.0–65.7 months). Radiation-induced tissue changes (22 out of 81 i.e. 27.2%) were documented on CT or MR images 6.3–33.8 months after radiosurgery (median time: 12.8 months). The actuarial risk at 2 years was 32.1% for the development of neuroradiological changes and 20.1% for the development of symptomatic tissue alteration. The coefficient of total volume receiving a minimum dose of 10 Gy (VTREAT10) reached statistical significance in a Cox proportional hazards model. These results demonstrate the particular vulnerability of normal brain tissue to single dose irradiation. Optimal conformation of the therapeutic isodose line to the 3D configuration of the target volume may help to reduce side effects.

Keywords: Radiosurgery; LINAC; risk prediction; arteriovenous malformation.

Introduction

Radiosurgery performed either with a modified linear accelerator or with the gamma knife is an attractive tool in the treatment of cerebral arteriovenous malformations. In recent years, a growing number of neurosurgical and radiation oncology centres have used this technique in addition to or as alternative to microsurgical resection. The large number of publications on the subject has also reflected the importance of this treatment modality.

However, little is known about the particular risks of single dose irradiation in patients suffering from an AVM. The main purpose of this analysis is the definition of risk factors and the comparison of the authors' results with already existing risk prediction models.

Patients

Eighty-one patients treated between June 1990 and August 1995 at the University of Cologne for an AVM with stereotactic single dose irradiation using a modified linear accelerator (LINAC) were selected for retrospective analysis of risk factors. The following selection criteria were applied: (a) Follow-up times of at least 9 months (end of follow-up; June 1996). (b) Availability of complete treatment data. (c) Follow-up information including the results of neurological and neuroradiological examinations (computed tomography (CT) and/or magnetic resonance imaging (MRI)). Patients with perilesional oedema on preoperative CT or MR images were excluded.

Methods

Clinical and Neuroradiological Criteria

The reference point was the date of radiosurgery. Endpoints of the study were radiation-induced changes on postoperative CT and MR images, date of last follow-up examination, patient's death, date of surgical intervention or spontaneous intracerebral haemorrhage. Radiation-induced tissue reactions were assumed if signal changes on follow-up CT or MR images indicated the occurrence of perilesional oedema either alone or in combination with a typical ring shaped contrast enhancement, the latter indicating localised blood-brain barrier (BBB) breakdown. The patient's clinical status as categorised in terms of new symptoms or improvement, and decrease or stabilisation of already documented symptoms was correlated with the results of image evaluation. Follow-up data were obtained using a standardised form either by examination of outpatients or by communication with the patients, their relatives and referring physicians.

Definitions and Statistical Analysis

Treatment parameters were labelled therapeutic dose (DOSEMIN) and the number of applied isocenters (ISOCEN). Besides DOSEMIN, the maximum dose inside the target volume (DOSEMAX) and the highest dose applied to perilesional brain tissue (MAXBRAIN) were assessed.

Integral dose volume histograms (DVH) were computed for the volume of the treated lesion (DVH_{target}) and the volume of tissue which was covered by the 10 Gy isodose-line (DVH_{10}). Two different volumes were calculated for all selected patients from DVHs: (a) Treatment volume (VTREAT): total volume covered by DOSEMIN. (b) VTREAT10: total volume covered by the 10 Gy isodose-line. The decision for 10 Gy as threshold value was based upon their own clinical observations in a few initial patients who developed symptomatic radiation necrosis. In these cases the rim of pathological contrast enhancement was nearly identical with the 10 Gy isodose line [16].

In most patients, the target volume (VTARGET) was assessed by measuring the maximum diameters (d_{ap1}, d_{lat1}) and the rectangular corresponding diameters (d_{ap2}, d_{lat2}) of the nidus on plane angiograms (anterior-posterior view and lateral view), which were taken intra-operatively under stereotactic conditions. The volume was then calculated from the three highest values using the formula: $V_{target} = \pi/6 \times d_{ap1} \times d_{lat1} \times (d_{ap2} \text{ or } d_{lat2})$. In patients treated from March 1995 to August 1995 the angiograms (anterior-posterior view and lateral view) were scanned into the computer and the nidus was delineated directly on the computer screen. Using this 2-dimensional information the software generated a 3-dimensional cubic target volume.

Factors relevant for the induction of tissue changes following radiosurgery were obtained from the Cox regression analysis [1]. Significant predictor variables were calculated using the proportional hazards model (forward stepwise selection). Results of this analysis are given as *p*-values. Additionally relative risks and 95% confidence intervals are given for those parameters which, in a full model, were significant predictor variables. Neuroanatomical localisation was described using three categories: (a) "Lobar" lesions situated in the cerebral grey or white matter. (b) Vessel malformations of the "midline" were located close to the ventricular system, septal area, and the splenium, or inside basal ganglia, diencephalon, and brainstem. (c) Lesions of the "posterior fossa" were extended in the cerebellum.

Treatment Planning and Irradiation Technique

The different hardware and software components of the treatment planning and irradiation appliances have been published previously [7, 8, 12–15]. In summary, after fixation of the patient's head in a modified, CT-compatible Riechert-Mundinger stereotactic frame, CT examination [15] and angiography were performed intra-operatively under stereotactic conditions. CT data were transferred to a microcomputer. Until February 1995 the diameter of the nidus and co-ordinates of isocenters were taken from plane angiograms. Beginning in March 1995 the angiograms were scanned into the computer and these parameters were assessed on the computer screen. Target points and width of the collimators were adjusted with respect to target volume and three dimensional configuration of the lesion and were calculated together with the depth dose distribution on the computer screen [13]. The treatment plan was controlled three dimensionally by the display of any significant isodose line to the CT images. In the authors' system [8, 12], beam convergence is achieved by use of 10 arcs of Linac table rotation in steps of 18° and rotation of the gantry from 20°–160°. Spherical fields from 5–45 mm in diameter can be irradiated with dose gradients from 10% (large fields) to 25% (small fields) per mm distance from the tumour surface. In order to achieve an ellipsoid modification of the originally spherical irradiation volume for dose conformation, a reduced number of arcs (6–9 arcs) and/or variations of the gantry rotation were applied.

Results

Patients and Treatment Parameters

Forty-one female and forty male patients ranged in age from 11–74 years (median: 37.1 years). The mean follow-up dated from radiosurgery until one of the endpoints of this study was 28.9 months (range: 9.0–65.7 months). Fifty-three vessel malformations were located in the lobar or cortical regions, 22 in the midline, and six in the posterior fossa.

The median therapeutic dose (DOSEMIN) applied to the surface of the nidus was 20.0 Gy (range: 8.0–25.0 Gy), the maximum dose inside the target volume (DOSEMAX) ranged from 13.3–57.0 Gy (median 27.4 Gy). In all patients, DOSEMIN was normalised to the 80% isodose line. Target volumes ranged from 0.1–49.9 cc (mean volume: 7.8 ± 1.1 cc). The therapeutic dose was applied with 1–5 isocenters. Sixty-five out of 81 AVM's (80.2%) were covered with one or two isocenters.

Neuroradiological Evaluation

Radiation induced tissue changes were documented on CT and/or MR images 6.3–33.8 months after radiosurgery (RS) (median time: 12.8 months). The total rate of complications was 27.2% (22 out of 81 lesions) with an actuarial risk at 2 years for the development of radiation-induced neuroradiological changes of 32.1% (Fig. 1). Twenty-three percent of the side effects (5/22 patients) were seen within 10

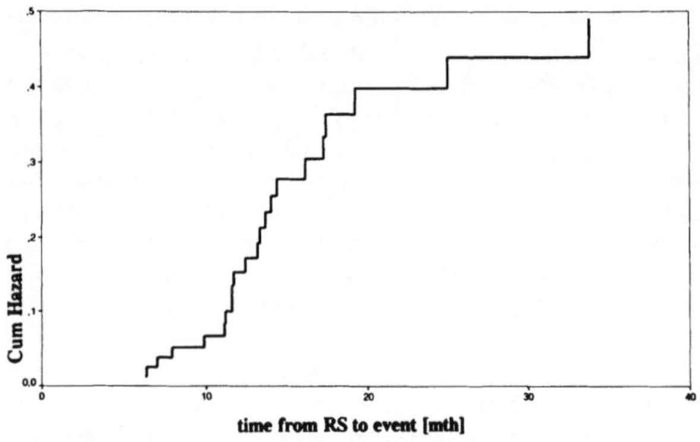

Fig. 1. The cumulative hazard for the occurrence of radiation-induced tissue changes (81 patients). The actuarial risk at 2 years was 32.1%

months after treatment, 73% (16/22 patients) within 16 months after treatment, and the remaining 4% thereafter. In evaluated patients, neuroradiological examinations demonstrated perilesional oedema in 3, a typical ring-shaped enhancement in 6, and in 13 patients oedema together with enhancement. Depending on location, the rate of image changes was 28.3%; 15 out of 53 patients with pratentorial/cortical location, 22.7% (5/22 patients) in the midline and 33% (2/6 patients) in the posterior fossa.

Clinical Data

Radiation-induced tissue changes were associated with deterioration in the clinical status in 16.1% of the evaluated patients (13 out of 81). In these patients, worsening was attributable to ring enhancement and oedema. The neurological deficits were as follows: hemiparesis (4 patients), visual field cuts (1 patient), paramnesia (1 patient), and diplopia (1 patient). One out of 13 patients had symptoms from both hemiparesis and visual field deficit. Another patient suffered from severe headache. The deterioration was permanent in 7 patients and improved in two cases. Newly occurring seizures (4 patients) could be controlled successfully with anticonvulsive medication. The actuarial risk at 2 years for the development of symptomatic neuroradiological changes was 20.1%.

In one patient, the new symptoms were not directly related to the treatment but to rebleeding which occurred 10 months after radiosurgery. In 4.9% of the cases (4 out of 81), improvement of preoperatively existing symptoms was found during follow-up despite neuroradiological changes.

Cox Regression Analysis

The variables DOSEMIN, DOSEMAX, VTARGET, VTREAT, VTREAT10, number of applied isocenters, age and localisation were considered in Cox regression analysis. The only variable which reached statistical significance in a proportional hazards model was VTREAT10 ($p = 0.0023$, relative risk: 1.0322, 95% χ: 1.0114–1.0535). If stratified to different volumes, no event was observed when VTREAT10 was equal to or lower than 10 cc. In contrast, all events occurred in patients with a VTREAT10 exceeding 10 cc. In addition, the technique of treatment planning seemed to influence the outcome: All complications were seen in patients in whom field size and coordinates of the isocenters were adjusted directly onto the images of plane angiograms. In 16 patients treated after February 1995, in whom the treatment planning software generated a cubic VOI on CT-images from the 2-dimensional data given by scanned angiograms, no complication was found up to follow-up. The follow-up time of this subgroup ranged from 9–16 months.

Discussion

Clinical Data

In the authors' own analysis the total rate of radiation induced neuroradiological changes was 27.2% (22 out of 81 patients) with an actuarial risk at 2 years of 32.1%. The actuarial risk at 2 years for the development of symptomatic oedema and/or contrast enhancement was 20.1%.

Serial post-irradiation MR images of 72 patients as well as clinical data were used by Flickinger *et al.* for an analysis of factors responsible for image changes and symptomatic complications after gamma knife radiosurgery of AVMs [4]. Twenty of 72 patients (27.8%) developed post radiosurgical image changes and 9 out of 20 patients (45%) developed symptoms. The actuarial risk at 2 years was 31% for the development of image changes in general and 14% for symptomatic image changes. Despite smaller target volumes (mean volumes: 3.75 cc [4] vs. 7.8 cc (the authors')) these data are in accordance with the present findings.

The comparatively high risk of the radiosurgical treatment of AVMs has been demonstrated by Flickinger et al. in a more recently published analysis [6]. In addition to patients with vessel malformations, those suffering from meningioma (55 patients) and acoustic neuroma (84 patients) were evaluated for risk factors. In a χ^2 test, the incidence of post-radiosurgical image changes differed statistically in a highly significant manner between AVM patients (31%) and tumour patients (8%). Although in multivariate logistic regression analysis the variable "histology" did not reach statistical significance, a *p*-value of 0.051 indicated that it might be an important coefficient.

The higher risk in AVM is explained by the fact that these lesions are completely surrounded by healthy brain tissue. Additionally, in most of the authors' patients, the vessel malformation was located in a critical area of the brain. Thus any significant radiation dose outside the prescribed target volume poses a potential risk for damage of healthy tissue. A second important point might be the technique of treatment planning. Until recently, in this series, the definition of the target volume in AVMs (i.e., demarcation of the nidus) had to be performed on plane angiographic images. Thus, in 65 out of 81 patients the treatment planning was 2-dimensional rather than 3-dimensional and, in general, overdose to normal brain tissue could not be avoided completely. All observed complications were related to this group of patients. In 16 patients, in whom the treatment planning was performed 3-dimensionally with an upgraded version of software no event has been observed. However, the comparatively short follow-up time of these patients does not yet allow a final evaluation.

Cox regression analysis demonstrated that the variable "volume covered by the 10 Gy isodose line (VTREAT10)" is a potential risk predictor for single dose radiosurgery in AVM patients. Flickinger *et al.* [4] described three factors which in univariate analysis correlated with postradiosurgical image changes: volume, risk predictions from the exponential version of the integrated logistic formula and the number of applied targets. Only the parameter "treatment volume" was statistically significant after a multivariate approach.

Flickinger's results are, in general, not contradictory to the authors' findings. With increasing treatment diameters the volume of normal brain tissue covered by the therapeutic dose is of increasing relevance for the outcome [3]. In a model estimation, assuming that a cubic target was irradiated with a single spherical field, the volume of normal tissue receiving the therapeutic dose increases with the cube of the diameter with larger treatment diameters (≥ 35 mm) [3]. If comparatively large target volumes are treated, as occurred in this study then a certain volume of tissue adjacent to the target is irradiated with a radiation dose above tissue tolerance (a correlation which is expressed by VTREAT [10]).

Risk Prediction Models

In 1979, Kjellberg established a schedule for risk estimation, plotting isoeffect lines for different proton beam diameters in a graph log radius of volume vs. log dose [9]. The threshold values for radiation-induced necrosis varied from 50 Gy for 7 mm beams to 10.5 Gy for 50 mm beams, with a linear relationship between the logarithm of beam diameter and the logarithm of therapeutic dose (the 1% isoeffect line). Integrating the dose-volume data points of 74 patients treated for an AVM with single proton beam irradiation, 6 of 8 patients with symptomatic complications were distributed above and 2 of 8 patients below the first percentile for isoeffective doses [10]. The calculated risk for symptomatic complications was 2.7% (2 out of 74 patients). In order to compare the authors' results with this analysis, field diameters and corresponding therapeutic doses of all 81 patients with AVMs were subjected to Kjellberg's risk estimation plot. Because in Kjellberg's analysis radiation necrosis was related to symptomatic patients, only those patients were considered at risk in whom ring shaped contrast enhancement plus oedema were combined with deterioration of the clinical status (13 patients). As demonstrated in Fig. 2, the majority of these patients (10 out of 13) were projected below the 1% isoeffect line resulting in a risk for symptomatic complications of 12.3% (10 out of 81 patients). This value is much higher than the risk probability calculated for Kjellberg's analysis.

In addition, when the dose/volume data of Flickinger's series [4] were incorporated in Kjellberg's schedule [11] the calculated risk (3 out of 72 patients, 4.2%) was somewhat different. This variability demonstrates that the 1% isoeffect line as threshold value is questionable, an aspect which has already been discussed by others [11].

The second approach for risk prediction has been described by Flickinger in 1989 [2]. Similar to Kjellberg's schedule, the integrated logistic formula predicts the risk of brain necrosis, Ling *et al.* revised the validity of this model [11]. Using treatment parameters

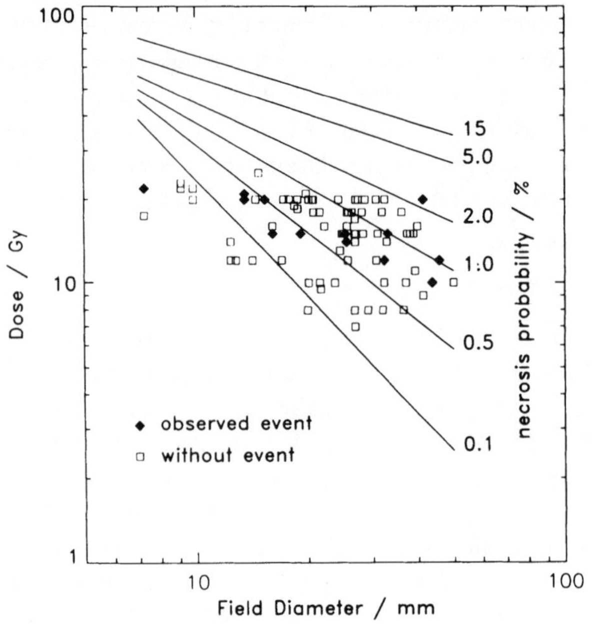

Fig. 2. Comparison of dose and field diameter of 81 patients, in whom an arterio-venous-malformation was treated with Linac-radiosurgery with Kjellberg's isoeffect lines predicting the risk for single dose radiosurgery with protons at various beam diameters [9]. Thirteen patients with clinically symptomatic neuroradiological pathologies were marked with (♦)

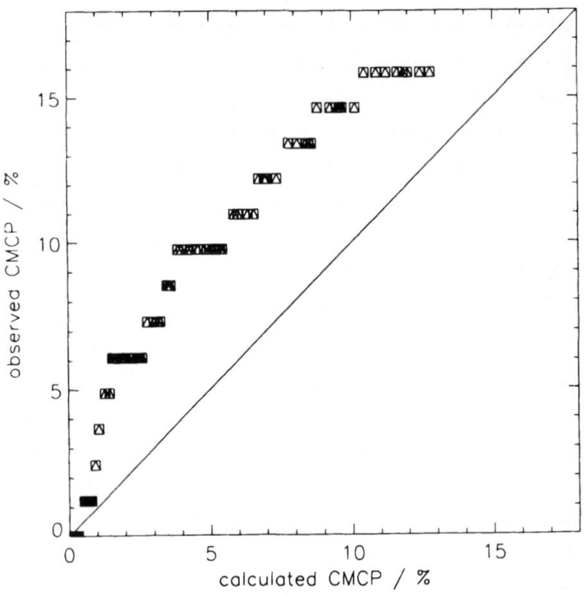

Fig. 3. Scatterplot of the observed cumulative mean complication probabilies (CMCP) for AVM patients with symptomatic complications vs. calculated CMCPs. According to Ling *et al.* [11] the displayed parameters are defined as observed CMCP: $n/N \times 100\%$ (n = cumulative number of complications, N = total number of patients or treated tumours in the study); and calculated CMCP: $Si(Pi)/N$ (Pi = calculated integral logistic probability for the nth patient). The calculated values (□) are based upon the integrated logistic formula [3].

which were given for 72 AVM-patients in a figure of Flickinger's original risk analysis [4], they plotted the calculated cumulative mean complication probability (CMCP) against the observed CMCP. If compared with the calculated probabilities (calculation was performed according to the integrated logistic formula), projection of the observed data points was in fact close to the 45° line, but a better fit could be achieved with a corrected line [11]. The same mathematical manoeuvre performed with the authors' data is shown in Fig. 3. Only patients with post-radiosurgical imaging changes, which represent "radiation necrosis" (ring enhancement plus oedema) were at risk. For calculation of the risk probability a generalised version of the integrated logistic formula was used [5]. The values for the different constants ($D_{50} = 11.78$ Gy, $V_{total} = 1367$ cc, $k = 1/0.054$) were taken from the literature [2, 5]. As before, to achieve a good fit of data points the slope of the 45° line has to be increased by about 15° resulting in a 60° line. Thus, probabilities calculated with the integrated logistic formula have to be corrected by a factor of about 1.3. These differences between calculated and observed incidence can be interpreted as an underestimation of the risk of single dose irradiation in AVM patients if the integrated logistic model is applied.

In conclusion, the authors' results clearly demonstrate that not only dose and target volume influence the outcome after single dose radiosurgery. Radiation of brain tissue adjacent to the target volume is also of major importance.

Despite differences in the power of risk prediction, all risk analyses performed so far proved the particular vulnerability of normal brain tissue to single dose irradiation. Thus, the primary aim of treatment planning should be the avoidance of overdose of tissue adjacent to the target volume. This challenge can be realised through careful dose conformation either by use of already available technical possibilities (i.e., in Linac-based radiosurgery application of multiple isocenters together with variations of table and/or gantry rotation) or by application of recently developed system components like the micromultileaf collimator. In AVMs, a true 3D instead of 2D treatment planning is of particular importance and will help to reduce the rate of side effects significantly.

References

1. Cox DR (1972) Regression models and life tables. JR Stat Soc (B) 34: 187–220
2. Flickinger JC (1989) An integrated logistic formula for prediction of complications from radiosurgery. Int J Radiat Oncol Biol Phys 17: 879–885
3. Flickinger JC, Lunsford LD, Kondziolka D (1993) Radiosurgical dosimetry: principles and clinical implications. In: De Salles AAF, Goetsch SJ (eds) Stereotactic surgery and radiosurgery. Medical Physics, Madison, Wisconsin, pp 293–306
4. Flickinger JC, Lunsford LD, Knodziolka D, Maitz AH, Epstein AH, Simons SR, Wu A (1992) Radiosurgery and brain tolerance: an analysis of neurodiagnostic imaging changes after gamma knife radiosurgery for arteriovenous malformations. Int J Radiat Oncol Biol Phys 23: 19–26
5. Flickinger JC, Schell MC, Larson DA (1990) Estimation of complications for Linear accelerator radiosurgery with the integrated logistic formula. Int J Radiat Oncol Biol Phys 19: 143–148
6. Flickinger JC, Kondziolka D, Kalend AM, Maitz AH, Lunsford LD (1996) Radiosurgery-related imaging changes in surrounding brain: multivariate analysis and model evaluation. In: Kondziolka D (ed) Radiosurgery, vol 1. Karger, Basel, pp 229–236
7. Gahbauer H, Sturm V, Schlegel W, Pastyr O, Zabel HJ, van Kaick G, Netzeband G, Scheer KE, Schabbert S (1983) Combined use of stereotactic CT and angiography for brain biopsies and stereotaxic irradiation. AJNR 4: 715–718
8. Hartmann GH, Schlegel W, Sturm V, Bernd K, Pastyr O, Lorenz WJ (1985) Cerebral radiation surgery using moving field irradiation at a linear accelerator facility. Int J Radiat Oncol Biol Phys 11: 1185–1192
9. Kjellberg RN (1979) Isoeffective dose parameters for brain necrosis in relation to proton radiosurgical dosimetry. In: Szikla G (ed) Stereotactic cerebral irradiation (INSERM Symposium no. 12). Elsevier/North Holland Biomedical Press, Amsterdam, pp 157–166
10. Kjellberg RN, Hanamura T, Davis KR, Lyons SL, Adams RD (1983) Bragg-peak proton beam therapy for arteriovenous malformations of the brain. N Engl J Med 309: 269–274
11. Ling CC, Lo YC, Larson DA (1995) Radiobiophysical aspects of stereotaxic radiation treatment of central nervous system disease. Sem Radiat Oncol 5: 192–196
12. Pastyr O, Hartmann GH, Schlegel W, Schabbert S, Treuer H, Lorenz WJ, Sturm V (1989) Stereotactically guided convergent beam irradiation with a linear accelerator: Localization – technique. Acta Neurochir (Wien) 99: 61–64
13. Schlegel W, Scharfenberg H, Doll J, Hartmann G, Sturm V, Lorenz WJ (1984) Three dimensional dose planning using tomographic data. In: IEEE Comp Society (eds) Proceedings of the Eighth International Conference on the Use of Computers in Radiation Therapy. IEEE, Silver Spring, pp 191–196
14. Schlegel WJ, Scharfenberg H, Sturm V, Penzholz H, Lorenz WJ (1981) Direct visualization of intracranial tumours in stereotactic and angiographic films by computer calculation of longitudinal CT-sections: a new method for stereotactic localization of tumour outlines. Acta Neurochir (Wien) 58: 27–35
15. Sturm V, Pastyr O, Schlegel W, Scharfenberg H, Zabel HJ, Netzeband G, Schabbert S, Berberich W (1983) Stereotactic computer tomography with a modified Riechert-Mundinger device as the basis for integrated neuroradiological investigations. Acta Neurochir (Wien) 68: 11–17
16. Voges J, Sturm V, Deuß U, Traud C, Treuer H, Schlegel W, Winkelmann W, Müller RP (1996) LINAC-Radiosurgery in pituitary adenomas – Preliminary results. Acta Neurochir (Wien) [Suppl] 65: 41–43

Correspondence: Jürgen Voges, M.D., Abteilung für Stereotaxie und funktionelle Neurochirurgie Universität Köln, Josef-Stelzmann-Str. 9, D-50931 Köln, Federal Republic of Germany.

Acta Neurochir (1997) [Suppl] 68: 124–126

Effect of LINAC Radiosurgery on Regional Cerebral Blood Flow, Glucose Metabolism and Sodium-Potassium AtPase in Skull Base Meningiomas and Metastasis

P. C. Warnke, A. Berlis, A. Weyerbrock, and C. B. Ostertag

Abteilung Stereotaktische Neurochirurgie, Neurozentrum, Freiburg, Federal Republic of Germany

Summary

Stereotactic radiosurgery is an elegant alternative to microsurgery in both skull base meningiomas and solitary brain metastasis. Though efficacy for both entities has been established prognostic variables pertaining to individual tumour biology have not yet been identified. Therefore the authors measured regional glucose utilisation, thallium-uptake and blood flow in 20 patients (10 meningiomas, 10 metastasis) before and after LINAC radiosurgery. Measurements were performed using SPECT and stable xenon-CT. The mean tumour dose given was 16.3 and 19.5 Gy in meningiomas and metastasis respectively. Metastatic tumours were hypermetabolic in comparison to contralateral normal brain and responders to radiosurgery showed a lower tumour/brain ratio than non-responders (1.43 vs 0.91 respectively, $p < 0.01$). Meningiomas did not exhibit hypermetabolism and therapeutic outcome was not related to glucose utilisation. Thallium-uptake, however, was closely related to therapeutic response in meningiomas (1.37 vs 2.2 in responders vs non-responders, $p < 0.01$). This relationship could not be established in metastatic lesions. Blood flow was widely distributed in both meningiomas and metastasis (26–72.8 and 30.2–70.8 ml/100 g/min). rCBF did not correlate with therapeutic outcome.

Using FDG-SPECT and thallium-201-SPECT the authors were able to distinguish between tumours likely to respond to stereotactic radiosurgery and those not prone to respond. Furthermore the methodology can be used to monitor therapeutic response in treated tumours before morphologic changes occur.

Keywords: Meningioma; brain metastasis; stereotactic radiosurgery; tumour metabolism.

Introduction

Stereotactic radiosurgery using linear accelerators or the Gamma-knife has evolved as an attractive treatment modality for small skull base meningiomas especially involving critical structures like the cavernous sinus [4, 8, 10]. The same pertains to small solitary brain metastases with a diameter of less than 3 cm [2, 5, 6]. For both pathological entities stereotactic radiosurgery can achieve an excellent tumour control rate and in a certain percentage of cases even a complete tumour response, thus becoming a less invasive alternative to microsurgery. Although large clinical series have established the clinical efficacy of stereotactic radiosurgery both in skull base meningiomas and metastasis, there is a lack of information concerning the effects of single fraction radiosurgery on tumour metabolism and physiology. The same applies to the effect of radiosurgery on metabolism and physiology of the surrounding healthy brain. Furthermore measurements of tumour metabolism have not been used in metastasis or meningiomas in order to identify responders on the basis of their metabolism or to predict tumour response based on the individual tumour metabolism. This approach seems worthwhile following as, in malignant gliomas, a clear relationship between tumour metabolism and outcome has been established and treatment responses have been evaluated by PET-measurements of tumour metabolism in a quantitative reproducible manner [1, 9]. In order to correlate the effects of radiosurgery with individual tumour metabolic measurements the authors prospectively evaluated patients with skull base meningiomas and metastases before and after radiosurgery in terms of their blood flow, their regional glucose utilisation and their sodium-potassium-AtPase activity.

Material and Methods

20 patients (10 meningiomas, 10 metastases) were prospectively enrolled into the study. Meningioma location was in the cavernous sinus ($N = 7$) or in the cerebello-pontine angle ($N = 3$). All patients underwent measurements of regional cerebral blood flow using stable xenon-CT. In each case regional glucose-utilisation ratio also was measured using a dedicated SPECT camera with a 511 keV collimator designed to image PET-emitters. Patients received 185 MBq 18-F-labelled deoxyglucose before and at 3 months intervals after stereotactic radiosurgery. Images were obtained with the Sie-

mens orbiter, SPECT-camera with a full-width half-maximum resolution of 8 × 8 mm. For image analysis a 64 × 64 matrix was used and a Butterworth-filter was employed to reconstruct tomographic images. Image analysis was performed as ratios between tumour and contralateral mirror-imaged brain. In addition each patient was examined using thallium-201 SPECT imaging to assess the sodium-potassium-AtPase activity. Thallium-201 is known to be actively transported into cells and thus a viability marker in oncology [3]. SPECT imaging again was performed using a Siemens orbiter camera and a Shepp-Logan-Hanning filter was employed for the construction of tomographic images.

The mean age of the meningioma patients was 56 years and for the patients with metastases 61 years. Median follow-up was 10.6 and 9.5 months respectively. The mean dose to tumour periphery was 16.3 Gy in meningioma patients and 19.5 Gy in patients with metastases. All treatments were performed with an 8 meV LINAC (Varian). Statistical analysis was performed using the paired t-test.

Results

Metastatic tumours showed – as had been expected from malignant tumours – a hypermetabolic glucose pattern as compared to normal brain and could be identified by deoxyglucose (FDG) SPECT. Contrary to that finding, most of skull base meningiomas with the exception of one malignant anaplastic grade III meningioma showed significantly lower glucose-utilisation rates than the contralateral normal brain structures. Figure 1 shows the relationship between base line glucose metabolism and tumour response as evaluated by volumetric MRI-analysis. Whereas in metastasis there was a significant difference in glucose metabolism between those that responded to radiosurgery by significant volume reduction as compared to those that did not respond, in meningiomas there was no such relationship between glucose metabolism and consequential tumour response after radiosurgery.

In terms of sodium/potassium AtPase, meningiomas showed a very prominent uptake of thallium-201 as compared to contralateral normal healthy brain. Although metastases showed a significant thallium-uptake as well this was conspicously lower than in meningiomas. Furthermore as shown in Fig. 2 thallium-uptake did not correlate to tumour response in metastases but did so quite significantly in meningiomas.

In addition, after radiosurgery in both metastases and meningiomas a significant drop in the ipsi- to contralateral ratio of FDG-utilisation could be seen, being more pronounced in metastases then in meningiomas and resulting in a drop of the ratio in metastases from 1.4 to 0.8 and in meningiomas from 0.92 to

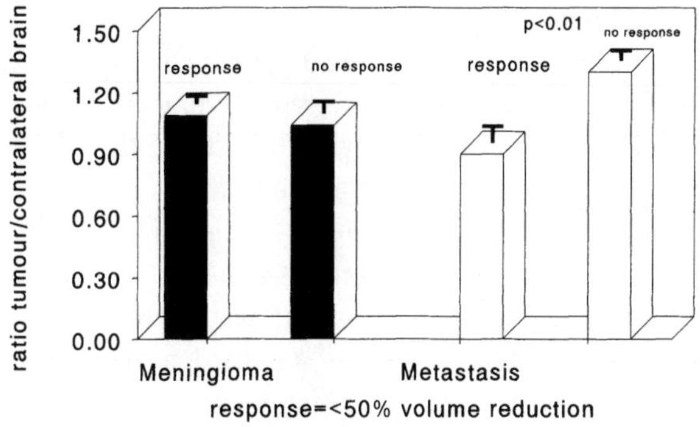

Fig. 1. Glucose utilisation ratios in meningiomas and metastases treated by stereotactic radiosurgery. Both groups are divided into responders and non-responders. A significant difference between subgroups is seen only in patients with solitary brain metastasis

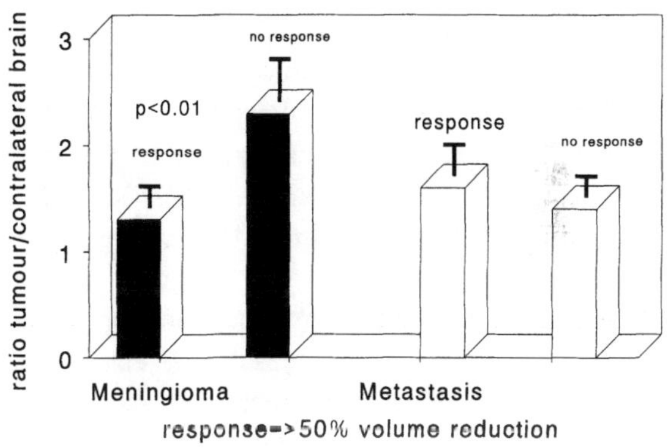

Fig. 2. Thallium-uptake ratios in meningiomas and metastases. Subdivision into responders and non-responders showed a significant difference in meningiomas whereas the difference in patients with metastases did not reach significance

0.71 ($p < 0.05$). Furthermore, in cases of meningioma involving the cavernous sinus the adjacent brain showed a significant drop of FDG-utilisation from 1.02 to 0.91 ($p < 0.05$) revealing a subtle effect of radiosurgery on metabolism of surrounding structures.

Blood flow in meningiomas was very heterogeneous and ranged between 26 and 72.8 ml/100 g/min. Blood flow did not predict tumour response. In metastasis blood flow ranged from 70.8 to 30.2 ml/100 g/min and also did not allow any prediction of tumour response after stereotactic radiosurgery.

Discussion

Stereotactic radiosurgery using linear accelerators is a powerful modern treatment modality for both small solitary brain metastases as well as skull base meningiomas adjacent to or involving critical structures e.g.

the cranial nerves. Whereas the tumour control rate in both cases is between 80 and 90%, the actual response rate defined as a 50% volume reduction, especially in meningiomas is only slightly higher than 50%. Using SPECT imaging and semi-quantitative metabolic imaging in a prospective manner the authors were able to distinguish between responders and non-responders both in meningiomas and metastases on the basis of either glucose metabolism of the individual tumour or thallium-uptake, which is supposed to reflect active membrane transport [7]. Whereas in the malignant phenotype (i.e. metastases) glucose metabolism was a good predictor of treatment outcome, this was not the case in meningiomas which were all hypometabolic compared to baseline measurements. In meningiomas thallium-uptake was best at predicting tumour response defined as a significant reduction of tumour volume. Both SPECT techniques also allowed the monitoring of tumour response in individual patients as well and showed necrotic changes in meningiomas after radiosurgery earlier than both CT and MRI imaging. This prospective series is continuing and, especially in brain metastases, will hopefully provide an answer to the question of whether radiosurgery is the ideal treatment for an individual solitary brain metastasis or whether microsurgical resection will allow for better control of the tumour. The same applies to skull base meningiomas where one could imagine that those tumours not responding to stereotactic radiosurgery and/or even progressing after radiosurgery can be identified prospectively and stratified for alternative treatments.

References

1. Alavi JB, Alavi A, Chawluk J, Kushner M, Powe J, Hickey W, Reivich M (1988) Positron emission tomography in patients with glioma. Cancer 62: 1074–1078
2. Alexander E, Moriarty TM, Davis RB, Wen PY, Fine HA, Black PM, Kooy HM, Loeffler JS (1995) Stereotactic radiosurgery for the definitive non-invasive treatment of brain metastases. J Natl Cancer Inst 87: 34–40
3. Brismar T, Collins VP, Kesselberg M (1989) Thallium-201-uptake relates to membrane potential and potassium permeability in human glioma cells. Brain Res 500: 30–36
4. Engenhart R, Kimmig BN, Höver KH, Wowra B, Sturm V, van Kaick G, Wannenmacher M (1990) Stereotactic single high dose radiation therapy of benign intracranial meningeomas. Int J Radiation Oncol Biol Phys 19: 1021–1026
5. Engenhart R, Kimmig BN, Höver KH, Wowra B, Romahn J, Lorenz WJ, van Kaick G, Wannenmacher M (1993) Long-term follow-up for brain metastases treated by percutaneous stereotactic single high-dose irradiation. Cancer 71: 1353–1361
6. Flickinger JC, Kondziolka D, Lunsford D, Coffey RJ, Goodman ML, Shaw EG, Hudgins WR, Weiner R, Harsh GR, Sneed PK, Larsson DA (1994) A multi-institutional experience with stereotactic radiosurgery for solitary brain metastasis. Int J Radiation Oncol Biol Phys 28: 797–802
7. Ishibashi M, Taguchi A, Sugita Y, Morita S, Kawamura S, Umezaki N, Shigemori M, Hayabuchi N (1995) Thallium-201 in brain tumors: relationship between tumor cell activity in astrocytic tumor and proliferating cell nuclear antigen. J Nucl Med 36: 2201–2206
8. Kondiziolka D, Lunsford D, Coffey RJ, Flickinger JC (1991) Stereotactic radiosurgery of meningeomas. J Neurosurg 74: 552–559
9. Patronas NJ, di Chiro G, Kufta C, Bairamian D, Kornblith PL, Simon R, Larson SM (1985) Prediction of survival in glioma patients by means of positron emission tomography. J Neurosurg 62: 816–822
10. Valentino V, Schinaia G, Raimondi AJ (1993) The results of radiosurgical management of 72 middle fossa meningeomas. Acta Neurochir (Wien) 122: 60–70

Correspondence: P. C. Warnke, M.D., Abteilung Stereotaktische Neurochirurgie, Neurozentrum, Breisacher Str. 64, D-79106 Freiburg, Federal Republic of Germany.

Acta Neurochir (1997) [Suppl] 68: 127–132

Potential Role of in vitro ^{1}H Magnetic Resonance Spectroscopy in the Definition of Malignancy Grading of Human Neuroepithelial Brain Tumours

C. M. Carapella[1], **G. Carpinelli**[2], **A. Knijn**[2], **L. Raus**[1], **F. Caroli**[1], and **F. Podo**[2]

[1] Department of Neurosurgery, Istituto Nazionale Tumori "Regina Elena", Roma and [2]Department of Cell Biology, Istituto Superiore di Sanità, Roma, Italy

Summary

The increasing sensitivity of neuro-imaging in the diagnosis of brain expanding lesions is not directly related to biopathological specificity and new technological approaches are under study. In particular Magnetic Resonance Spectroscopy (MRS) allows evaluation of some biochemical pathways whose metabolic alterations may be correlated with the nature and malignancy grading of primary brain tumours.

In the present study the author performed an in vitro high field ^{1}H MRS (9.4 and 14.1 T) analysis of specimens obtained from stereotactic biopsy or microsurgical removal of primary brain tumours. Different samples derived from heterogeneous areas and/or infiltrated perilesional regions were examined.

This study was principally focused on malignancy grading of gliomas and its correlation with the ratio (***R***) between the resonance band arising from choline containing compounds (between 3.14 and 3.35 ppm) and the total creatine signal (3.0 ppm). Analyses allowed significant discrimination between astrocytomas ($\boldsymbol{R} = 2.4 \pm 0.6$) and glioblastoma (GBM) ($\boldsymbol{R} = 4.4 \pm 1.3$) [$p < 0.002$]; however the results did not allow discrimination between differentiated and anaplastic astrocytomas.

The GBM showed the largest spread of values corresponding to their higher level of tissue heterogeneity and de-differentiation.

Studies on non astrocytic brain tumours indicated that even higher ***R*** values were exhibited by oligodendrogliomas, even in well differentiated forms ($p < 0.02$ with respect to GBM).

Moreover, preliminary observations indicated that signals arising from other metabolites may also contribute to a differential diagnosis of different oncotypes. Among these glycine appears particularly relevant, since higher levels were measured for this amino acid in GBM with respect to both astrocytomas and oligodendrogliomas.

Keywords: Magnetic resonance spectroscopy; brain tumours; glioma; metabolism.

Introduction

Brain tumours still represent a relevant diagnostic and therapeutic problem. Non-invasive neuro-imaging does not allow biopathological characterisation and biopsy procedures are still necessary to obtain accurate diagnosis and to select more efficient multimodality therapeutic strategies.

MRS could represent a useful method of obtaining biochemical characterisation of brain tumours and to study peculiar metabolic alterations associated with tumour growth and progression or induced by different antineoblastic treatments [5, 6, 16, 21].

In vitro and in vivo ^{1}H MRS has been extensively utilised to identify relevant spectral components and assess specific variations related to malignancy grading of brain tumours. By allowing a better spectral resolution, in vitro MRS studies provide quantitative analysis of a wide variety of metabolites [9, 24]. The major peaks commonly present in brain spectra include: N-acetylaspartate (NAA), an aminoacid derivative principally located in neurones; choline containing compounds, such as phosphorylcholine and glycerophosphorylcholine, involved in phospholipid synthesis and degradation; and creatine and phosphocreatine, which are related to energy metabolism.

In the present study the authors performed high-resolution ^{1}H MRS analyses at 9.4 and 14.1 tesla on biopsy specimens obtained from a series of primary brain tumours, with the aim of correlating tissue metabolism with the malignancy grading of neuroepithelial brain tumours and identifying metabolic markers helpful in differential diagnosis and in monitoring the outcome of clinical management.

Materials and Methods

The samples were obtained from neurosurgical specimens of patients affected by different brain tumours. MRS analyses were performed on a total of 74 samples, obtained either from stereotactic biopsies or from conventional microsurgical operations of tumour removal: 15 samples (7 patients) from well differentiated astrocytoma (AS); 13 samples (7 patients) from anaplastic astrocytoma (AA); 24 samples (16 patients) from glioblastoma (GBM); 13 samples (6 patients) from oligodendroglioma (OG); 3 samples (2 patients) from medulloblastoma (MDB); 4 samples (2 patients) from ependymoma; 2 samples (1 patient) from central neurocytoma. In this series 3 samples (2 patients) obtained from cerebellar haemangioblastoma were also included, in consideration of the relevant astrocytic component. Parallel samples were submitted to pathological examination, and classified according to WHO classification [11].

The specimen selection was guided by pre-operative MRI, CT or intra-operative ultrasound; tumour samples were selected from central tumour areas, trying to avoid areas with necrosis or other regressive events. When there was the possibility of obtaining multiple samples from the same tumour, stereotactic specimens were separately collected from perilesional or oedematous tissue, peripheral tumour areas and central tumour core. Normal brain tissue (2 samples) was obtained from two patients undergoing frontal lobectomy for radical removal of frontal AA.

After dissection, specimens were frozen in liquid nitrogen and then extracted with ethanol 70% by vol [18]. After centrifugation the supernatant was lyophilised and redissolved in deuterium oxide containing either sodium 2,2-dimethyl-2-silapentane-5-sulfonate or 3-trimethylsylylpropionate as internal standard. The pellet was utilised for protein assay according to Lowry [14].

^{1}H NMR spectra were obtained at both 14.1 T (600 MHz) and 9.4 T (400 MHz) by using Bruker AMX spectrometers.

Metabolite concentrations were determined from peak areas corrected by the appropriate saturation factors (obtained from the relative peak areas in fully relaxed spectra) and taking into account the number of protons contributing to each signal. All data were presented as means $\pm$ SD and the statistical significance was evaluated using a two-tailed Student t test; for p values the patient number was considered for the sample size.

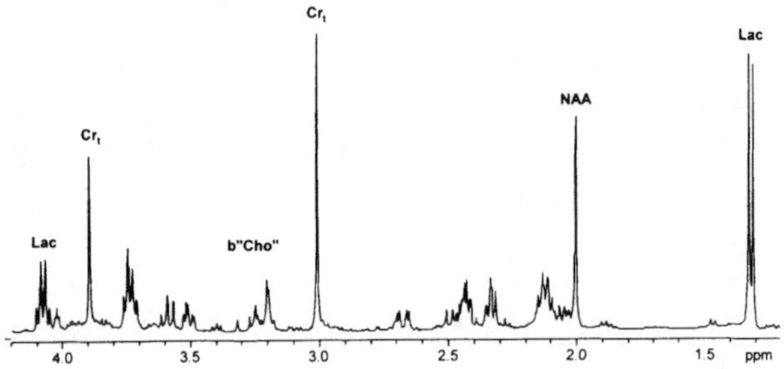

Fig. 1. In vitro spectrum obtained from normal brain tissue extract. *Lac* lactate; Cr_t, total creatine; *b"Cho"* choline-containing compounds; *myo-inositol* taurine; *NAA* N-acetylaspartate

Table 1. *b"Cho"/(Cr + PCr) Signal Area Ratio, in Healthy Brain and Brain Tumours, Determined by ^{1}H MRS Analyses of Bioptic Specimens at 14.1 Tesla*

Diagnosis	Patients	Samples	b"Cho"/ (Cr + PCr)
Control	2	3	0.8 ± 0.1
Differentiated astrocytoma	7	15	2.1 ± 0.9
Anaplastic astrocytoma	6	14	2.4 ± 0.6
Glioblastoma	16	23	4.4 ± 1.3
Oligodendroglioma	6	13	5.4 ± 2.2
Medulloblastoma	1	1	8.5
Medulloblastoma[a]	1	2	4.7; 3.9
Ependymoma	2	4	12.5 ± 1.7
Haemangioblastoma	2	3	6.4 ± 2.0
Neurocytoma	1	2	5.8; 8.2

[a] Treated with polychemotherapy prior to surgery.

Results

A typical spectrum from normal brain extract at 14.1 tesla is shown in Fig. 1. High resolution ^{1}H-MR spectral analysis allowed separate detection of several signals contributing to the in vitro resonance band b"Cho" (corresponding to the in vivo "Cho peak"), which includes signals from $-N^+(CH_3)_3$ of GPC (3.23 ppm), PCho (3.22 ppm) and Cho (3.20 ppm), H5 of Ino (multiplet signal centered at 3.25 ppm) and Tau ($-NCH_2-$ triplet centered at 3.26 ppm), with contribution from PEtn ($-NCH_2-$).

The data obtained from glial tumours were the most interesting, since their tissue extracts showed significant and reliable variations with respect to normal brain tissue and according to tumour malignancy grading.

In the present study, the ratio ***R*** between the integrated choline containing compounds (b"Cho") resonance and the total creatine peaks [b"Cho"/(Cr + PCr)] represented a most relevant parameter in ^{1}H MR spectral analysis (Table 1).

Analyses at 14.1 T showed that this ratio was elevated in glial tumours with respect to the normal brain tissue and significantly differed in glioblastoma (4.4 ± 1.3) from both differentiated and anaplastic astrocytomas (2.4 ± 0.6) [$p < 0.001$]. Similar results were also obtained from analyses performed at 9.4 T [1].

Moreover in multisample analyses performed on GBM cases regional variations in ***R*** values measured in either peripheral or central tumour areas were observed, according with tumour cell density and atypia.

In oligodendrogliomas the ***R*** value was significantly higher than in GBM (5.4 ± 2.2) even in well differentiated, non-anaplastic tumours [$p = 0.02$] (Fig. 2A). In mixed oligo-astrocytomas more heterogeneous spectral profiles from different samples dissected from the same tumour were observed.

The increase in the ***R*** value was not substantially

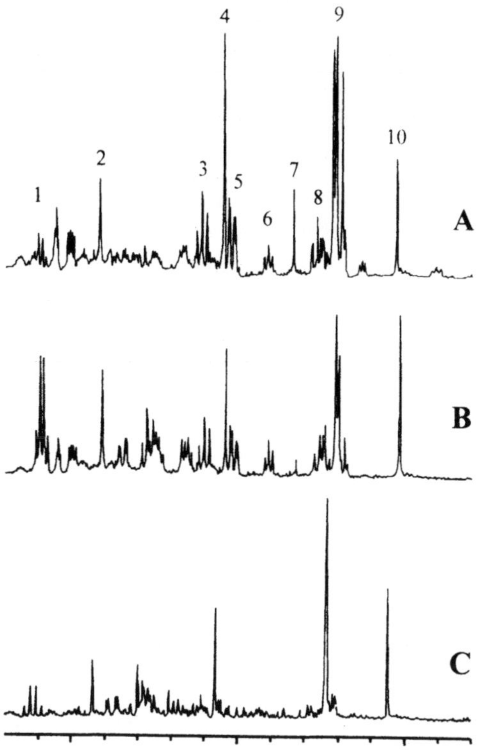

Fig. 2. ^{1}H NMR 600 MHz in vitro spectra obtained from biopsy specimens of: (A) oligodendroglioma; (B) well differentiated astrocytoma; (C) glioblastoma. Peak assignment: *1* lactate; *2* and *10* total creatine; *3* and *5* myo-inositol; *4* glycine; *6* taurine; *7* scyllo-inositol; *8* taurine + myo inositol; *9* choline-containing compounds

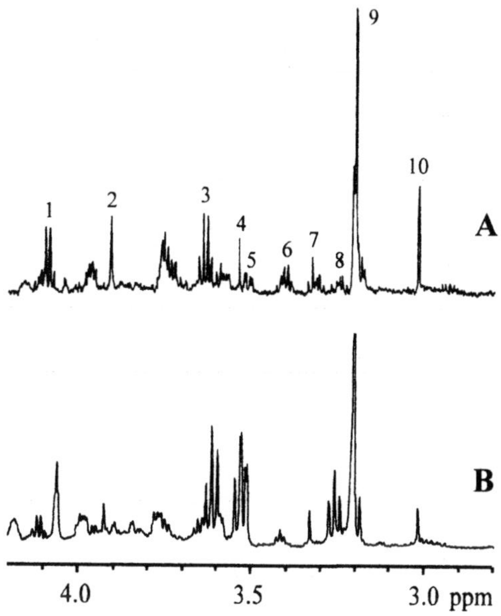

Fig. 3. ^{1}H NMR 600 MHz in vitro spectra obtained from biopsy specimens of: (A) neurocytoma; (B) ependymoma. Abbreviations: see Fig. 2

related to a decrease in the (Cr + PCr) peak area, because quantitative analyses indicated only moderate (if any) alteration in the level of these metabolites; more important was the elevation in the overall area of the b"Cho" resonance, which increased in accordance with malignancy grading in astrocytic tumours (Fig. 2B and C).

In these tumours other relevant spectral features were represented by glycine (Gly) and NAA signals. Gly was increased in GBM compared with AS and AA. Also the [Gly]/[Cr + PCr] ratio was increased in GBM (1.8 ± 1.00) with respect to AS + AA (0.49 ± 0.36). Scattered values were observed in OG, where differently from the [b"Cho"/(Cr + PCr)] ratio, in no case was the [Gly]/[Cr + PCr] value as high as in GBM samples.

The NAA signal was detected in AS samples obtained not only from peripheral but also from central tumour areas, while in more malignant tumours it was mainly present in peripheral tumour regions, probably associated with sample contamination from the surrounding normal brain tissue [23].

Regarding the other types of tumours considered in the present study, the few cases analysed so far did not allow the reaching of similar conclusions on the significance of ***R*** value with respect to tumour malignancy grading.

Similarly to GBM, two cases of ependymoma also showed elevated ***R*** values, principally due to an enhanced b"Cho" peak intensity and, to lesser extent, to a decrease in total creatine. Very low levels of Gly were present in these specimens (Fig. 3B).

In one case of medulloblastoma a high level of ***R*** was measured, essentially due to an increased area of the b"Cho" resonance. In another case of recurrent MDB, treated with polychemotherapy prior to surgery, a general reduction of all MRS signals was observed, with the exception of a very high level of taurine (Fig. 4).

In two samples derived from a central neurocytoma, in spite of the benign biopathological nature of the tumour, very high ***R*** values were found (5.8 and 8.2), associated with spectral profiles very similar to those of AA (Fig. 3A).

Finally, three samples of haemangioblastoma also exhibited elevated ***R*** values, associated with an increase in Gly, probably due to a striking astrocytic reaction present in the peripheral tumour areas.

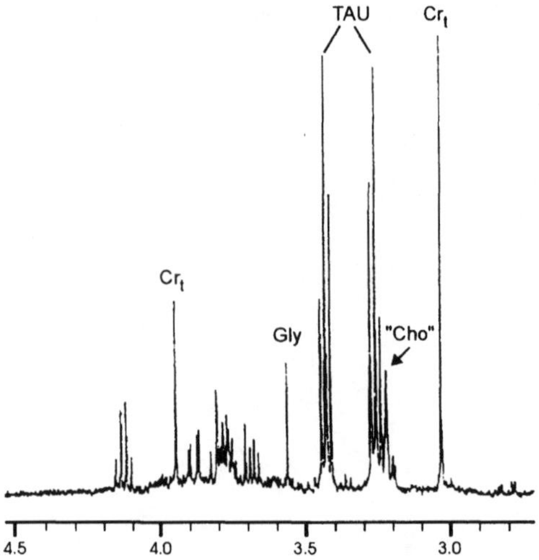

Fig. 4. ^{1}H NMR 600 MHz in vitro spectra obtained from biopsy specimen of medulloblastoma treated with polychemotherapy prior to surgery. *Tau* taurine; "*Cho*" choline-containing compounds; Cr_t total creatine

Discussion

The role of MRS in the characterisation of brain tumours is under study in many clinical and experimental trials. Currently in vivo data do not seem to permit a definite pre-operative evaluation of tumour malignancy grading, due to the overlapping data obtained from low- and high-grade glial tumours and the risk of contamination from brain adjacent tissue [15].

For this reason in vitro analyses, performed at much higher magnetic fields than those utilised in the clinical practice (1.5–2.0 T), appear particularly helpful for identifying spectral alterations specifically related to tumour growth and progression and for assessing the relevance of other metabolites undetectable under the conditions of spectral resolution allowed by in vivo methods. In vitro studies are in fact useful in the identification and quantification of different proton resonances, even though some metabolic alterations may occur during sample handling and tissue extraction. In particular, lactate is expected to increase during and following tissue dissection, due to tumour hypoxia, while PCr is easily hydrolysed into Cr. Regarding the latter point, however, it should be noted that total creatine (Cr + PCr) peak should be unaffected by this degradation mechanism and in practice reflect the total Cr_t pool present in the tissue, provided that the extraction yield is sufficiently high.

The results of this study point to a significant discrimination between astrocytomas and glioblastoma, based on the difference in the value of the ***R*** ratio, [b"Cho"/(Cr + PCr)]. The increase in this value, observed also in previous in vivo and in vitro studies [6, 9, 10, 15, 17, 22], was generally associated with moderate (if any) decrease in signal intensity of total creatine, but was mainly due to large increases in the b"Cho" signal intensity, primarily Cho and GPC, in tumour tissues compared with healthy brain.

It is well described that in many clinical and experimental tumour systems alterations in the levels of phospholipid metabolites are correlated with cell growth and proliferation, although the specific role of these compounds in the metabolic activity of tumour cells has not yet been elucidated [2, 4, 13]. In brain neuroepithelial tumours, which present a low growth fraction also in more malignant oncotypes, it is more difficult to separate different tumour forms and correlate modulations in the levels of phospholipid metabolites with tumour cell proliferation.

It was not possible to discriminate well differentiated from anaplastic astrocytomas on the basis of the ***R*** ratio. This appears to be in accordance with biomolecular studies showing specific genetic alterations in astrocytic tumours, associated with tumour progression, and separate variations for GBM [25].

Interesting results were obtained from ^{1}H MRS analyses of OG which showed increased levels of the [b"Cho"/(Cr + PCr)] ratio even in well differentiated tumour forms. This phenomenon was associated with specific pathological features of moderate cell density and the presence of mitoses [20].

Regarding other metabolites detected in ^{1}H MRS spectra, glycine might offer, in larger series, interesting diagnostic and prognostic indications. The level of this amino acid, in fact, exhibited relevant alterations in GBM with respect to both AS and AA. It is well known that Gly is one of the major inhibitory neurotransmitters in mammalian brain. The presence of a Gly cleavage system in astrocytes, but not in neurones [19] indicates that astrocytes are the main site of Gly degradation in the central nervous system. On the other hand, astrocytes also possess receptors for Gly uptake. It is suggested that the excess of Gly is transported to the astrocytes and then degraded. A high activity of the Gly cleavage system in astrocytes results in the low levels of Gly usually observed under healthy conditions. Different enzymatic alterations have been described to explain the elevated Gly levels found in some diseases [19]; the higher levels of this amino acid in GBM may be due to replacement of healthy astrocytes by tumour cells and/or to alterations in the Gly cleavage system. Moreover, activation of serine methyltransferase, with consequent increase in Gly levels, has been described in C6 glioma cells, which could also contribute to the Gly elevation observed in human GBM [3, 7–10, 12, 19]. On this basis a high level of Gly could be supposed to be present in less differentiated or in anaplastic tumours.

The authors' preliminary observations on other oncotypes did not allow them to establish a clear correlation between ***R*** and tumour malignancy grading. In some cases it seems that the [b"Cho"/(Cr + PCr)] ratio cannot be assumed as a potential marker of malignancy. Indeed high ***R*** values were also found in benign tumours such as central neurocytoma and cerebellar haemangioblastoma, characterised by high cell density levels.

In conclusion, ^{1}H MRS techniques might represent an interesting method to evaluate the metabolic activity of neuroepithelial brain tumours, to assess the presence and the relevance of peculiar metabolic alterations linked to malignancy grading and tumour progression, such as the variation in the [b"Cho"/(Cr + PCr)] ratio. Other signals, derived from different metabolites (Gly, NAA), may also assume relevance in differential diagnosis between different oncotypes.

This evidence provides strong indications for the possible development, with the continuous advancement in MR technology, of novel, non-invasive protocols of in vivo MRS with the aim of obtaining better diagnostic definition, selecting new clinical therapeutic protocols and evaluating the results determined by different antiblastic treatments.

Acknowledgement

We acknowledge support by CNR PF ACRO and AIRC (Milan) and technical assistance by Mr. M. Giannini.

References

1. Carpinelli G, Carapella CM, Palombi L, Raus L, Caroli F, Podo F (1996) Differentiation of glioblastoma multiforme from astrocytomas by in vitro H-MRS analysis of human brain tumors. Anticancer Res 16: 1559–1564
2. Carpinelli G, Podo F, Di Vito M, Proietti E, Gessani S, Belardelli F (1984) Modulations of glycerophosphorylcholine and phosphorylcholine in Friend erythroleukemia cells upon in vitro-induced erythroid differentiation: ^{31}P NMR study. FEBS Lett 176: 88–92
3. Davidoff RA, Shank RP, Graham LT, Aprison MH, Werman R (1967) Is glycine a neurotransmitter? Nature 214: 680–683
4. de Certaines JD, Larsen VA, Podo F, Carpinelli G, Briot O, Henriksen O (1993) In vivo ^{31}P MRS of experimental tumors: Review paper. NMR Biomed 6: 345–365
5. Frahm J, Bruhn H, Gyngell ML, Merboldt KD, Hanicke W, Sauter R (1989) Localized high resolution proton NMR spectroscopy using stimulated echoes: initial applications to human brain in vivo. Magn Reson Med 9: 79–93
6. Gill S, Thomas DGT, Van Bruggen N, Gadian DG, Peden CJ, Bell JD, Cox IJ, Menon DK, Iles RA, Bryant DJ, Coutts GA (1990) Proton MR spectroscopy of intracranial tumors: in vivo and in vitro studies. J Comput Assist Tomogr 14: 497–504
7. Henn FA (1976) Neurotransmission and glial cells: a functional relationship? J Neurosci Res 2: 271–282
8. Johnson JW, Ascher P (1987) Glycine potentiates the NMDA response in cultured mouse brain neurons. Nature 325: 529–531
9. Kinoshita Y, Kajiwara H, Yokota A, Koga Y (1994) Proton magnetic resonance spectroscopy of brain tumors: an in vitro study. Neurosurgery 35: 606–614
10. Kinoshita Y, Kajiwara H, Yokota A, Koga Y (1993) Proton magnetic resonance spectroscopy of astrocytic tumors: an in vitro study. Neurol Med Chir (Tokyo) 33: 350–359
11. Kleihues P, Burger PC, Scheithauer BW (1993) Histological typing of tumours of the central nervous system. WHO Blue Book, 2nd ed. Springer, Berlin Heidelberg New York Tokyo, pp 1–37
12. Kohl RL, Perez-Polo JR, Quay WB (1980) Effect of methionine, glycine and serine hydroximethyltranspherase activity in rat glioma and human neuroblastoma cells. J Neurosci Res 5: 271–280
13. Leach M, Le Moyec L, Podo F (1992) MRS of Tumours: basic principles. In: de Certaines JD, Bovée WMMJ, Podo F (eds) MR spectroscopy in biology and medicine. Pergamon, London, pp 295–344
14. Lowry OH, Rosebrough NJ, Lewis Farr A, Randall RJ (1951) Protein measurement with the folin phenol reagent. J Biol Chem 193: 265–275
15. Negendank W, Sauter R, Brown TR, Evelhoch JL, Falini A, Gotsis ED, Heerchap A, Kamada K, Lee BCP, Mengeot MM, Moser E, Padavic-Shaller KA, Sanders JA, Spraggins TA, Stillman AE, Terwey B, Vogl TJ, Wicklow K, Zimmerman RA (1996) Proton magnetic resonance spectroscopy in patients with glial tumor: a multicenter study. J Neurosurgery 84: 449–458
16. Negendank W (1992) Studies of human tumors by MRS: a review. NMR Biomed 5: 303–324
17. Nicklas WJ, Browning ET (1988) Amino acid metabolism in glial cells: homeostatic regulation of intra- and extracellular milieu by C6 glioma cells. J Neurochem 30: 163–171
18. Podo F, Carpinelli G, Di Vito M, Giannini M, Proietti E, Fiers W, Gresser I, Belardelli F (1987) Nuclear magnetic resonance analysis of tumor necrosis factor-induced alteration of phospholipid metabolites and pH in Friend leukemia cell tumors and fibrosarcomas in mice. Cancer Res 47: 6481–6489
19. Sato K, Yoshida S, Fujiwara K, Tada K, Tohyama M (1991) Glycine cleavage system in astrocytes. Brain Res 567: 64–70
20. Schiffer D and Vigliani MC (1993) Prognostic factors in oligodendrogliomas. Crit Rev Neurosurg 3: 59–65
21. Segebarth CM, Balériaux DF, Luyten PT, Den Hollander JA (1990) Detection of metabolic heterogeneity of human intracranial tumors in vivo by ^{1}H-NMR spectroscopic imaging. Magn Reson Med 13: 62–76
22. Shimizu H, Kumabe T, Tominaga T, Kayama T, Hara K, Ono Y, Sato K, Arai N, Fujiwara S, Yoshimoto T (1996) Non-invasive evaluation of malignancy of brain tumors with proton MR spectroscopy. Am J Neuroradiol 17: 737–747

23. Tohyama T, Lee VMY, Trojanowski J (1993) Co-expression of low molecular weight neurofilament protein and glial fibrillary acidic protein in established human glioma cell lines. Am J Pathol 142: 823–892
24. Usenius JP, Vainio P, Hernesniemi J, Kauppinen RA (1994) Choline-containing compounds in human astrocytomas studied by ^{1}H NMR spectroscopy in vivo and in vitro. J Neurochem 63: 1538–1543
25. von Deimling A, Louis DN, Schramm J, Wiestler OD (1994) Astrocytic gliomas: characterization on a molecular genetic basis. Rec Res Cancer Res 135: 33–42

Correspondence: Carmine M. Carapella, M.D., Department of Neurosurgery, Istituto Nazionale Tumori "Regina Elena", Viale Regina Elena, 291, 1-00161 Roma, Italy.

Acta Neurochir (1997) [Suppl] 68: 133–138

Stereotactic Brain Biopsy Guided by Positron Emission Tomography (PET) with [F-18]Fluorodeoxyglucose and [C-11]Methionine

B. Pirotte, S. Goldman[1], Ph. David[2], D. Wikler[1], Ph. Damhaut[1], A. Vandesteene[3], I. Salmon[4], J. Brotchi, and M. Levivier

Department of Neurosurgery, [1]PET/Biomedical Cyclotron Unit, Departments of [2]Neuroradiology, [3]Anaesthesiology and [4]Pathology, Université Libre de Bruxelles, Erasme Hospital, Brussels, Belgium

Summary

The aim of the present study was to compare the contribution of the labelled tracers [C-11]methionine (Met) and [F-18]-fluorodeoxyglucose (FDG) in positron emission tomography (PET)-guided stereotactic biopsy of non resectable brain lesions. Twenty-five patients underwent combined Met-PET-, FDG-PET- and computerized tomography (CT)- or magnetic resonance (MR)-guided stereotactic biopsy according to a previously described technique for stereotactic FDG-PET. Met-PET and FDG-PET images were analyzed to determine which tracer offers the best information to guide at least one stereotactic biopsy trajectory. Histological diagnosis was obtained in all patients (23 tumours and 2 non-tumorous lesions). All tumours had an area of abnormal Met uptake and were biopsied under PET-guidance. FDG uptake in the tumour was higher than in the grey matter and was used for target selection in 12 of 23 tumours. Eleven of them were located in the basal ganglia or the brainstem. Met was used for target selection in 11 of 23 tumours where there was no FDG uptake or where FDG uptake was equivalent to that of the grey matter. Ten of them were located in the cortex. Two non tumoral lesions had no Met uptake and were biopsied under CT- or MR-guidance only. Forty-three out of 53 stereotactic trajectories obtained in these 25 patients were based on PET-defined targets and had an area of abnormal Met uptake. These trajectories always yielded a diagnosis of tumour. Moreover, all tumorous trajectories had an area of abnormal Met uptake. Finally, all non-diagnostic trajectories (n = 4) were CT/MR-defined because there was no area of abnormal Met uptake. These results suggest that patients who can benefit the most from Met-PET guidance could be selected preoperatively. In conclusion, this work shows that Met is a good alternative to FDG for target selection in PET-guided stereotactic brain biopsy.

Keywords: Stereotactic biopsy; positron emission tomography; brain tumour; [F-18]fluorodeoxyglucose; [C-11]methionine.

Introduction

Because brain tumours are histologically heterogeneous, computerized tomography (CT)- or magnetic resonance (MR)-guided stereotactic brain biopsy does not not always yield the actual diagnosis or grading [3–5, 10, 11]. Since positron emission tomography (PET) provides useful, independent and complementary metabolic information on brain tumours [1, 8, 12, 21], the authors have previously developed a technique allowing routine integration of PET data in the planning of stereotactic brain biopsy [16]. They originally used [F-18]-labelled fluorodeoxyglucose (FDG) as radiotracer. The selection of targets on stereotactic FDG-PET-generated images allows direct biopsies accurately in the abnormal metabolic foci of brain tumours. The authors have shown that FDG-PET-guided stereotactic brain biopsy increases the diagnostic yield of the technique [17].

In their hands, FDG-PET-guided biopsy has, however, some limitations. Indeed, targetting may be difficult when there is no or minor FDG uptake, such as in low-grade tumours. Also, when a hypermetabolic lesion is in close relationship with the cortical or subcortical grey matter, tumorous and normal FDG uptake are difficult to differentiate. Therefore, [C-11]-methionine (Met) was tested as an alternative tracer for stereotactic PET guidance. The aim of the present study was to evaluate the relative contribution of Met and FDG in a series of patients who underwent PET-guided stereotactic brain biopsy with both tracers.

Methods and Material

Since June 1991, the authors routinely perform PET-guided stereotactic brain biopsy in patients suspected of having a non-resectable brain tumour based on a preoperative neuroimaging work-up [17]. Their current series comprises more than 100 cases. Between July 1992 and April 1996, a non-consecutive series of 25 patients with either non-enhanced lesion suspected of low-grade histology or contrast-enhanced lesion located in the cortical/subcortical grey matter (including the basal ganglia and the brainstem) underwent biopsy guided by combined FDG-PET and Met-PET performed in stereotactic conditions. There were 16 men and 9 women whose ages ranged between 2 and 79 years (mean 52.6 years). Twenty-four patients were previously untreated and one presented with a recurrent lesion.

For data acquisition, the technique of combined stereotactic PET with Met and FDG was adapted from their previous experience with FDG-PET-guided stereotactic brain biopsy [16, 17]. Placement of the stereotactic frame, data acquisition including stereotactic PET with Met and FDG as well as CT or MR, surgical planning and the biopsy procedure were performed the same day. All patients gave their informed consent and the procedure was in accordance with the ethical guidelines of their institution.

After placement of the CT- and MR-compatible base ring (Fischer ZD-Neurosurgical Localizing Unit, Howmedica Leibinger, Freiburg, Germany), stereotactic CT or MR with intravenous contrast enhancement was obtained. For stereotactic PET, a clamp specifically designed to secure the head ring to the Siemens couch (Howmedica Leibinger, Freiburg, Germany) was used. In order to create a fiducials reference system compatible with PET, the commercial MR localizers with minor modifications were used as previously described [16]. After the transmission scan, the patient was first injected intravenously with 10 to 15 mCi of Met. Images used for stereotactic calculation were acquired between 20 to 40 minutes after injection of the tracer. Eighty minutes after Met injection, the patient was injected with 6 to 9 mCi. Images used for stereotactic calculation were acquired between 40 to 60 minutes later. The authors PET camera (CTI/Siemens 933/08/12 tomograph, Knoxville, Tennessee, U.S.A.) allowed simultaneous acquisition of 15 slices about 6.5 mm-thick, with a full width at half-maximum resolution of about 5 mm.

The surgical planning began with analysis of the PET images. Areas of abnormal metabolism used for target selection were either zones of FDG or Met uptake that were higher than the surrounding normal appearing brain tissue or foci of relative increase of FDG or Met uptake in a hypometabolic lesion. If the PET images revealed such areas, the plane that best displayed the abnormal FDG or Met uptake was selected and a pixel located in the centre of this zone was interactively pointed at on visual inspection. The coordinates of that pixel were calculated and set as a target for biopsy. The targets selected on PET images with one tracer were then projected onto the corresponding PET slice acquired with the other tracer to analyse and compare the local uptake of both tracers. These targets were also projected onto the corresponding stereotactic CT or MR slice to control the reliability and the safety of the target selection and of the trajectory.

Whenever possible, 2 targets were selected in order to sample different metabolic areas of the tumour. FDG-PET images were used first for target selection when they gave more information than Met-PET images or when both tracers were equivalent, because of previous experience with stereotactic FDG-PET [17]. When the area of highest FDG uptake was smaller than the limits of the lesion visualized on the corresponding slice of Met-PET, another target was selected on the Met-PET, outside the area of increased FDG uptake. When Met-PET images gave more information than FDG-PET images, Met-PET was used for target selection. In patients where there is no obvious abnormal FDG or Met uptake that can be used to select a target for biopsy, surgery is planned using CT or MR data only.

In all patients, serial stereotactic biopsies were performed along each trajectory, following the technique described by Kelly *et al.* [15]. For all biopsy specimens, smear preparation and formalin-fixed samples were analyzed after appropriate staining [16, 17, 22, 23]. For the present study, glial tumours were classified using a three-tier system: low-grade glioma astrocytoma (LGA), anaplastic astrocytoma (AA) and glioblastoma (GB); non-glial tumours, whether neoplastic or not, were also included; if non-tumorous samples made of gliotic reactional tissue were found, they were classified as non-diagnostic (ND).

For each patient, a histological diagnosis was established. Then, the diagnosis obtained in each biopsy trajectory was recorded separately, regardless of the patient's final diagnosis. In order to evaluate the role of Met-PET in target selection, the authors retrospectively classified biopsy trajectories in 3 groups, according to their metabolic characteristics: FDG-PET-guided trajectory, Met-PET-guided trajectory or CT-MR-guided trajectory. For that purpose, they first looked at whether Met uptake was increased [Met(+)] or not [Met(−)]. In Met(+) trajectories, they further looked at whether FDG-PET was involved in the surgical planning. Indeed, as described above, FDG-PET images were used for target selection when they gave more information than Met-PET images or when both tracers were equivalent (FDG-PET-guided trajectory). On the other hand, when Met-PET data were superior to those of FDG-PET, Met-PET was used for target selection (Met-PET-guided trajectory). In Met(−) trajectories, target selection was based on CT or MR only (CT-/MR-guided trajectory).

Table 1. *Tumorous FDG Uptake in 23 Tumours with [C-11]-Methionine Uptake*

Diagnosis	Tumour FDG > grey matter FDG	Tumour FDG = grey matter FDG	Tumour FDG = 0
GB	5	2	—
AA	4	2	2
LGA	—	—	5
PNHL	1	—	—
Metastasis	2	—	—
Total	12	4	7

GB glioblastoma; *AA* anaplastic astrocytoma; *LGA* low-grade astrocytoma; *PNHL* primary non-Hodgkin's lymphoma.

Results

Histological diagnosis was obtained in all patients. Diagnoses included 7 GB, 8 AA, 5 LGA, 1 primary non-Hodgkin's lymphoma (PNHL), 2 metastases, 1 ischaemic stroke and 1 post-radiation gliosis without tumour recurrence.

All tumours (n = 23), had an area of abnormal Met uptake. Among them, 11 tumours were biopsied based on Met-defined targets and the other 12 tumours based on FDG-defined targets. These 23 tumours may be divided in 3 groups according to their level of FDG uptake (Table 1). When tumorous FDG uptake was higher than in the grey matter, i.e. the tumour was clearly visible on FDG-PET, it was used for target selection. In this group were found 5 GB, 4 AA, 1 PNHL and 2 metastases. When tumorous FDG uptake was equivalent to that of the surrounding grey matter, a target could not easily be defined on FDG-PET and therefore Met-PET was used for target selection. This was the case in 2 GB and in 2 AA. Finally, when no FDG uptake was found, targets were also selected on Met-PET as in 2 AA and all 5 LGA. Thus, Met was the only tracer which allowed the definition of a target for biopsy in 11 of these 23 tumours (48%). These corresponded to 6 high-grade tumours and to 5 LGA. In the present series, there were only 2 non-tumorous lesions and they had no Met uptake. They were biopsied on CT- or MR-defined targets.

In this series, 13 lesions were located in the cortical area (Table 2). There were 2 non-tumorous lesions and 11 tumours (3 GB, 3 AA and 5 LGA). The 2 non-tumorous lesions were Met(−) and biopsy was guided on CT- or MR-enhanced areas. In the 11 cortical tumours, Met was used for target selection in 10 (91%) while FDG was used only in one GB. The 10 cortical tumours biopsied on Met-PET included 2 lesions that were not enhanced on CT or MR (1 LGA and 1 AA). The 12 other lesions were located in the deep-seated grey matter. Nine were located in the basal ganglia and 3 in the brainstem (Table 3). They were all malignant tumours and showed CT or MR enhancement. In 11 of them (92%), FDG was used for target selection because its uptake was higher than in the grey matter. However, in 7 cases, a second trajectory was performed in an area of high Met uptake outside the limits of high FDG uptake and all yielded tumorous tissue. In the twelfth case (thalamic AA), tumorous FDG uptake was equivalent to that of the grey matter and Met-PET was used to guide the biopsy.

A total of 53 stereotactic trajectories were performed (2.1 trajectories per patient). Forty-three trajectories were based on PET-defined targets (Table 4). The other 10 were based on CT- or MR-defined targets. All 43 PET-guided trajectories were Met(+) and always yielded tumorous tissue (Table 4). These 43 Met(+) trajectories were analyzed for their FDG uptake (superior or equivalent to that of grey matter or absent). In 16 trajectories, tumorous FDG uptake was higher than in the grey matter. This group included 6 GB, 7 AA, 1 PNHL and 2 metastases samples. The targets used to define these trajectories were all CT- or MR-enhanced. Fifteen of them (94%) were in the basal ganglia or the brainstem. In 11 other trajectories, tumorous FDG uptake was equivalent to that of the grey matter. This group included 6 GB and 5 AA samples. Eight targets corresponded to enhanced areas on CT or MR and 3 to non-enhanced areas. Finally, 16 trajectories had very low or no tumorous FDG uptake and trajectories were guided on Met-PET. They included 2 GB, 4 AA and all LGA (n = 10) samples. All hypodense or hyposignal targets on CT or MR were in this group. Thus, Met was superior to FDG in differen-

Table 2. *FDG Uptake in 13 Lesions Located in the Cortex*

Diagnosis	Tumour FDG > grey matter FDG	Tumour FDG = grey matter FDG	Tumour FDG = 0
GB	1	2	—
AA	—	1	2
LGA	—	—	5
Post-Rad	—	—	1
Ischaemia	—	—	1
Total	1	3	9

GB glioblastoma; *AA* anaplastic astrocytoma; *LGA* low-grade astrocytoma; *Post-Rad* post-radiation gliosis.

Table 3. *FDG Uptake in 12 Lesions Located in the Basal Ganglia or the Brainstem*

Diagnosis	Tumour FDG > grey matter FDG	Tumour FDG = grey matter FDG	Tumour FDG = 0
GB	4	—	—
AA	4	1	—
LGA	—	—	—
PNHL	1	—	—
Metastasis	2	—	—
Total	11	1	—

GB glioblastoma; *AA* anaplastic astrocytoma; *LGA* low-grade astrocytoma; *PNHL* primary non-Hodgkin's lymphoma.

Table 4. *Diagnostic Yield and [C-11]Methionine Uptake of 53 Biopsy Trajectories*

Diagnosis	Met(+) trajectories	Met(−) trajectories
GB	14	—
AA	16	—
LGA	10	—
PNHL	1	—
Metastasis	2	—
Post-Rad	—	4
Ischaemia	—	2
Non-diagnostic	—	4
Total	43	10

Met(+) uptake of [C-11]methionine; *Met(−)* no uptake of [C-11] methionine; *GB* glioblastoma; *AA* anaplastic astrocytoma; *LGA* low-grade astrocytoma; *PNHL* primary non-Hodgkin's lymphoma; *Post-rad* post-radiation gliosis.

tiating tumorous tissue from surrounding and to define target for biopsy in 27 of the 43 trajectories (63%).

There are 10 trajectories that had neither Met nor FDG uptake [Met(−)] and that were based on CT or MR defined targets. All these Met(−) trajectories yielded non-tumorous tissue. They included 2 ischaemic, 4 post-radiation gliosis and 4 non-diagnostic samples.

Among the 4 non-diagnostic samples, 3 of them were targets with no contrast enhancement on CT, one showed a discrete but significant enhancement on CT. It is worth noting that all these non-diagnostic trajectories were obtained in patients where the diagnosis was always given in another trajectory guided on PET [Met(+)].

Discussion

[C-11]methionine is a marker of amino acids uptake and protein synthesis which has already been studied in neurooncology [2, 7, 9, 18–20]. This PET tracer has several advantages: 1) it is considered as efficient and more sensitive than FDG in delineating tumorous zones, 2) its uptake is reported in low-grade glial tumours, 3) its uptake is low in the grey matter, and 4) the biological behaviour of this tracer in neoplastic tissues shows that its accumulation in tissues seems representative of the active transport of amino acids.

In the present study, the authors have combined the use of Met and FDG for PET-guided stereotactic brain biopsy. This work confirms and extends their previous results with the use of stereotactic PET guidance [16, 17] in that the technique is feasible routinely, it does not bring any major discomfort to the patient, even with 2 consecutive PET, and it improves the diagnostic yield of stereotactic brain biopsy [17]. Moreover, these results show that Met may be a good alternative to FDG for target selection.

Indeed, with Met-PET guidance, histological diagnosis was obtained in all patients. The 4 non-diagnostic samples were obtained exclusively from trajectories defined on CT or MR in an area where there was no Met uptake. Because CT or MR were abnormal in those areas (hyposignal or contrast-enhancement), one cannot rule out that biopsy guidance limited to CT/MR data in those 4 patients would have jeopardized the final diagnosis. This high diagnostic value of Met-PET is also illustrated by the fact that, in this series of patients, all tumours presented with an area of increased Met uptake. This study confirms that, in some locations, high grade tumours really present limitations to FDG in target definition. Moreover, this experience with both tracers in stereotactic conditions shows that in all tumour locations, even those where FDG have limitations, Met was easily used for target selection. Therefore, Met-PET appears superior to FDG-PET in some respects. In 11 of the 23 tumours, which were all located in grey matter areas, Met was the only tracer usable for target selection. This was the case in high-grade tumours located in the grey matter, where tumorous and normal FDG uptake were difficult to differentiate as well as in low-grade tumours where there was no FDG uptake. Indeed, in this series, the highest focus of Met uptake was used for target definition in 5 LGA. In those LGA, Met seemed more contributive than FDG because no FDG uptake was found and because all tumours were in close contact with the cortex. However, LGA do not always present in cortical locations and Met uptake in LGA is not a constant finding. Moreover, one could argue that FDG is particularly efficient in detecting the anaplastic component in lesions suspected of low grade histology on CT/MR [13].

When the tumour was located in the cortex, target definition was not easy with FDG in the majority of the cases (10 out of 11) whereas, when the tumour was seated inside subcortical grey matter, FDG was useful for target selection in 11 out of 12 cases. Met seemed therefore superior to FDG for target selection in enhanced or non-enhanced tumours located in the cortex. These results should be confirmed for non-enhanced lesions in subcortical grey matter. Met did not prove its superiority in deep-seated enhanced tumours. Interestingly, the two cases of enhanced non-tumorous lesion in the cortical area indicate that absence of Met uptake could suggest, before the biopsy, a non-tumorous diagnosis. With regard to stereotactic biopsies in the brainstem, the short experience of combined Met- and FDG-PET-guidance is still too limited to draw any conclusion.

A study on patients in which PET images with two tracers are acquired in stereotactic conditions can only be conducted during a limited period. Using two tracers in routine PET-guided stereotactic biopsies leads to a time-consuming and costly imaging procedure that should not be performed repetitively when not needed. In this study, the authors have evaluated the contribution of the two tracers to determine whether only one of them could be selected a priori, for example, on the basis of CT or MR data.

It has previously been shown that there is a relationship between the uptake of FDG and tumour malignancy [13, 17]. Because in the present study, Met uptake was increased in all tumours, whether benign or malignant, one can argue that Met-PET was not discriminating enough to direct the biopsy to the most malignant area of the tumour, as is possible by FDG-PET [17]. At visual analysis, however, it was found that areas of highest tracer uptake usually corresponded on equivalent FDG-PET and Met-PET images. Furthermore, a correlation was recently found between Met uptake and FDG uptake in samples from stereotactic biopsy of malignant brain tumours [14].

In conclusion, this work shows that Met is a good alternative to FDG for target selection in PET-guided stereotactic brain biopsy. These data suggest that a priori, on preoperative CT/MR, the cases could be selected where Met could be preferred to FDG. Indeed, Met-PET guidance is more efficient in non-enhanced lesions suspected of being low-grade, which usually have a low FDG uptake and in enhanced cortical lesions because it is difficult to differentiate between tumorous and cortical FDG uptake. In the case of enhanced lesions located in the basal ganglia, this experience shows that FDG is sufficient and could be used alone in the large majority of cases. Finally, multiple-tracer stereotactic PET combined with stereotactic biopsy offers a unique opportunity to accurately compare tracers' characteristics and accordingly provides useful information for the understanding of the role of PET in neurooncology [13, 14].

Acknowledgement

Supported by research grants 9.4503.91 from the Belgian National Lottery and 3.4509.92 from the National Funds for Scientific Research (F.N.R.S., Belgium).

References

1. Alavi J, Alavi A, Chawluk J, Kushner M, Powe J, Hickey W, Reivich M (1988) Positron emission tomography in patients with glioma. A predictor of prognosis. Cancer 62: 1074–1078
2. Bergstrom M, Ericson K, Hagenfeldt L, *et al* (1987) PET study of methionine accumulation in glioma and normal brain tissue: competition with branched chain amino acids. J Comput Assist Tomogr 11: 208–213
3. Black PM (1991) Brain tumors (Second of two parts). N Engl J Med 324: 1555–1564
4. Chandrasoma PT, Smith MM, Apuzzo MLJ (1989) Stereotactic biopsy in the diagnosis of brain masses: Comparison of results of biopsy and resected surgical specimen. Neurosurgery 24: 160–165
5. Choksey MS, Valentine A, Shawdon H, Freer CER, Lindsay KD (1989) Computed tomography in the diagnosis of malignant brain tumours: Do all patients requires biopsy? J Neurol Neurosurg Psychiatry 52: 821–825
6. Coleman RE, Hoffman JM, Hanson MW, Sostman HD, Schold SC (1991) Clinical application of PET for the evaluation of brain tumors. J Nucl Med 32: 616–622
7. Derlon JM, Bourdet C, Bustany P, *et al* [11C]L-methionine uptake in gliomas (1989) Neurosurgery 25: 720–728
8. Di Chiro G (1986) Positron emission tomography using [18F] fluorodeoxyglucose in brain tumors. A powerful diagnostic and prognostic tool. Invest Radiol 22: 360–371
9. Ericson K, Lilja A, Bergstrom M, *et al* (1985) Positron emission tomography with ([11C]methyl)-L-methionine, [11C]D-glucose, and [68Ga]EDTA in supratentorial tumors. J Comput Assist Tomogr 9: 683–689
10. Feiden W, Steude U, Bise K, Gündisch O (1991) Accuracy of stereotactic brain tumor biopsy: Comparison of the histologic findings in biopsy cylinders and resected tumor tissue. Neurosurg Rev 14: 51–56
11. Glantz MJ, Burger PC, Herndon II JE, Friedman AH, Cairncross JG, Vick NA, Schold Jr SC (1991) Influence of the type of surgery on the histological diagnosis in patients with anaplastic gliomas. Neurology 41: 1741–1744
12. Glantz MJ, Hoffman JM, Coleman RE, Friedman AH, Hanson MW, Burger PC, Herndon II JE, Meisler WJ, Schold Jr SC (1991) Identification of early recurrence of primary central nervous system tumors by [18F]fluorodeoxyglucose positron emission tomography. Ann Neurol 29: 347–355
13. Goldman S, Levivier M, Pirotte B, Brucher J-M, Wikler D, Damhaut P, Stanus E, Brotchi J, Hildebrand J (1996) Regional glucose metabolism and histopathology of gliomas. A study based on positron emission tomography-guided stereotactic biopsy. Cancer 78: 1098–1106
14. Goldman S, Levivier M, Pirotte B, Brucher J.-M, Wikler D, Damhaut P, Dethy S, Brotchi J, Hildebrand J (1996) Regional methionine and glucose uptake in high grade gliomas: a comparative study on PET-guided stereotactic biopsy. J Nucl Med, in press
15. Kelly PJ, Daumas-Duport C, Kispert DB, Kall BA, Scheithauer BW, Illig JJ (1987) Imaging-based stereotactic serial biopsies in untreated intracranial glial neoplasms. J Neurosurg 66: 865–874
16. Levivier M, Goldman S, Bidaut LM, Luxen A, Stanus E, Przedborski S, Balériaux D, Hildebrand J, Brotchi J (1992) Positron emission tomography-guided stereotactic brain biopsy. Neurosurgery 31: 792–797
17. Levivier M, Goldman S, Pirotte B, Brucher JM, Baleriaux D, Luxen A, Hildebrand J, Brotchi J (1995) Diagnostic yield of stereotactic brain biopsy guided by positron emission tomography with [18F]fluorodeoxyglucose. J Neurosurg 82: 445–452
18. Mineura K, Sasajima T, Kowada M, Uesaka Y, Shishido F (1991) Innovative approach in the diagnosis of gliomatosis cerebri using carbon-11-L-methionine positron emission tomography J Nucl Med 32: 726–728
19. Mosskin M, von Holst H, Bergström M, Collins VP, Eriksson L, Johnström P, Norén G (1987) Positron emission tomography with 11C-methionine and computed tomography of intracranial tumours compared with histopathologic examination of multiple biopsies. Acta Radiol 28: 673–681
20. Ogawa T, Shishido F, Kanno I, *et al* (1993) Cerebral glioma – evaluation with methionine PET. Radiology 186: 45–53
21. Patronas NJ, Di-Chiro G, Kufta C, *et al* (1985) Prediction of

survival in glioma patients by means of positron emission tomography. J Neurosurg 62: 816–822
22. Salmon I, Rorive S, Camby I, Decaestecker Ch, Pirotte B, Rombaut K, Haot J, Pasteels JL, Brotchi J, Kiss R (1995) Stereotactic biopsies from astrocytic tumors – Diagnostic information contributed by the quantitative chromatin pattern description. Analyt Quant Cytol Histol 17: 332–343
23. Salmon I, Levivier M, Camby I, Rombaut K, Gras T, Pasteels JL, Brotchi J, Kiss R (1993) Assessment of nuclear size, nuclear DNA content and proliferation index in stereotactic biopsies from brain tumours. Neuropathol Appl Neurobiol 19: 507–518

Correspondence: Marc Levivier, M.D., Ph.D., Department of Neurosurgery, Erasme Hospital, University of Brussels, 808, route de Lennik, B-1070 Brussels, Belgium.

Acta Neurochir (1997) [Suppl] 68: 139–143

Glioma Cells Transduced with Selection Transgenes May Not Form Gliomas in vivo and Can Also Inhibit Glioma Formation by Admixed Wild Glioma Cell Lines

I. R. Whittle, W. L. Kimber, M. Li, H. S. Bell, and **J. W. Ironside**[1]

Department of Clinical [1]Neurosciences and Neuropathology Laboratory, Western General Hospital, Edinburgh, Scotland, UK

Summary

Following in vitro lipofection transfection of the rat glioma cell line A15A5 with the plasmid transgene CMV/HyTK, which confirms hygromycin resistance and ganciclovir sensitivity, a series of experiments was planned in which the "bystander" phenomenon would be evaluated using the rodent implantation glioma model. However examination of the brain of rodents in which the A15A5-HyTK cells were implanted showed no evidence of glioma growth. Furthermore, rodents having intracerebral implantation of (i) wild A15A5 and A15A5HyTK cells in a 50/50 mix, (ii) wild A15A5 and A15A5HyTK cells in a 90/10 mixture and (iii) wild C6 and A15A5HyTK cells in a 50/50 mix all failed to grow macroscopic tumours by 15–17 days irrespective of whether the animals had been administered ganciclovir (GCV) in the week before sacrifice. Neuropathological and immunocytochemical analysis of the implantation sites showed no difference between the GCV and saline treated groups of animals for any implantation cell mix. These observations confirm previous results that suggest transduction of malignant rodent glioma cell lines with a variety of selection, oncogenic and marker genes significantly impairs their in vivo tumorigenic potential compared to the wild type cell lines. This study also demonstrates that even without GCV treatment the transduced cells inhibit, by an unknown mechanism(s), the tumorigenicity of other non transfected malignant cells. The implications of this study for gene therapy of human malignant glioma are discussed.

Keywords: Glioma; bystander effect; gene therapy.

Introduction

The "bystander" effect was first described by Moolten and Wells [10] when they noticed that the toxicity of ganciclovir (GCV) therapy was much greater than that predicted by the number of cells transduced with herpes simplex viral thymidine kinase (HSV-TK). Subsequent in vitro studies showed that HSV-TK transduced cells can cause the death of co-mixed wild tumour cell lines following GCV administration when as little as 3–10% of the total tumour cells were HSV-TK positive [5, 13, 16]. These findings have been confirmed in vivo, using a variety of tumour models, with regression occurring after GCV administration when between 10–70% of the tumour cells were HSV-TK positive [3, 4, 11, 14, 15]. In these experimental models it has been postulated that the bystander effect may also enhance the immune response and impair neovascularisation [1, 5, 14]. The bystander effect is particularly relevant to human gene therapy directed against malignant glioma, since in situ hybridisation studies suggest only 0.6% of glioma cells are transfected by retroviral genome released from vector producing cells (Oldfield E, Personal communication, 1995).

Although studies evaluating the bystander effect on glioma cells have been performed in vitro few qualitative and quantitative studies have been performed in immunocompetent rodents using mixtures of transduced and wild cell types [14, 16]. In this series of experiments, using the rodent implantation glioma model in adult Wistar rats, a TK^+ glioma cell line was coimplanted with a wild glioma cell line of similar and different types. After a period of 8–10 days, when the tumour would normally be well established, the rodents were divided into saline and GCV groups and treated for 7 days, after which the animals were sacrificed. From previous studies by Wu and colleagues [16], who used a similar experimental paradigm in mice using K1735 C19 melanoma cells, the assumption was that neuropathological analysis would show the saline treated animals had large tumours whilst those treated with GCV would have tumours with variable amounts of tumour necrosis and tumour regression. The authors assumed the size and viability of the residual tumour would be related to the proportion to TK^+ cells in the primary inoculum, and whether the animal had been treated with GCV or saline. However, the results provide further evidence that expression of a transgene by certain malignant cell lines significantly alters their in vivo malignancy and influences through unknown mechanisms the malignancy of admixed wild glioma cell lines.

Methods

A15A5 cells were a gift from Dr Geoffrey Pilkington, Institute of Psychiatry, London. The C6 cell line was obtained from the European Centre for Cell Cultures, Porton Down. Both cell lines were cultured in Hams F12 with 10% foetal calf serum, added glutamine, penicillin, streptomycin and fungizone. All cultures were performed at 37° and 5% carbon dioxide. A clone of A15A5 cells was established that had been stably transfected with the plasmid transgene CMV/HyTK [7] using the cationic liposome lipofectin (Gibco-BRL). The CMV/HyTK plasmid contains an expression cassette in which a hygromycin phosphotransferase gene has been fused in frame with the herpes simplex virus type 1 thymidine kinase gene under control of a cytomegalovirus promoter. Expression of this cassette results in production of fusion protein which confers both resistance to hygromycin and sensitivity to GCV. A15A5HyTK cells were selected by continuous culture in hygromycin (100 ug/ml), and the presence of the transgene in the hygromycin selected clones confirmed by Southern blotting (Fig. 1). The A15A5HyTK cells had an IC_{50} to GCV of circa 1–2 uM whereas the IC_{50} for wild type A15A5 cells to GCV was > 100 uM (Fig. 2).

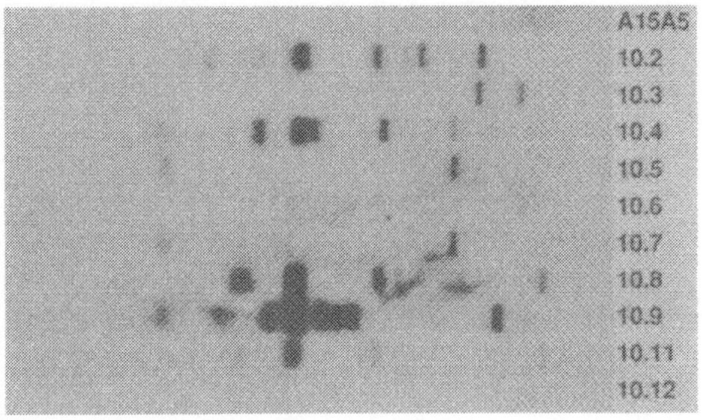

Fig. 1. Southern Blot showing the presence of the plasmid HyTK DNA (dark lines) in several clones of A15A5 cells grown after hygromycin selection and digestion with the restriction enzyme EcoR1. The wild cell line (A15A5) is negative and there has been variable incorporation of the plasmid construct after transfection. Clone 10.2 was used for these experiments

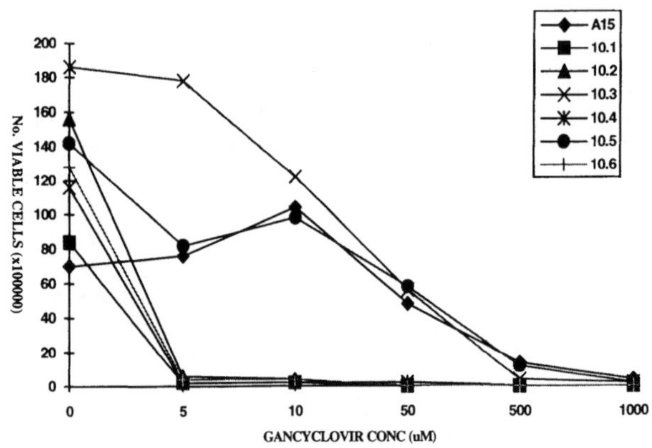

Fig. 2. The ganciclovir resistance of several clones of A15A5 cells transfected with the plasmid transgene CMV/HyTK. Most clones are killed by ganciclovir concentrations <5 uM however the wild cell type and clones 10.5 and 10.6 are relatively resistant to the effects of ganciclovir. Both these clones showed minimal transgene incorporation on the Southern Blot (Fig. 1)

Tumour Inoculation

Experimental gliomas were induced in rodents using standard implantation protocols. This has previously just been described [2, 8, 9, 17], but will be summarised here. Confluent cells were harvested using 0.1% trypsin and briefly stored in HamsF-12 media in an incubator at 37°C until use. Adult Wistar rats (250–350 g) were anaesthetised with pentabarbitone (45 mg/kg) and a retrocoronal burr hole was drilled 4 mm lateral to the midline. The animal was placed in a stereotactic frame and 10 μl of cells (approximately 10^6) injected into the rodent brain at a depth of 5.5 mm. For these experiments the following co-mixtures of cells were implanted (i) Pure A15A5HyTK cells; (ii) A15A5HyTK admixed with wild A15A5 in a ratio of 50 : 50; (iii) A15A5HyTK admixed with wild A15A5 in a ratio of 10 : 90; and (iv) A15A5HyTK admixed with wild C6 in a ratio 50 : 50.

The animals were allowed to recover from the implantation and given water and pellets ad libitum. The 8 animals comprising each experimental paradigm were divided into groups of 4 on day 7. Half were then given GCV 15 mg intra peritoneally bd whilst the other cohort was injected with a similar volume of saline. GCV treatment continued for 7 days and the animals were sacrificed between day 15 and day 17. This experimental protocol was approved by the Home Office under the Animals (Scientific Procedures) Act, 1986.

Tissue Processing and Immunocytochemistry

The brains were fixed overnight in 10% formalin and then sectioned into 2 mm coronal slices which were processed into paraffin wax blocks. Five micron thick sections were cut and mounted onto poly-L-lysine coated slides. Haematoxylin and Eosin staining was carried out for routine light microscopy. The immunocytochemical markers studied were GFAP (Dako, UK), S-100 and Vimentin and the proliferating cell marker PCNA (PC10, Dako, UK). In an attempt to assess host response the monoclonal antibodies ED1 and ED2 (Serotec, UK) which recognise macrophage epitopes and OX-6 which recognises a determinant of MHC Class II antigen presenting cells were also studied [17]. Sections were pretreated with Trypsin (0.1% solution in CaC12 – Tris buffered saline at 37°C, pH 7.6 for 30 minutes) before staining for Vimentin, ED1 and ED2. Sections were pretreated by microwaving (in 0.21% Citric Acid solution at pH 6.0 for 15 minutes, cooling over a further 20 minutes) before staining for OX-6. All primary antibody incubations were for 30 minutes at room temperature except for anti PCNA which was for 18 hours at 4°C. For visualisation the avidin-biotin-peroxidase (ABC) method was employed with 3,3′-diaminobenzidine (DAB; Vector, Peterborough, UK) as a peroxidase substrate. Sections were lightly counterstained with haematoxylin.

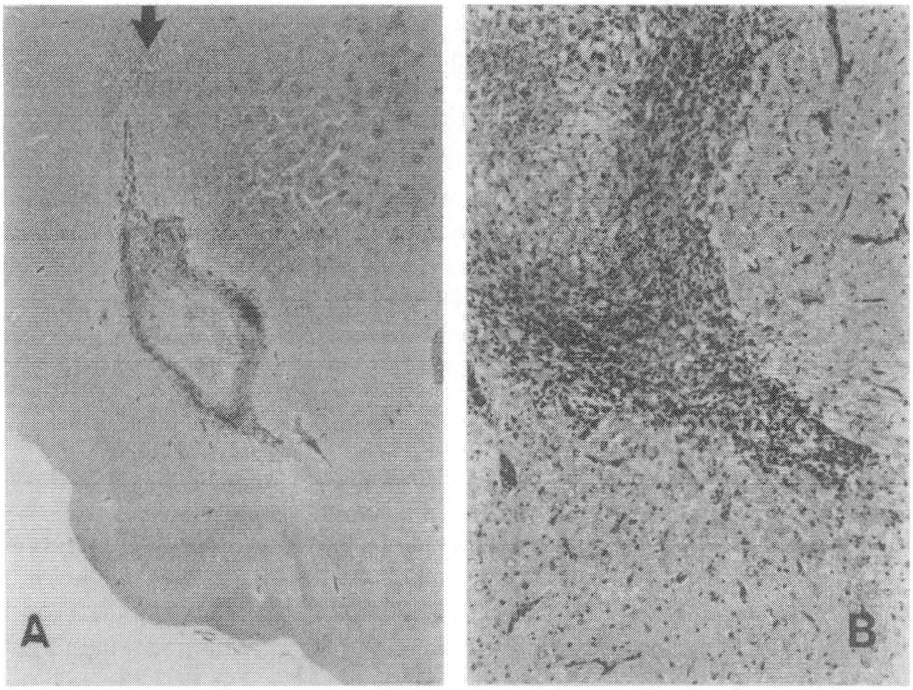

Fig. 3. Photomicrographs of a small brain tumour in an animal implanted 17 days previously with a mixture of C6 and A15A5HyTK cells and treated for one week with 15 mg ganciclovir bd. The macroscopic coronal view (A) shows a small tumour in the basolateral caudate region. The line of injection of the cells is shown by the arrow. The centre of the tumour is necrotic and there is surrounding perilesional brain oedema (H & E, ×40). Higher power study of the inferior pole of the tumour shows a wedge of viable tumour cells with vacuolation and necosis centrally. The viable tumour margin is invading the neuropil which is oedematous (H & E, ×200)

Results

There were no fatalities following implantation or GCV therapy and none of the animals exhibited any neurological deficit, behavioural abnormality or seizure disorder. Neuropathological examination of the brains revealed no macroscopic tumour present in any animal. In some areas there was cystic cavitation in the region of the implantated site, with mild ipsilateral ventricular dilation, but there was no midline shift in any animal. Most implantation sites could be seen following coronal section of the fixed brain and resembled a tear drop shape approximately 1 mm across and 2–3 mm in length (Fig. 3a).

Histological review of the implantation site revealed that in some animals small clumps of surviving glioma cells could be seen adjacent to a variably sized area of central necrosis that represented the inoculation site (Fig. 3b). All these animals with residual tumour cells had inoculums containing the C6 cell line. All animals having inoculums containing wild and transfected A15A5 cells had no viable tumour and the implantation site showed encephalomalacia often with cystic changes. In the neuropil adjacent to these areas there were perivascular and perilesional lymphocytic and macrophage infiltrates, intersitial vacuolation and in places there were microcystic areas with encephalomalacia. Intralesional and perilesional haemorrhages were not seen, although haemosiderin laden macrophages could be seen.

Immunocytochemical studies showed that most animals showed only scattered PCNA positive cells in the region of implant. However, where there were clumps of surviving tumour cells, the PCNA staining index varied from 5 to 15%. There was a dense perilesional GFAP positivity but the tumour/inflammatory/necrotic mass was GFAP negative. There was also prominent GFAP positivity in the corpus callosal fibres overlying the implantation site. There were numerous, intensively positive ED1 and ED2 staining cells within the tumour/inflammatory inoculum area and also in immediate perilesional brain. Areas of cortical damage related to the burrhole and implantation site also contained ED1 and ED2 positive cells but both the number of the cells and intensity of staining was less than that seen in the implantation site. OX-6 positivity was generally restricted to scattered cells within and around the inflammatory and residual tumour areas.

The inoculum site with the most cells staining for OX6 corresponded to the largest viable tumour mass. However subsequent in vitro studies showed that both the C6 and A15A5 cell lines are constitutively OX-6 positive. Except for the presence of small tumours in some of the animals implanted with the C6 cells (Fig. 3) the overall histological features and immunocytochemical features related to the tumour implantation sites were essentially identically in both the GCV and saline treated groups for all 4 experimental paradigms.

Discussion

This series of experiments was designed to evaluate the bystander effect in vivo and the toxicity of TK^+ cell lines on similar and different wild rodent glioma cell lines following GCV therapy. Because the authors did not have the laboratory facilities to transfect the glioma cells in vivo, and because they wished to evaluate the importance of cell type in this experimental paradigm, different proportions of transduced A15A5 cells were co-mixed with similar and dissimilar wild variants. The failure of tumours to grow in the GCV treated arms of the experiments was not an unexpected finding in view of previous reports on the potency of the bystander effect [3, 4, 14–16] and the sensitivity of the transfected cells to GCV. Much to the authors' surprise, particularly since they have concurrently successfully grown pure C6 (circa 95% take rate) and A15A5 (circa 75% take rate) and admixed C6/A15A5 (circa 80% take rate) gliomas following similar implantation protocols in adult Wistar rats [2, 8, 9, 17], no macroscopic tumours grew, although clumps of tumour cells survived, even in the saline (control) arm of these experiments.

The failure of the transduced A15A5 cells to form gliomas in vivo is consistent with previous observations using the same transgene in the rat 9L gliosarcoma [14]. These workers used in vivo infection of intracerebral 9L gliosarcomas with a replication defective retrovirus carrying the CMV/HyTK gene. However they also found inhibition of tumour growth with 9L tumour cells modified to express the selection neomycin phosphotransferase gene. Growth inhibition in vivo following transduction with either gene was independent of drug selection. Schwartz and colleagues who also use the rodent 9L gliocarcoma cell line showed that in vitro transfection with a range of oncogenes (neu, ras, PDGF-A, PDGF-B) and even the reporter beta-Gal gene, either singularly or in combination, could lead to significant changes in proliferative potential of the cell line following intracerebral implantation [12]. Tumours grown subcutaneously in the flanks of mice from C6 glioma cells transduced with a variety of selection and marker genes also have been shown in vivo to have considerable differences in proliferative capacity compared to the wild cell type [13]. Decreased in vivo malignancy has also been demonstrated for Walker 256 cells transduced with HSV-TK, in a leptomeningeal carcinomatosis model in rodents [15]. The C19 cell line transduced with HSV-TK was also not tumorigenic when implanted intracerebally in mice whereas the wild cell type caused death within a median 20 day post implantation [16]. Most recently transduction of the G1261 glioma cell line with either the interleukin 2 (IL-2) or gamma interferon (γ-IFN) genes was associated with longer term survival following intracerebral implantation in mice than that seen with the wild cell type [6]. In the latter experiment some of the survival benefit may be related to the boosted immune function related to IL-2 and γ-IFN secretion. Overall therefore, it would appear that transduction with a variety of genes may not impair in vitro growth or doubling time [12–14] but may cause a significant reduction in in vivo tumorigenicity. The mechanism underlying this decreased in vivo malignancy is conjectural. It would not appear to be related to the method of transfection of the transgene since retroviral, liposomal and adeno associated viral transfection methods have been used. Similarly the HSV-TK genes transfected have utilised a range of promoters and plasmid constructs. It may be that the mechanism involves a failure of tumour neovascularity together with an enhancement in tumour cell immunogenicity [1, 5, 14]. The immunogenicity of the transduced cells may be related to the type of promoter and marker genes used.

The major unexpected finding in this study was that the co-mixed wild C_6 cells did not progress to form large tumours even in the saline arm of these experiments. Tumour cells did however survive in some animals and it may be that if the animals had been sacrificed at a later time larger tumours would have been encountered. The transduced cells have somehow altered, at least temporarily, either the proliferation capacity of the admixed C_6 cell line or induced higher rates of necrosis or apoptosis. Failure of non-transduced cells to proliferate is consistent with the findings of Tapscott and colleagues who noted that in vivo retroviral gene therapy, using a variety of selection genes, in the rat 9L gliosarcoma model did not require parenteral GCV administration [14]. Co-implantation of the wild C19 melanoma cell line with C19 TK positive cells in a 1–10 mix again resulted in a modest, albeit statistically insignificant, prolongation of animal survival that was independent of GCV therapy [16]. Impairment of tumour neovascularity with or without a nonspecific boost to the host immune system may explain this finding. The immunocytochemical findings in this study did not however show any significant differences in the number of infiltrating ED1 or ED2 positive cells at the implantation site between any of the experimental groups. The intensity of ED1 and ED2 positivity also did not vary between groups. The macroscopic appearance of coronal sections of the brain and the qualitative and quantitative nature of the immune response measured using the immunocytochemical markers was very similar to that described after GCV therapy in rats with transduced 9L gliosarcoma [1]. Similar features were also found after implantation of with pure A15A5, C6 and F98 cells, 50/50 mixes of C6/F98 cells and A15A5/C6 cells [17].

The potential implications of the observation that transduced glioma cells are inherently less malignant in vivo and also down regulate the malignancy of adjacent wild tumour cell lines has major implications for human gene therapy. The initial human gene therapy studies in humans using mouse vector cells secreting retroviral HSV-TK with later parenteral GCV administration showed mixed results. One of the major findings, however, was that the transfection efficiency of the retrovirus was extremely low. It may be, that if more effective ways of transducing glioma cells can be found, the replicative potential of the nontransduced glioma cells may also be significantly impaired and perhaps its immunogenicity enhanced so that survival may be longer.

Acknowledgements

Wendy Kimber was a Brain Tumour Research Fellow, 1994–95; Dr M Li was a British Council Fellow 1994–95. This work was supported by the British Council and the Melville Trust. Prof David Porteous, MRC Human Genetics Unit, Edinburgh provided laboratory facities, encouragement and useful advice.

References

1. Barba D, Hardin J, *et al* (1994) Development of anti-tumor immunity following thymidine kinase-mediated killing of experimental brain tumors. Proc Natl Acad Sci USA 91: 4348–4352
2. Beaumont A, Clarke M, Whittle IR (1996) The effects of malignant glioma on the EEG and seizure thresholds; an experimental study. Acta Neurochir (Wien) 138: 370–381
3. Culver KW, Ram Z, Walbridge S *et al* (1992) In vivo gene transfer with retroviral vector producer cells for treatment of experimental brain tumors. Science 256: 1550–1552
4. Freeman SM, Abboud C, Whartenby K *et al* (1993) The "bystander effect": Tumor regression when a fraction of the tumor mass is genetically modified. Cancer Res 53: 5274–5283
5. Kramm CM, Sena-Esteves M *et al* (1995) Gene therapy for brain tumours. Brain Pathol 5: 346–381
6. Lichtor T, Glick RP *et al* (1995) Prolonged survival of mice with glioma injected intracerebrally with double cytokine-secreting cells. J Neurosurg 83: 1038–1044
7. Lupton SD, Brunton LL, Kalberg VA *et al* (1991) Dominant positive and negative selection using a hygromycin phosphotransferase-thymidine kinase fusion gene. Mol Cell Biol 11: 3374–48
8. Malcolm G, Kelly PA, Whittle IR *et al* (1995) Experimental implantation glioma using the A15A5 cell line. J Neurol Neurosurg Psychiatry 58: 390–191
9. MacArthur D, Malcolm G, Ironside JW, Whittle IR (1995) Can experimental models of implantation glioma be improved? Br J Neurosurg 9: 251–252
10. Moolten FL, Wells JM (1990) Curability of tumors bearing herpes thymidine kinase genes transferred by retroviral vectors. J Natl Cancer Inst 82: 297–300
11. Samejima Y, Meruelo D (1995) "Bystander killing" induces apoptosis and is inhibited by forskolin. Gene Ther 2: 50–58
12. Schwartz MS, Morris J, Sarid J (1991) Overexpression of oncogene products can cause tumor progression without parenchymal infiltration in the rat brain. Cancer Res 50: 3595–3601
13. Takamiya Y, Short MP, Ezzadine ZD *et al* (1992) Gene therapy of malignant brain tumors: a rat glioma line bearing the herpes simplex virus type a-thymidine kinase gene and wild type retrovirus kills other tumor cells. J Neurosci Res 33: 493–503
14. Tapscott SJ, Miller AD *et al* (1994) Gene therapy of rat 9L gliosarcoma tumors by transduction with selectable genes does not require drug selection. Proc Natl Acad Sci USA 91: 8185–8189
15. Vrionis FD, Wu JK, Qi P *et al* (1996) Tumor cells expressing the herpes simplex virus-thymidine kinase gene in the treatment of Walker 256 meningeal neoplasia in rats. J Neurosurg 84: 250–257
16. Wu JK, Cano WG, Sven AG *et al* (1994) Bystander tumoricidal effect in the treatment of experimental brain tumours. Neurosurgery 35: 1094–1103
17. Whittle IR, Macarthur DC, Malcolm GP *et al* (1996) Can experimental implantation models of rodent glioma be improved? A study of pure and mixed glioma cell line tumours. Acta Neurochir (Wien) submitted

Correspondence: Ian R Whittle, Ph.D., FRCS Ed., Western General Hospital, Department of Clinical Neurosciences, Crewe Road, Edinburgh, EH5 2XU, U.K.

Index of Keywords

Springer-Verlag
and the Environment

WE AT SPRINGER-VERLAG FIRMLY BELIEVE THAT AN international science publisher has a special obligation to the environment, and our corporate policies consistently reflect this conviction.

WE ALSO EXPECT OUR BUSINESS PARTNERS – PRINTERS, paper mills, packaging manufacturers, etc. – to commit themselves to using environmentally friendly materials and production processes.

THE PAPER IN THIS BOOK IS MADE FROM NO-CHLORINE pulp and is acid free, in conformance with international standards for paper permanency.

SPRINGER NATURE

GPSR Compliance

The European Union's (EU) General Product Safety Regulation (GPSR) is a set of rules that requires consumer products to be safe and our obligations to ensure this.

If you have any concerns about our products, you can contact us on ProductSafety@springernature.com

In case Publisher is established outside the EU, the EU authorized representative is:

Springer Nature Customer Service Center GmbH
Europaplatz 3
69115 Heidelberg, Germany

Kolibri 360 GmbH
Ferdinand-Jühlke-Straße 7
99095 Erfurt, Deutschland
produktsicherheit@kolibri360.de